The University of Texas
M. D. Anderson Symposium on Fundamental Cancer Research

Volume 38

IMMUNOLOGY AND CANCER

Published for
The University of Texas System Cancer Center,
M. D. Anderson Hospital and Tumor Institute, Houston, Texas,
by the University of Texas Press, Austin

The University of Texas
M. D. Anderson Symposium on Fundamental Cancer Research

VOLUME 38

Immunology and Cancer

Edited by

Margaret L. Kripke, Ph.D.
Kathryn O'Connor Research Professor
of Immunology
Department of Immunology

Philip Frost, M.D., Ph.D.
Professor of Medicine and Cell Biology
Department of Cell Biology

THE UNIVERSITY OF TEXAS
M. D. ANDERSON HOSPITAL AND TUMOR INSTITUTE AT HOUSTON
HOUSTON, TEXAS

University of Texas Press, Austin

Library of Congress Cataloging-in-Publication Data
Symposium on Fundamental Cancer Research (38th :
  1985 : Houston, Tex.)
  Immunology and cancer.
  (UT M. D. Anderson Symposium on Fundamental Cancer
Research ; v. 38)
  "A compilation of the proceedings of the University
of Texas M. D. Anderson Hospital and Tumor Institute
at Houston's 38th Annual Symposium on Fundamental
Cancer Research, held February 26–March 1, 1985,
in Houston, Texas"—T.p. verso.
  Includes bibliographies and index.
  1. Cancer—Immunological aspects—Congresses.
2. Immunotherapy—Congresses. I. Kripke, Margaret L.
II. Frost, Philip, 1940– . III. M. D. Anderson
Hospital and Tumor Institute at Houston. IV. Title.
V. Series: UT M. D. Anderson Symposium on Fundamental
Cancer Research (Series) ; v. 38. [DNLM: 1. B Lympho-
cytes—congresses. 2. Cell Communication—congresses.
3. Neoplasms—immunology—congresses. 4. T Lymphocytes
—congresses. W3 SY5177 38th 1985i / QZ 200 S985 1985i]
RC268.3.S958 1985   616.99'4079   85-26441
ISBN 0-292-73841-2

Materials appearing in the book prepared by individuals as part of their official
duties as U.S. Government employees are not covered by copyright.

This volume is a compilation of the proceedings of The University of Texas
M. D. Anderson Hospital and Tumor Institute at Houston's 38th Annual Symposium
on Fundamental Cancer Research held February 26–March 1, 1985, in Houston,
Texas. The volume is indexed in the *Index Medicus* MEDLINE database and its
subsets.

The material contained in this volume was submitted as previously unpublished
material, except in the instances in which credit has been given to the source from
which some of the illustrative material was derived.

Great care has been taken to maintain the accuracy of the information contained in
this volume; however, the Editorial Staff, The University of Texas, and the University
of Texas Press cannot be held responsible for errors or for any consequences arising
from the use of the information contained herein.

Contents

Immune Responses to Cancer

Immunologic Effector Mechanisms

Immunological Approaches to Cancer Therapy

The Wilson S. Stone Award Lecture

Preface

One of the most rapidly advancing areas of biomedical research concerns the nature and regulation of the immune system. Recent findings on the genetic and biochemical bases for immunologic recognition have revolutionized our understanding of the principles governing the immune system and have made us aware of the intricacies involved in its regulation. However, these rapid advances have not been paralleled by similar progress in cancer immunology. Our understanding of immune responses to tumor antigens and their regulation during carcinogenesis and tumor growth has not kept pace with current progress in basic immunology.

The 38th Annual Symposium on Fundamental Cancer Research, "Immunology and Cancer," was designed to address this deficiency and to review and discuss the recent advances that have been generated in several areas of basic immunology. These concern the organization of genetic information coding for molecules involved in immunologic recognition (antibodies, class I and class II antigens, T cell receptors), networks that control immune responsiveness, a better understanding of the ontogeny and differentiation of lymphoid cells, and identification of effector molecules that mediate various steps in immunologic reactions (lymphokines, cytokines, suppressor and augmenting factors).

The Symposium had three components—a review of these recent scientific advances, a review of our current understanding of the immune response against cancer in light of this new information, and a discussion of immunologic approaches to cancer therapy. Based on the presentations and discussions at the Symposium, this monograph brings to light the gap between basic immunology and tumor immunology and points to areas where bridging of these two disciplines can occur. We hope that this information will stimulate analyses of how our better understanding of the nature and regulation of the immune system might be applied to cancer prevention, detection, and treatment.

MARGARET L. KRIPKE

PHILIP FROST

Acknowledgments

The editors would like to thank the many individuals who unselfishly provided advice and assistance at every stage during the planning and execution of the symposium. We thank the Symposium Organizing Committee members from The University of Texas System Cancer Center, Drs. James M. Bowen, Frederick F. Becker, and Evan M. Hersh, and the external advisory committee, Drs. James P. Allison and Osias Stutman, for their assistance in planning the meeting. We also thank the session chairmen, Drs. Susan Rich, Stewart Sell, Robert Good, Eva Lotzová, and Osias Stutman, for their guidance during the meeting.

We are especially grateful for the cosponsorship of the National Cancer Institute and the American Cancer Society, Texas Division, Inc. In addition, we extend our appreciation for the generous support of Hoffmann-La Roche, Inc., Smith, Kline and French Laboratories, Triton Biosciences, Inc., Schering Corporation, Bristol-Myers Co., E. I. du Pont de Nemours & Co., Merrell Dow Research Institute, Becton Dickinson Immunocytometry Systems, Genentech, Inc., Lilly Research Laboratories, Merck Sharp & Dohme Research Laboratories, Syntex USA, Inc., and The Upjohn Co.

Finally, we owe special thanks to Mr. Jeff Rasco and the staff of UT M. D. Anderson Hospital Conference Services and Ms. Frances Goff for providing assistance throughout the symposium and to the Department of Public Information and Education for its assistance to us and the professional and public media.

IMMUNE RECOGNITION
BY T AND B CELLS

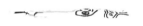

Symposium on Fundamental Cancer Research, Vol. 38.
© 1986 by The University of Texas System Cancer Center.

1. The Structure and Function of the T3-Ti Molecular Complex on Human T Lymphocytes

Ellis L. Reinherz,* Hans Dieter Royer, † Thomas J. Campen, †
Dunia Ramarli, † Hsiu-Ching Chang, † and Oreste Acuto †

*Division of Tumor Immunology, Dana-Farber Cancer Institute and the Departments
of *Medicine and † Pathology, Harvard Medical School, Boston, Massachusetts
02115*

T lymphocytes, unlike B lymphocytes, predominantly recognize antigen in the context of membrane-bound products of the major histocompatibility complex (MHC) (Benacerraf and McDevitt 1979, Schlossman 1979, Zinkernagel and Doherty 1975, Corradin and Chiller 1979, Hunig and Bevan 1981, Cerottini 1980). This "dual" recognition is important for activation of T cells that have cytotoxic effector function, as well as immunoregulatory activities. With regard to the cytotoxic effector function, T cells can lyse specific target cells, including those that have been infected with viruses and carry viral antigens (Doherty 1980, Quinnan et al. 1982, Wallace et al. 1982, Meuer et al. 1983d). Moreover, they regulate the activity of cells within the immune system, such as T cells, B cells, and macrophages, as well as hematopoietic stem cells, fibroblasts, osteoblasts, and other cell types outside the lymphoid system (Gershon 1974, Pick et al. 1979, Waldmann 1978, Cantor and Gershon 1979, Lipton et al. 1980, Reinherz and Schlossman 1980a,b, 1981). Characterization of T cell receptors encoding various specificities could be particularly valuable for an understanding of the molecular events in the cellular interactions underlying these activities.

Given that T lymphocytes precisely recognize antigens, discriminative surface structures restricted in their expression to individual T cell clones (clonotypic) must exist. The recent development of technologies for continual propagation of clonal populations of human T lymphocytes in vitro (Morgan et al. 1975, Kurnick et al. 1979, Bonnard et al. 1980, Sredni et al. 1980, Meuer et al. 1982c) has provided a new basis for identification of such clonotypic recognition determinants. Thus, clonal human T cell populations of predefined specificities have been used as immunogens to produce a series of clone-specific murine monoclonal antibodies. These anticlonotypic antibodies identify a novel class of 90-kDa heterodimers, termed Ti, that are membrane associated with the previously described 20- and 25-kDa T3 glycoproteins present on all mature human T lymphocytes (Meuer et al. 1983a,c).

With this approach, it is possible to provide compelling evidence for the notion that each T lymphocyte, regardless of subset derivation, specificity, or regulatory activity, uses an analogous T3-associated Ti heterodimer (one α and one β subunit) as its receptor for antigen and MHC. The subunits of the Ti heterodimer are products of gene segments that rearrange in T lineage cells to give rise to an active set of Ti_α and Ti_β genes. The mechanism by which triggering of the T3-Ti molecular complex produces a clonal T cell population and its linkage to an interleukin (IL) 2–dependent autocrine pathway will also be discussed.

T4$^+$ AND T8$^+$ CYTOTOXIC T LYMPHOCYTES THAT RECOGNIZE DIFFERENT MHC GENE PRODUCTS

A number of human T cell lineage-restricted surface glycoproteins have been defined by monoclonal antibodies. For example, each mature T lymphocyte expresses the 20- and 25-kDa T3 glycoprotein. The glycoproteins appear in the late intrathymic ontogeny at the time immunologic competence occurs and play a central role in T cell function (Reinherz et al. 1980a,d, 1982, van Wauwe et al. 1980, Chang et al. 1981, Burns et al. 1982, Umiel et al. 1982). Moreover, among T3$^+$ T lymphocytes, two subsets were found that exhibit unique regulatory and effector activities. On the basis of their unique 62-kDa and 76-kDa membrane markers, these were termed T4$^+$ and T8$^+$, respectively (Reinherz and Schlossman 1980a,b, 1981, Reinherz et al. 1979a). The T4$^+$ subset, which represented approximately two thirds of peripheral T cells, provided inducer-helper activities for T-T, T-B, and T-macrophage interactions, whereas the T8$^+$ subset (one third of peripheral T cells, reciprocal to T4$^+$ T cells) was principally a suppressor (Reinherz et al. 1980b, 1979b). Although both subsets of cells proliferated in response to alloantigen (foreign cell surface determinants) in mixed lymphocyte culture (MLC), most of the cytotoxic effector function was detected in the T8$^+$ population. Moreover, development of cytotoxicity by T8$^+$ cells, in general, required interactions with T4$^+$ cells or their soluble products. In contrast, only a minor component of the cytotoxic effector function resided within the T4$^+$ subset, and this was maximal when T4$^+$ cells alone were sensitized in MLC (Reinherz et al. 1979a).

To characterize individual cytotoxic effector lymphocytes (CTL) in humans, we developed a strategy to clone and propagate antigen-specific T cell populations in vitro (Meuer et al. 1982c). This involved in vitro expansion with IL 2, a T cell–specific growth factor, and frequent restimulation with a specific alloantigen. As expected from the above data with purified T cells, the majority of cytotoxic T cell clones were derived from the T8$^+$ subset.

The specificity of T4$^+$ and T8$^+$ clones and subclones was also characterized. T8$^+$ clones killed targets that shared class I MHC antigens (HLA-A,B,C) with the original stimulator cells, whereas cytotoxic T4$^+$ clones were directed at class II MHC antigens (Ia related). These results indicated that the vast majority of T4$^+$ and T8$^+$ T lymphocytes had receptors for different classes of MHC antigens (T8 class I and T4 class II correlation) (Meuer et al. 1982b,c, Krensky et al. 1982, Biddison et al. 1982). Analogous findings have been reported from studies with autoreactive T cell clones as well.

EFFECTS OF MONOCLONAL ANTIBODIES DIRECTED AT MONOMORPHIC STRUCTURES ON ANTIGEN-SPECIFIC FUNCTION

The association between the surface phenotype, that is, surface glycoproteins, of CTL and the class of MHC molecules that are recognized implied that the subset-restricted structures, T4 and T8, might be required to facilitate selective lysis of different target antigens. To determine if individual anti-T4 and anti-T8 antibodies influenced killing function, cytotoxic T cell clones were preincubated with T cell–specific monoclonal antibody or with medium alone prior to the cell-mediated lympholysis (CML) assay. It was found that anti-T8 did not diminish the level of killing by MHC class II–restricted T4$^+$ clones, but markedly decreased cytotoxicity mediated by the MHC class I–restricted T8$^+$ clones (Meuer et al. 1982c, Reinherz et al. 1981c). In contrast, anti-T4 preincubation resulted in a greater than 80% reduction of cytotoxicity by the T4$^+$ clones, but had no effect on killing by the T8$^+$ clones. In addition, anti-T3, unlike anti-T4 and anti-T8, inhibited the killing by both T4$^+$ and T8$^+$ clones. Moreover, anti-T3 was unique among antibodies that define other mature T cell surface structures, since other antibodies did not inhibit the cytotoxic capacity of all clones, even when used in saturating concentrations. Thus, the observed inhibition was not simply a function of antibody binding to a clonal effector population.

These results implied that at least several surface molecules were important in CML: T3 and T4 molecules on T4$^+$ clones and T3 and T8 molecules on T8$^+$ clones (Meuer et al. 1982a). Since other studies showed that CML was restored by lectin approximation of killer and target cells, even in the presence of monoclonal antibodies to these molecules, it appeared that T3, T4, and T8 were involved in recognition events rather than in the lytic mechanism. The observation that the target cell specificity of CTL clones was abrogated by lectin approximation further supported the notion of T3, T4, and T8 involvement in recognition.

Antigen-specific CTL clones that recognize autologous B lymphoblastoid lines transformed by Epstein-Barr virus (EBV) are also governed by a series of recognition elements identical to those of the clones directed at allogeneic

targets (Wallace et al. 1982, Meuer et al. 1983b,d). Specifically, CTL expressing the T8 phenotype recognize the autologous B lymphoblastoid line in the
context of class I MHC molecules. Anti-HLA antibodies block CTL effector
function at the target level, and anti-T8 antibodies abrogate the ability of these
class I–specific killers to kill. In contrast, T4+ CTL recognize Ia (class II)
determinants on the autologous lymphoblastoid cell and are inhibited by
anti-T4 but not anti-T8 antibodies. As with the allogeneic CTL, anti-T3 antibody preincubation inhibits the killing ability of both T4+ and T8+ effector
T cells. Because these clones fail to lyse autologous B cells not infected with
EBV or B cell blasts stimulated with pokeweed mitogen (PWM), such T4+
and T8+ effectors seem to recognize virally encoded surface glycoproteins in
association with class II or class I molecules, respectively. Thus, they exhibit
either a class II or a class I MHC restriction. At present, however, these viral
proteins have not been identified.

THE T3 MOLECULAR COMPLEX MODULATION FROM
THE T CELL SURFACE

The appearance of 20- and 25-kDa T3 surface molecules in late intrathymic
ontogeny at the time immunologic competence occurred and their critical role
in T lymphocyte function suggested that T3 was closely linked to an important recognition receptor or to a cell-cell interaction molecule (van Wauwe et
al. 1980, Chang et al. 1981, Burns et al. 1982, Reinherz et al. 1980d, 1982,
Umiel et al. 1982). Antibodies directed against T3 were unique in their abilities to block the induction phase (MLC) and the effector phase (lysis) of
CML, to inhibit T lymphocyte proliferative responses to soluble antigen, and
to induce mitosis in resting T cells. In the third case, activation was accompanied by release of various T cell lymphokines including IL 2 and gamma
interferon (Meuer et al. 1983e, Acuto et al. 1983b).

   Given the central role of the T3 molecules in human T cell function and the
known rapid surface receptor loss (modulation) that occurs with a variety of
hormone and growth factor receptors after ligand binding, we examined the
capacity of anti-T3 to induce modulation of T3. Preincubation of peripheral
blood T cells or T cell clones with anti-T3 for 18 hours at 37°C resulted in loss
of cell surface T3 antigen (Reinherz et al. 1982, Meuer et al. 1982a). In contrast, anti-T3–modulated cells were unaffected in their expression of cell surface T4 or T8 antigen. Modulation of T3 antigen with anti-T3 antibody had
no effect on the viability of T cell clones. Furthermore, once anti-T3 was removed from cell culture supernatants, T3 antigen was reexpressed within 48
hours (Reinherz et al. 1982).

FUNCTIONAL EFFECTS FROM ANTI-T3 ANTIBODY–INDUCED MODULATION OF THE T3 SURFACE COMPLEX ON ANTIGEN-SPECIFIC HUMAN T CELL CLONES

One could argue that the inhibitory effects of anti-T3 monoclonal antibodies (Chang et al. 1981, Reinherz et al. 1982, Meuer et al. 1982a) on CTL function were indirect and occurred as a consequence of antibody-induced agglutination of cells or of steric blockade of still undefined but functionally important surface determinants. However, since anti-T3 led to T3 modulation by selective shedding of both the T3 antigen and the anti-T3 antibody directed toward it without altering cell viability or changing the density of other T cell antigens (including T1, T4, T8, T11, T12, and Ia), it was possible to examine the lytic activity of T3-modulated cells in the absence of surface-bound monoclonal antibodies that could otherwise affect steric blockade (Reinherz et al. 1982, Meuer et al. 1982a).

Anti-T3 modulation of T4 and T8 clones markedly reduced cytotoxic effector function to less than 25% of the maximum. Perhaps more important is that cytotoxic function increased to approximately 60% of the maximum when T4 and T8 clones were tested one day after modulation and had achieved maximal levels two days after modulation. Given the fact that 48 hours were required to complete T3 antigen reexpression after anti-T3 modulation of T4 and T8 clones, this reestablishment of cytotoxic T lymphocyte effector function appeared to be temporally related.

Since many cytotoxic T lymphocyte clones display specific proliferative responses when confronted with alloantigen, we also determined whether anti-T3 modulation influenced antigen recognition (Reinherz et al. 1982). Anti-T3–modulated clones had a significantly reduced proliferative response to the alloantigen in comparison with unmodulated clones. In contrast, they mounted a greater proliferative response to IL 2 than the unmodulated clones did. Taken together, these studies suggested that modulated loss of T3 surface molecules interferes with T cell antigen recognition and that this is a specific effect, since IL 2 responsiveness is enhanced. Thus, the functional consequences of anti-T3–induced modulation could not be explained on the basis of a nonspecific diminution of cell responsiveness. The relevance of enhanced IL 2 responsiveness after anti-T3 modulation will be discussed later.

CLONOTYPIC SURFACE STRUCTURES INVOLVED IN ANTIGEN-SPECIFIC HUMAN T CELL FUNCTION

Given that T lymphocytes recognize antigen in a precise fashion, there had to exist, in addition, discriminative surface recognition structures unique to individual T cell clones. To delineate such clonotypic molecules, we produced

TABLE 1.1. *Monoclonal Antibodies Influencing T Cell Function*

Monoclonal Antibody	Molecular Mass (kDa)	Functional Effect of Monoclonal Antibody		
		Antigen-Induced Proliferation	CTL Function	IL 2 Response
Anti-T3	20–25	Decreased	Decreased	Increased
Anti-T4	58	None or decreased	Decreased	None
Anti-T8	72	None or decreased	Decreased	None

CTL = cytotoxic T lymphocytes; IL 2 = interleukin 2.

monoclonal antibodies against several human cytotoxic T cell clones and developed a screening strategy that selected for such anticlonotypic antibodies.

Unlike anti-T3, which blocked the cytotoxic effector functions of all clones, anticlonotypic (termed anti-Ti) antibodies selectively blocked killing of the clone to which they were directed. Also, in contrast to anti-T3, anticlonotypic antibodies only blocked the antigen-specific proliferative capacity of that individual clone. Pretreatment of a clone with the appropriate anti-Ti antibody did, however, augment the clone's proliferative response to human IL 2. These functional effects are summarized in Table 1.1 and are compared with those of other antibodies. Pretreatment of a given clone with an irrelevant anticlonotypic antibody had no effect on T cell function, even when clones were derived from the same individual. Hence, the anti-Ti antibodies have been termed non–cross-reactive.

Ti AND T3 ASSOCIATED IN THE CELL MEMBRANE

The observation that anti-T3, as well as anti-Ti, antibody specific for a given clone could inhibit both antigen-specific proliferation and CTL effector function of this clone and could enhance its IL 2 responsiveness suggested a relationship between the cell surface structures defined by these antibodies. This was borne out by immunofluorescence studies in which anti-T3–induced modulation of T3 also resulted in loss of anti-Ti reactivity. This was not a nonspecific effect, since the T8 or T4 antigen density was not influenced by this process (Meuer et al. 1983c).

Given the strong evidence that the clonotypic structures were involved in antigen recognition and membrane association with T3, it was important to quantitate the number of surface Ti and T3 molecules on representative T cell populations. Three points emerged from this analysis. First, the number of T3 and Ti molecules on each of the clonal populations was similar despite some interclonal variation in the absolute number of T3 and Ti molecules (30,000–40,000). This finding suggested a stoichiometric relationship in which one T3 molecule is linked to one Ti molecule in the cell membrane. Second, on the clonal populations, the density of the associative recognition structures T4 and T8 was far greater (118,000 and 175,000 binding sites per cell, respectively) than T3 and Ti. Third, in contrast to T3 (and presumably Ti), which is expressed to a similar degree on the resting T lymphocytes and T cell clones, there were three to four times fewer T4 and T8 molecules on resting lymphocytes of the appropriate subset derivation (30,000 and 60,000, respectively) than on the respective activated clonal populations (Meuer et al. 1983a). Thus, T cell activation may result in expression of additional T4 and T8 molecules. This probably offers one explanation for their critical involvement in clonal effector function. In contrast, the number of antigen receptors defined by anti-T3 and anti-Ti remains comparable and hence fully expressed in the resting state before antigen binding.

Ti: A 90-kDa DISULFIDE–LINKED HETERODIMER

Since all of these studies demonstrated that a close functional and phenotypic relationship existed between 20- and 25-kDa T3 glycoproteins and the Ti clonotype, it was important to define biochemically the surface molecules detected by anti-Ti monoclonal antibodies. Thus, solubilized membrane preparations were obtained from two representative ^{125}I-labeled clones, $CT4_{II}$ and $CT8_{III}$; antigens defined by anti-Ti antibodies were precipitated and separated electrophoretically on sodium dodecyl sulfate (SDS) polyacrylamide gels (Meuer et al. 1983a). As shown in Figure 1.1, the molecule precipitated by anti-Ti_1 (specific anticlonotype) from ^{125}I-labeled $CT8_{III}$ cells appears as two bands and consists of a 49-kDa α chain and a 43-kDa β chain in reducing conditions (lane a). Moreover, in nonreducing conditions, this structure appears as a single band at 90 kDa (lane c). In contrast, anti-Ti_1 does not immunoprecipitate material from the ^{125}I-labeled $CT4_{II}$ clone (lanes f, h). This is not surprising, since anti-Ti_1 reacts with $CT8_{III}$ but not with $CT4_{II}$ by indirect immunofluorescence. In a reciprocal fashion, anti-Ti_2 precipitates material from ^{125}I-labeled $CT4_{II}$ (lanes e, g) but not $CT8_{III}$ (lanes b, d). The former appears as two bands of apparent 51 kDa and 43 kDa on SDS polyacrylamide gel electrophoresis (PAGE) under reducing conditions (lane e) and 90 kDa under nonreducing conditions (lane g). Thus, although the Ti_2 and Ti_1 antigens are comparable in molecular characteristics and are derived from T cell clones of the same individual, they express unique structures that can be defined by non–cross-reactive monoclonal antibodies. This, together with the fact that neither antibody reacted with peripheral T cells or with a total of 80 clones derived from the same donor, further suggested that the Ti_2 and Ti_1

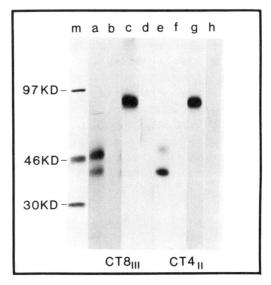

FIGURE 1.1. Isolation and characterization of Ti_1 and Ti_3 molecules. Immuno-precipitations were performed using the clonotypic antibodies anti-Ti_{1B} or anti-Ti_{2A} (both IgM) covalently linked to CnBr-activated Sepharose 4B. Before electrophoresis, immunoprecipitates were washed three times with RIPA solution. Sodium dodecyl sulfate polyacrylamide gel electrophoresis (SDS-PAGE) was performed under reducing (R) and nonreducing (NR) conditions in a 12.5% polyacrylamide gel according to a modification of the Laemmli procedure followed by autoradiography. The following ^{14}C methylated molecular weight markers (New England Nuclear, Boston, MA) were used (m): carbonic anhydrase (30,000); ovalbumin (46,000); phosphorylase b (97,000). Lanes a–d: $CT8_{III}$; lanes e–h: $CT4_{II}$. a, anti-Ti_{1B} (R); b, anti-Ti_{2A} (R); c, anti-Ti_{1B} (NR); d, anti-Ti_{2A} (NR); e, anti-Ti_{2A} (R); f, anti-Ti_{1B} (R); g, anti-Ti_{2A} (NR); h, anti-Ti_{1B} (NR).

antigens detected clone-specific rather than allotypic or isotypic determinants on Ti molecules.

More recently, we have described three additional clone-specific monoclonal antibodies that detect similar 90-kDa disulfide–linked heterodimers. Slight differences in molecular weight were noted among all the different α chains. Whether these variations reflect different posttranslational modifications or protein size differences is still unclear. Biosynthetic labeling of Ti molecules also indicated that they are synthesized by T cells rather than merely absorbed from culture medium.

To determine whether the T3-associated disulfide-linked Ti heterodimer was also the receptor for antigen on inducer clones, we produced an anti-clonotypic monoclonal antibody (termed anti-Ti_{4A}) against the class II MHC–restricted ragweed antigen-specific clone RW17C. Not surprisingly, the surface structure defined by anti-Ti$_{4A}$ comodulated with T3 following incubation of RW17C cells with either anti-Ti$_{4A}$ or anti-T3 monoclonal antibodies (Meuer et al. 1982a).

To characterize the surface structure recognized by anti-Ti$_{4A}$ on RW17C, we performed immunoprecipitation experiments with membrane preparations externally labeled with [125]I (Meuer et al. 1983b,e). As shown in Figure 1.2, anti-Ti$_{4A}$ precipitates two bands under reducing conditions on SDS-PAGE, one at 52 kDa and a second at 41 kDa (lane C). It appears as a single band at about 90 kDa under nonreducing conditions (lane F). These molecular weight species were not present in control immunoprecipitates (lanes A, D) or in

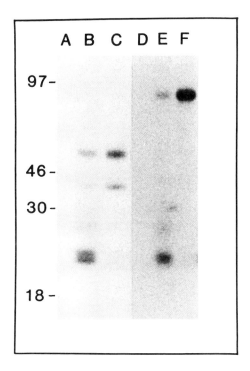

FIGURE 1.2. Characterization of Ti$_{4A}$ and T3$_C$ surface structures. RW17C cells (30 × 10⁶) were surface labeled with 1 mCi of Na[125]I (NEN) and immunoprecipitated with the monoclonal antibodies anti-T6, anti-Ti$_{4A}$, and anti-T3$_C$ that were covalently linked to CnBr-activated Sepharose 4B. Sodium dodecyl sulfate polyacrylamide gel electrophoresis was performed under reducing and nonreducing conditions in a 10% polyacrylamide gel, according to a modification of the Laemmli procedure. The following ^{14}C methylated molecular weight markers (NEN) were used: phosphorylase B (97,400); ovalbumin (46,000); carbonic anhydrase (30,000); lactoglobulin A (18,300). Lanes A–C show reducing conditions: A, anti-T6; B, anti-T3$_C$; C, anti-Ti$_{4A}$; D–F show nonreducing conditions; D, anti-T6; E, anti-T3$_C$; F, anti-Ti$_{4A}$.

anti-Ti$_{4A}$ from ^{125}I-labeled clones with specificities different from RW17C, for example, T15A (not shown). In contrast to anti-Ti$_{4A}$, anti-T3 precipitated four bands on SDS-PAGE under reducing conditions from RW17C (lane B). The major protein band was 20 kDa with three additional bands at 25 kDa, 41 kDa, and 52 kDa. Moreover, the two bands of higher-molecular-mass proteins were identical in size to those found in anti-Ti$_{4A}$ immunoprecipitates from RW17C (lane C), which suggests that they may be related. Further support for this notion came from the observation that, like Ti$_{4A}$ under nonreducing conditions, the 52-kDa and 41-kDa upper bands detected by anti-T3$_C$ appeared as a band at about 90 kDa (lane E). Note that the 20-kDa and 25-kDa species within the anti-T3 precipitate were similar under reducing and nonreducing conditions. These findings are analogous to those previously obtained with the above series of human cytotoxic T cell clones. The observation that anti-Ti$_{4A}$ (lanes C, F) as well as other anti-Ti antibodies did not precipitate detectable material in the range of the 20- to 25-kDa T3 molecule implied that binding of the monoclonal antibody anti-Ti$_{4A}$ may dissociate the clonotypic structure from the 20- and 25-kDa molecules. Given the above T3 association and the subunit composition of Ti$_{4A}$, it appears that the clonotype on an MHC-restricted antigen-specific inducer clone is very similar in molecular characteristics to the clonotypes found on CTL clones. Although not shown, clonotypes on T8[+] suppressor T lymphocytes are also T3-associated disulfide-linked heterodimers.

PEPTIDE VARIABILITY OF Ti MOLECULES OF DIFFERENT
T CELL CLONES

Comparison by two-dimensional isoelectric focusing and SDS gel electrophoresis of Ti molecules immunoprecipitated from two representative CTL clones, CT4$_{II}$ and CT8$_{III}$, showed that the α subunits of Ti$_1$ and Ti$_2$ had distinct isolectric points (pI 4.4 versus 4.7) as did the two β subunits (pI 6.0 versus 6.2). Both α and β subunits resolved into a series of closely migrating spots (Acuto et al. 1983b). Prolonged treatment of immunoprecipitated Ti molecules with neuraminidase, which cleaves off sialic acid residues from complex oligosaccharides, reduced both α and β subunits to virtually a single spot at unique pI. This indicated that the observed microheterogeneity was due to glycosylation (Acuto O, Reinherz EL unpublished data). Moreover, our unpublished results demonstrated that the polymorphism detected by anti-Ti$_1$ and anti-Ti$_2$ antibodies resided in the peptide moiety of the Ti molecules. Similar analysis of T3, T4, and T8 molecules derived from clones of differing specificities revealed no such evidence of molecular variability.

Based on the above results, we speculated that Ti molecules, similar to the immunoglobulin receptor, may be composed of constant and variable domains. To test this hypothesis directly, we determined comparative two-dimensional peptide maps on isolated ^{125}I-labeled Ti subunits following digestion with proteolytic enzymes (Acuto et al. 1983b). The tryptic peptide maps of the α chains from clones CT4$_{II}$ and CT8$_{III}$ were similar but distinct. At least one major and one minor peptide was identical in both clones. Moreover, the major peptide was also shared by the Ti$_\alpha$ subunit isolated from a thymic tumor (REX), and this implied that constant domains are preserved among Ti molecules even when derived from genetically unrelated individuals (Acuto et al. 1983a).

PARTIAL N-TERMINAL AMINO ACID SEQUENCING OF THE Ti$_\beta$ SUBUNIT

Peptide maps and two-dimensional analysis showed that a 94-kDa disulfide-linked heterodimer existed on the surface of the REX line. This structure was isolated by monoclonal antibodies and was homologous to both α and β subunits of Ti molecules from other IL 2–responsive T cell clones. The advantage of the T3$^+$ REX line growth over clone growth prompted us to exploit the former for large-scale purification of Ti-receptor molecules. To this end, microgram amounts of the heterodimer were isolated by immune affinity chromatography from REX cell membrane and α and β subunits separated by preparative SDS-PAGE. Given the large variability that is observed within the β subunit on peptide map analysis, it was of interest to obtain data on the primary structure of this molecule (Acuto et al. 1984). Unambiguous amino acid analysis was possible for 17 residues out of 20 cycles in a gas-liquid-solid phase protein sequencer. A rabbit antiserum raised against synthetic peptide containing the amino acid sequence from residues 2–11 conjugated to bovine serum albumin as a carrier immunoprecipitated the isolated denatured β chain from REX Ti. This result confirmed that the protein sequence was indeed that of the Ti$_\beta$ subunit. In order to determine whether there were homologies between this N-terminal sequence (residues 2–11 as well as residues 2–20) and known proteins, a computer search employing the Dayhoff protein data bank was utilized. Homologies with the first framework of the variable region of the Ig λ and κ light chains were found. Lambda homology was evident in a search employing residues 2–11, whereas κ homology was obvious when residues 2–20 were used. In fact, 44 of 66 matches were made with human and mouse light-chain first framework of the variable region.

GENES ENCODING THE T CELL RECEPTOR

By using a novel technique of complementary DNA (cDNA) cloning known as subtractive hybridization, two groups very recently described the isolation of human and mouse cDNA clones that encoded putative membrane proteins uniquely expressed in T cells and identified genes that were rearranged in these same cells (Yanagi et al. 1984, Hedrick et al. 1984a,b). Comparison of the Ti_β subunit N-terminal sequence that we obtained and the predicted gene product from the human cDNA clone demonstrated an identity of all residues that could be analyzed. Specifically, the N-terminal amino acid sequence began at residue 22 of the predicted protein, indicating that the first 21 residues belong to the leader signal peptide. The predicted gene protein has a remarkable homology to the human Ig λ light chain in both N-terminal and C-terminal regions and particularly in the area of the cysteine residues. This too agrees with the finding from the N-terminal amino acid sequence of the Ti_β subunit.

The identity of 17 of 17 amino acids in these sequences and the fact that the molecular weights of the predicted polypeptide encoded by the human cDNA protein (35,000) and the membrane form of the Ti_β subunit (43,000) are very close strongly supports the notion that this cDNA clone is the gene for the β subunit of the human Ti molecule. Any differences in molecular weight between the predicted protein and the observed protein likely result from glycosylation. In this regard, it is worthy of note that the human Ti_β subunit is a glycoprotein and at least two potential glycosylation sites for complex oligosaccharides have been identified on the human cDNA gene product. Analysis of the murine T cell–specific cDNA clone revealed, in addition, that the putative protein encoded by the gene contained an N-terminal variable and a C-terminal constant region, which agreed with our own peptide map data. The high degree of homology between the C-terminal regions in the human and mouse clones (80% between residues 134 and 306) and a lack of homology of the α and β subunits at the protein level indicate that the mouse equivalent of the Ti_β subunit has also been cloned.

To characterize the structure of the predicted protein encoded by one such Ti_β cDNA clone, pβREX, a Kyte-Doolittle plot was generated (Figure 1.3) (Kyte and Doolittle 1983). This analysis is based on a water-vapor transfer free energy values exterior-interior distribution of amino acid side chains. Data are expressed as hydropathicity plots, in which peaks above the X axis represent hydrophobic residues (internally buried) and amino acids below the X axis represent hydrophilic residues (exposed). Amino acid positions are numbered according to the N-terminal amino acid sequence data as 1–291. Several features are worthy of comment. First, amino-terminal residues −21 to −1 constitute an extremely hydrophobic portion of the sequence, consistent with the fact that it is the leader sequence. Second, while the carboxy terminal 257–286 sequence is hydrophobic, the residues 287–291 (Lys-Arg-Lys-Asp-Phe) are hydrophilic and heavily charged. This finding predicts that residues 257–286 define a transmembrane region of the molecule and that amino acids 287–291 compose a characteristic cytoplasmic tail similarly found on a large number of transmembrane proteins. Third, the alternating hydrophobic-hydrophilic regions throughout the molecule are characteristic

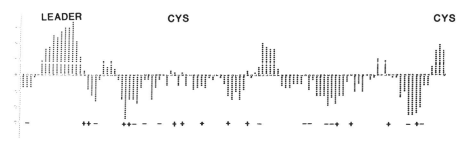

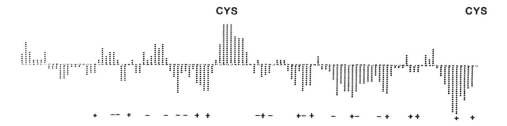

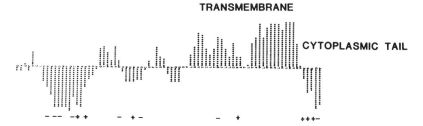

FIGURE 1.3. Hydrophobicity plot of the Ti_β subunit. The weighting system of Kyte and Doolittle was used to delineate hydrophobic regions of the β REX sequence and predict its transmembrane region. The first, second, and third rows correspond to residues 1–90, 91–210, 211–291, respectively. Values are as described by Hendrick et al. (1984b). Charged residues are indicated by $+$ and $-$ Cysteine residues at position 21 and 90 likely define the boundaries of one surface domain and those at 145 and 210 a second domain.

of globular membrane proteins, including Ig (Kabat et al. 1983). Fourth, the positions of cysteine residues within the Ti_β molecule are analogous to those found in Ig. Thus, the pair of cysteines in positions 21 and 90, as well as 145 and 210, are separated by approximately the same number of residues as those cysteines that form intrachain disulfide bonds in Ig molecules (69 and 65 residue spans, respectively) and likely form disulfide loops defining two distinct Ti_β domains. Moreover, the cysteine located at position 245, just N-terminal to the transmembrane region, is in an analogous position to the cysteine of the Ig light chain that forms an interchain disulfide bond to the Ig heavy chain

(Kabat et al. 1983). Whether the cysteine in position 189 also might participate in interchain disulfide bonding is not known, but it appears likely, given the fact that rabbit Ig heavy chains are covalently associated by more than one cysteine residue.

Analysis of a number of Ti_β cDNA nucleotide sequences and this predicted protein sequence suggested that the gene products were strikingly similar to Ig insofar as they contain variable (V), constant (C), joining (J), and diversitylike (D) elements (Figure 1.4). That the rearrangement of germ line Ti_β segments was detected in all functional, mature T cell populations further supported this view (Royer et al. 1984b). Comparison of genomic clones from murine liver DNA and functional T cell populations has led to an understanding of the germ line arrangement of Ti_β elements and signal sequences that result in somatic recombination (Siu et al. 1984a.). Similar organization is found for the human Ti_β locus.

As shown in Figure 1.5, the genomic organization of the constant region locus, which encodes the Ti_β subunit, consists of two tandem sets of segments termed $D_{\beta 1}$-$J_{\beta 1}$-$C_{\beta 1}$ and $D_{\beta 2}$-$J_{\beta 2}$-$C_{\beta 2}$. The two constant regions are remarkably

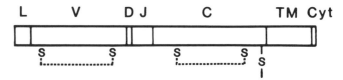

FIGURE 1.4. Predicted primary structure of the β-chain subunit after translation from cDNA sequence. The variable region leader (L), variable domain (V), diversity (D), and joining (J) elements are shown. As part of the constant region (C), a hydrophobic transmembrane segment (TM) and the cytoplasmic part (CYT) are indicated. Potential intrachain sulfhydryl bonds (S-S) are shown as well as the single SH group (S), which can form a sulfhydryl bond with the α subunit.

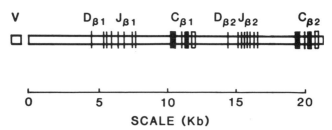

FIGURE 1.5. Scheme of the genomic organization of human β-chain genes. V indicates the V_β gene pool located 5' at an unknown distance of the $D_{\beta 1}$ (diversity) element, $J_{\beta 1}$ cluster and C_β constant region gene. Farther downstream, a second $D_{\beta 2}$ element, $J_{\beta 2}$ cluster and $C_{\beta 2}$ constant region gene are indicated. Distances are noted by kb (kilobases).

similar; they differed only by six amino acids in the translated region. They are, however, dissimilar in the 3′ untranslated region (Yoshikai et al. 1984). Each constant region in the mouse molecule, in turn, is composed of four distinct exons: a first exon encoding an external domain of approximately 125 amino acids; a mini exon encoding six amino acids, including a cysteine thought to form a disulfide bridge to the Ti_α subunit; a third exon encoding 36 amino acids, most of which constitute the hydrophobic transmembrane region; and a fourth exon encoding the cytoplasmic tail and 3′ untranslated region. The transmembrane and cytoplasmic exons are the only coding regions of the molecule where amino acid differences are noted. In contrast, the 3′ untranslated region of the $C_{\beta 1}$ and $C_{\beta 2}$ loci are less than 50% homologous (Yoshikai et al. 1984).

There is a cluster of J segments on the 5′ side of each C_β region. In the murine system, seven J elements have been located on the 5′ side of the C regions, of which only six appear to be functional. Moreover, a D element occurs on the 5′ side of each of the J_β clusters (Siu et al. 1984b). The presence of such D elements was anticipated from the nucleotide sequencing data, which indicated that eight nucleotides between the V and J segments could not be accounted for. Figure 1.5 also indicates that V gene segments are located upstream of $D_{\beta 1}$ at an unknown distance. Rearrangements in T cell receptor genes occur during intrathymic ontogeny. In this process, the D gene segment is brought into a location adjacent to a given J element with deletion of intervening J components. Subsequently, an upstream V segment is repositioned to a site immediately to the 5′ side of the DJ segment. Thus, a contiguous V-D-J sequence is formed that is separated from the C exons by an intervening sequence (Siu et al. 1984a).

In the Ig system, germ line V_H, D_H, and J_H elements are flanked by recombination sequences separated in space by one or two turns of the DNA helix (Early et al. 1980). A feature of the recognition sequences for Ig V_H and V_L gene rearrangement is that a one-turn element is always joined to a two-turn recognition sequence. This rule of one- and two-turn joining is found in the Ti_β gene family as well. Thus, on the 3′ side of V_β and 5′ side of J_β genes are segments with two-turn and one-turn recognition signals, respectively, whereas the D_β gene segment has a one-turn recognition signal on its 5′ side and a two-turn recognition signal on its 3′ side (Siu et al. 1984b). This organization would permit several types of V_β gene formations consistent with the one- to two-turn joining rule: V_β gene segments could join directly to J_β gene segments; V_β-D_β-J_β joining may occur and involve a single D gene segment or several D_β gene segments. Thus, additional combinatorial joining possibilities exist within the Ti_β gene family.

Similar analysis based on biochemistry and molecular cloning of the human and murine Ti_α subunit indicated that these molecules contain an NH_2-terminal V domain, probably created by joining of dispersed germ line genes.

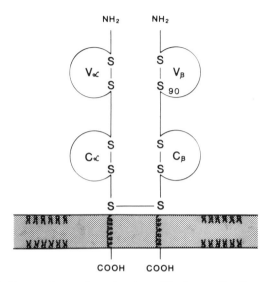

FIGURE 1.6. Proposed secondary structure of the human T cell receptor α and β chains. Starting at the amino terminus (NH$_2$), the α and β chains have variable regions (V$_\alpha$ and V$_\beta$), which form a domain stabilized by an intrachain S-S bond between cysteines. In a similar way, the constant region domains are formed by intrachain S-S bonds. The subunits are held together by an interchain S-S bond close to the cell membrane. Both chains have a hydrophobic transmembrane segment and a short cytoplasmic tail at their carboxy terminus.

Moreover, the Ti$_\alpha$ subunit, like the Ti$_\beta$ subunit, bears homology to Ig heavy and light chains (Saito et al. 1984, Chien et al. 1984, Hannum et al. 1984, Fabbi et al. 1984). Thus, it is likely that variable regions of the Ti$_\alpha$ and Ti$_\beta$ chains will interact to form a single combining site (Figure 1.6). To date, all evidence has indicated that functional isotypes (helpers versus suppressors) are not encoded in the T cell receptor subunits themselves (Royer et al. 1984b).

THE ONTOGENY OF THE T CELL RECEPTOR

Earlier studies delineated three discrete stages of human intrathymic differentiation based upon surface expression of multiple T lineage–specific glycoproteins (stage I: T10$^+$T3$^-$T4$^-$T6$^-$T8$^-$; stage II: T10$^+$T3$^-$T4$^+$T6$^+$T8$^+$; and stage III: T10$^+$T3$^+$T4$^+$[T4$^-$]T6$^+$T8$^+$[T8$^-$]) (Reinherz and Schlossman 1980a, van Wauwe 1980, Royer et al. 1984a). Of note was the finding that T3 appeared on a minor population of cells and only during late intrathymic ontogeny (stage III). To determine whether clonotypic structures were expressed on T lineage cells during thymic differentiation, we produced monoclonal antibodies to REX (T10$^+$T3$^+$T4$^+$T6$^-$T8$^+$) (Reinherz et al. 1980c). The results of SDS-PAGE and peptide map analyses indicated that a homologous T3-associated heterodimer was synthesized and expressed by REX. In addition, similar Ti-related molecules appeared during intrathymic ontogeny in parallel with surface T3 expression. This expression could be documented by the presence of disulfide-linked heterodimers on Goding map analysis of ^{125}I-labeled membranes from T3$^+$ but not T3$^-$ thymocytes.

The presence of Ti-related, disulfide-linked heterodimers, as defined by two-dimensional gel analysis on T3$^+$ thymocytes and T3$^+$ T cell tumors, was not surprising, given the unique association of Ti with the T3 molecule and the fact that these T3$^+$ cells are derived in the late stages of intrathymic and postthymic differentiation. The fact that T3$^-$ T acute lymphoblastic leukemia cells or thymocytes derived from stage I or early stage II compartments lack Ti strengthened the implication that the Ti antigen receptor is intimately linked to T3 expression during ontogeny. This result provided a structural

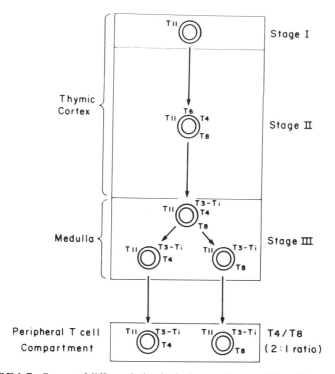

FIGURE 1.7. Stages of differentiation in the human thymus. Three discrete stages of thymic differentiation are defined based on the sequential expression of T cell differentiation antigens and the T3-Ti molecular complex.

TABLE 1.2. *Relationship of Ti$_\beta$ Gene Rearrangement to Surface Ti Expression*

Stage	Phenotype	Surface Ti	Ti Gene Rearrangement
I	T11$^+$T3$^-$T6$^-$	−	−
II	T11$^+$T3$^-$T6$^+$	−	+
III	T11$^+$T3$^+$T6$^-$	+	+

basis for the observation that immunologic competence (such as responsiveness to alloantigens in MHC) was acquired only among the population of thymocytes that expressed surface T3 (Figure 1.7) (Umiel et al. 1982).

It seemed likely that surface Ti expression on thymocytes was preceded by DNA rearrangements analogous to those occurring in Ig heavy-chain genes prior to surface Ig expression during B cell differentiation (Early et al. 1980). To obtain further information about the ontogeny of the T cell antigen and MHC receptor, a Ti$_\beta$ subunit cDNA probe and heteroantisera specific for the Ti$_\alpha$ and Ti$_\beta$ subunits were utilized to characterize human T lineage cells. Analysis of thymic tumors and normal thymocytes at both the DNA and protein levels demonstrated that Ti$_\beta$ gene rearrangement was evident in stage II (T11$^+$T6$^+$T3$^-$) and stage III (T11$^+$T6$^-$T3$^+$), but not stage I (T11$^+$T6$^-$T3$^-$) thymocytes. In contrast, surface expression of Ti$_\alpha$ and Ti$_\beta$ molecules was exclusively restricted to stage III thymocytes. Thus, human T lineage ontogeny is characterized by an orderly series of differentiation steps wherein Ti$_\beta$ gene rearrangement precedes surface expression of the T3-Ti molecular complex (Table 1.2) (Royer et al. 1984a). Recent data also indicate that Ti$_\alpha$ gene rearrangement occurs duing intrathymic ontogeny, probably after Ti$_\beta$ gene activation. Although the T3 molecule has not been defined in the murine system, there are disulfide-linked dimers analogous to Ti that are expressed on murine thymocytes and T-T hybridomas (Allison et al. 1982, Haskins et al. 1983). Future analysis of these structures will indicate whether their ontogeny is identical to that of Ti in humans.

ANTIGENLIKE EFFECTS OF MONOCLONAL ANTIBODIES DIRECTED AT T CELL RECEPTOR STRUCTURES

If anti-Ti monoclonal antibodies define variable regions of the T cell receptor, then under the appropriate conditions, anti-Ti antibodies might induce clonal T cell activation in a fashion analogous to that of antigen itself. Because the alloantigens that serve as receptor ligands are membrane bound and likely interact via multipoint surface attachment and because anticlonotypic monoclonal antibodies, by themselves, were not mitogenic, we investigated the functional effects of purified monoclonal antibodies bound to a solid surface support (Sepharose beads) (Meuer et al. 1983e).

A number of important points emerged from these experiments: (1) antigen, Sepharose-linked anti-Ti, and Sepharose-linked anti-T3 caused very similar functional effects, initiating clonal proliferation and secretion of lymphokines including IL 2, (2) triggering a single clonally unique epitope appears to be sufficient to induce antigen-specific functions and to substitute for antigen plus MHC determinant, (3) multimeric interaction between ligand and antigen receptor was an essential requirement for the initiation of clonal T cell responses because non-surface–linked monoclonal antibodies do not mediate these effects, (4) the T4 and T8 surface structures, although critical for MHC-restricted CTL effector function, could not be triggered by monoclonal antibodies to induce clonal proliferation or lymphokine secretion, and (5) these clones produced and responded to IL 2 (Meuer et al. 1984).

A MODEL OF ANTIGEN RECOGNITION BY T CELLS

From these studies, it is possible to construct a unifying model of antigen recognition by T lymphocytes. The structure responsible for dual recognition (antigen and MHC) consists of the clonally unique Ti molecule, which is associated with the T3 glycoproteins. In addition, depending on the subset derivation of the individual T lymphocyte, T4 or T8 glycoproteins serve as "ancillary" binding structures for an invariant portion of class II or I MHC gene production, respectively. The T4 and T8 glycoproteins do not appear to be critical for T cell activation and may therefore be considered stabilizing elements that facilitate the cell-cell contact necessary for efficient target-cell lysis by CTL. This might be particularly important for killer-target cell interactions, as well as triggering primary immune responses prior to clonal selection of high-affinity antigen-responsive cells. However, it seems likely that at the clonal level, some effector cells exist that display high-affinity Ti-T3 receptors for specific antigens and thus do not require T4 or T8 in order to interact with stimulator and target cells. Such T cell clones have been reported recently (Spits et al. 1983). Given the extent of T cell diversity, one might also expect to find an occasional clone viewing antigen plus MHC gene product only with its high affinity Ti-T3 antigen receptor and in apparent contradiction to the T4 class II and T8 class I correlation.

T3-Ti ANTIGEN RECEPTOR COMPLEX TRIGGERING IN CLONAL T CELL PROLIFERATION

Upon binding to the surface of a clone, monoclonal antibodies to either T3 or Ti induced rapid loss of the T3-Ti complex and inhibited all antigen-specific functions of a given clone. However, at the same time, these antibodies

produced a markedly enhanced clonal proliferative response to IL 2. Moreover, when coupled to Sepharose, the appropriate surface-linked anti-Ti and
anti-T3 antibodies were able to induce IL 2 secretion and clonal proliferation,
analogous to the physiologic ligand (antigen) itself (Meuer et al. 1983e).
These findings suggested that clonal proliferation resulting from triggering
the T3-Ti antigen receptor might be mediated through the growth factor IL 2.
IL 2 is a 15-kDa sialoglycoprotein that interacts with activated T cells through
specific membrane receptors distinct from the T3-Ti complex and induces T
cell growth when it binds to the surface (Robb et al. 1981, Smith et al.
1980a,b, Uchiyama 1981, Leonard et al. 1982, Depper et al. 1983).

As expected, the IL 2–driven proliferative responses of clones in either an
unmodulated or anti-Ti modulated state could be abrogated by anti–IL 2 receptor antibodies or anti–IL 2 antibodies ($\geq$90% inhibition). Moreover, these
same studies showed that the enhanced in vitro proliferative response to IL 2
by anti-Ti– or anti-T3–modulated T cell clones was a consequence of rapid
induction (within hours) of IL 2 receptors (6- to 10-fold increase). Perhaps
more important is that similar increases in IL 2 receptor expression and T3-Ti
modulation were triggered by the appropriate combination of antigen and
MHC.

That triggering of the T structure should result in endogenous IL 2 production, enhanced IL 2 receptor expression, and clonal proliferation appeared
more than coincidental and suggested that stimulation of clonal proliferation
through antigen receptor triggering was due to release and subsequent binding
of endogenous IL 2 (an autocrine mechanism). Thus, one would anticipate
that clonal proliferation after antigen receptor triggering and cross-linking
could be inhibited by anti–IL 2 or anti–IL 2 receptor antibodies. This was
precisely the case (Meuer et al. 1984).

Therefore, it appears that T cell proliferation occurs as a series of complex
and precisely orchestrated events, as outlined in Figure 1.8. Resting T cell
clones or T cells express few or no IL 2 receptors but display a maximal number of surface antigen receptors (stage 1). However, T3-Ti receptor triggering
by the appropriate antigen plus MHC gene product or Sepharose-bound anticlonotypic monoclonal antibodies results in modulation of the T3-Ti complex
(stage 2), thus diminishing the number of surface antigen receptors and rapidly
inducing surface IL 2 receptor expression (stage 3). Furthermore, such activation also leads to endogenous IL 2 production, secretion, and subsequent
binding to IL 2 receptors on the same clones (stage 4). Once a critical number
of IL 2 receptors have bound IL 2, DNA synthesis and cell mitosis occur
(stage 5). Finally, in the absence of continued antigenic stimulation, there is
reexpression of surface T3-Ti antigen receptor complex and, reciprocally, a
reduction in the number of IL 2 receptors (stage 1).

The view that is emerging regarding the relationship of the T3-Ti antigen
receptor to the IL 2 receptor points to a mechanism whereby external stimuli

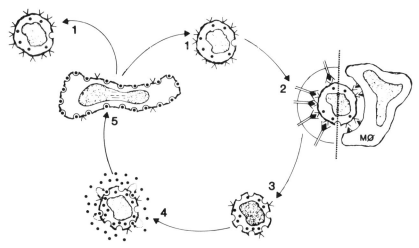

FIGURE 1.8. Schematic model of T cell proliferation mediated by an IL 2–dependent autocrine mechanism. Stage 1: Resting T cells or T cell clones. Stage 2: T3-Ti triggering. Stage 3: IL 2 receptor and antigen receptor modulation resulting from T3-Ti triggering. Stage 4: Activation via T3-Ti. Stage 5: DNA synthesis and mitosis occur. IL 2 (•), IL 2 receptors (∿), antigen receptors (∨), antigen/MHC-restricing element (▲), surface-bound anti-T cell receptor antibodies (Ƴ).

(i.e., antigens) direct the magnitude and extent of T cell clonal proliferation by means of the IL 2 hormone-receptor system. Immunologic specificity is ensured by the antigen dependence of the IL 2 receptor expression, and yet, the reciprocal appearance of T3-Ti and IL 2 receptors presumably leaves the cell in a state of responsiveness to either the hormone or the antigen ligand. However, the transient expression of the IL 2 receptors themselves serves as a fail-safe system to eliminate any possibility of uncontrolled growth through an IL 2–dependent mechanism. Whether alteration of this mechanism results in tumor growth in vivo, as suggested by studies on continuously growing, IL 2–producing primate tumor lines of T cell lineage, remains to be determined, but appears to be likely (Gootenberg et al. 1981).

The present construct clearly implies that T cell proliferation is mediated through an autocrine network in which antigen receptor triggering leads to IL 2 receptor expression, IL 2 production, IL 2 release, and subsequent IL 2 receptor occupancy, which ultimately promotes cell division. It does not necessarily follow that all T cells produce and respond to their own IL 2. In fact, one would predict that the failure of certain cells to proliferate in response to antigenic stimulus occurs as a consequence of their inability to produce sufficient amounts of endogenous IL 2, although such cells would, in all likelihood, be triggered to express IL 2 receptors. Furthermore, even for IL

2–producing T cells, exogenous sources of IL 2 would amplify clonal proliferation. However, the present results are clearly different from those anticipated from the conventional endocrine notion that suggests that one cell type produces IL 2 while a different one responds to it.

IMPLICATIONS OF THE MOLECULAR DEFINITION OF THE T3-Ti T CELL RECEPTOR COMPLEX FOR HUMAN DISEASE

Functional and structural studies indicate that the T3-Ti T cell antigen receptor complex consists of at least five polypeptide chains: the polymorphic α and β subunits of the Ti molecule and the invariant glycosylated 20-kDa and 25-kDa and nonglycosylated 20-kDa T3 subunits (Figure 1.9). The specificity of the anticlonotypic antibodies for the Ti molecule and unique peptides resulting from proteolysis of different Ti heterodimers implies that variable regions exist within both Ti_α and Ti_β subunits. Hence, the subunits presumably serve as ligand binding sites. In contrast, the 20- and 25-kDa T3 molecules are likely necessary for transducing signals from the surface into the cytosol following allosteric changes created by ligand-Ti binding. This transduction appears to be associated with sodium- and calcium-dependent plasma membrane–mediated depolarization (Weiss et al. 1984). The observation that the 20-kDa subunit (glycosylated) has a long cytoplasmic tail, whereas the Ti_α and Ti_β subunits do not, further supports the notion that one or more of the T3 subunits function in signal transaction. Whether the T3 subunits themselves represent ion channels, as shown for other receptors, e.g., acetyl choline, is not known. However, since the nonglycosylated 20-kDa subunit of T3 is hydrophobic, this subunit represents a candidate for an ion channel.

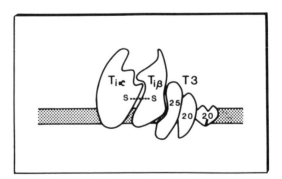

FIGURE 1.9. Subunit composition of the human T cell receptor. Ti_α and Ti_β subunits are held together by S-S bonds and are associated with the 25-kDa chain of the T3 molecule. The α and β subunits are anchored in the cell membrane with their transmembrane segments. The T3 complex consists of two additional subunits of 20 kDa.

Structural or functional defects of the T3-Ti T cell activation system could result in a number of immunodeficient states. Release of cells lacking the T3-Ti complex either prematurely or as a consequence of aberrations of T cell maturation would lead to an immunoincompetent state. The lymphoid cells of most patients with severe combined immunodeficiency, for example, lack surface T3 expression and hence have not acquired T cell antigen receptors (Reinherz et al. 1981a). In contrast, other patients demonstrate phenotypically mature (T3$^+$) inducer T cells, but the cells fail to respond to antigens or mitogens (Reinherz et al. 1981b). These cells likely display defects in transmembrane signaling or aberrant function of the IL 2–dependent autocrine pathway. Additional functional and biochemical analyses of such patients shall provide insight into the precise level of dysfunction. Whether functional abnormalities of T4$^+$ inducer cells in patients with acquired immunodeficiency syndrome (AIDS) or other viral diseases is related to defects in T cell receptor activation pathway is not known, but it appears likely, particularly in view of recent reports suggesting that anti-T3 antibody fails to activate T cells of patients with AIDS.

While congenital or acquired defects in the T cell activation system may account for the devastating effects of immunodeficiency disorders, understanding the molecular basis of T cell activation via the T3-Ti complex could help the design of selective immunosuppressive therapies. We already know, for example, that cyclosporin A inhibits antigen-specific T cell proliferation (Pawelec and Wernet 1983) but not IL 2–induced proliferation. Thus, it may inhibit T3-Ti signal transduction leading to T cell proliferation. Human T cell clones and antireceptor monoclonal antibodies should provide ideal systems with which to test the effects of various experimental drugs for their potency in inhibiting T cell activation.

The ability to produce anticlonotypic antibodies has important diagnostic and therapeutic implications for autoimmune disorders. In diseases such as multiple sclerosis (MS), dermatomyositis, and rheumatoid arthritis, it is likely that a single dominant clone initiates destruction of the target organ. Anticlonotypic monoclonal antibodies specific for such effector or regulatory cells could provide a rapid and reliable means to monitor disease activity. Moreover, the anticlonotypes may provide a powerful selective therapeutic strategy for elimination of these cells. Because cross-reactive anticlonotypic antibodies exist in many experimental antibody systems, it is also conceivable that anticlonotypic reagents to "renegade" T cell clones in one MS patient would react with those in other MS patients.

The ability to define cell surface antigens that appear at specific stages of human T cell differentiation has allowed for the orderly dissection of T cell malignant processes. In fact, these T cell diseases reflect the same degree of heterogeneity and maturation present in normal T cell ontogeny. Whereas the tumor cells in most cases of acute T cell lymphoblastic leukemia arise from an early T3⁻ thymocyte or prothymocyte compartment, the tumors from patients with acute lymphoblastic lymphoma, T cell chronic lymphatic leukemia, adult T cell leukemia, Sézary syndrome, and mycosis fungoides are derived from a mature T cell compartment bearing the T3 molecule. Since T3 is coordinately expressed with a Ti receptor structure, anticlonotypic reagents may be diagnostically and therapeutically useful in these T cell malignancies as well.

SUMMARY

Recent studies using cloned antigen-specific T lymphocytes and monoclonal antibodies directed at their various surface glycoprotein components have led to identification of the human T cell antigen receptor as a surface complex composed of a clonotypic 90-kDa Ti heterodimer and the invariant 20- and 25-kDa T3 molecules. Approximately 30,000–40,000 Ti and T3 molecules exist on the surface of human T lymphocytes. These glycoproteins are acquired and expressed during late thymic ontogeny, thus providing the structural basis for immunologic competence. The Ti_α and Ti_β subunits bear no precursor-to-product relationship and are encoded by separate germ line V, D, J, and C segments, which rearrange during intrathymic differentiation to form an active gene set. Triggering of the T3-Ti receptor complex induces a rapid increase in free cytoplasmic Ca^{2+} and gives rise to specific antigen-induced proliferation through an autocrine pathway involving endogenous IL 2 production, release, and subsequent binding to IL 2 receptors.

REFERENCES

Acuto O, Fabbi M, Smart J, et al. 1984. Purification and N-terminal amino acid sequencing of the β subunit of a human T cell antigen receptor. Proc Natl Acad Sci USA 81:3851.

Acuto O, Hussey RE, Fitzgerald KA, et al. 1983a. The human T cell receptor: Appearance in ontogeny and biochemical relationship of the α and β subunits on IL-2 dependent clones and T cell tumors. Cell 34:717.

Acuto O, Meuer SC, Hodgdon JC, et al. 1983b. Peptide variability exists within the α and β subunits of the T cell receptor for antigen. J Exp Med 158:1368.

Allison JP, McIntyre RW, Bloch D. 1982. Tumor specific antigen and murine T lymphoma defined with monoclonal antibody. J Immunol 129:2293.

Benacerraf B, McDevitt H. 1979. Histocompatibility-linked immune response genes. Science 175:273.

Biddison WE, Rao PE, Thalle MA, et al. 1982. Possible involvement of the OKT4 molecule in T cell recognition of class II HLA antigen: Evidence from studies of cytotoxic T lymphocytes specific for SB antigens. J Exp Med 156:1065.

Bonnard GD, Yasaka K, Macad RD. 1980. Continued growth of functional human T lymphocytes: Production of human T cell growth factors. Cell Immunol 51:390.

Burns GF, Boyd AE, Beverley PCI. 1982. Two monoclonal anti-human T lymphocyte antibodies have similar biologic effects and recognize the same cell surface antigen. J Immunol 124:1451.

Cantor H, Boyse EA. 1977. Regulation of cellular and humoral immune responses by T cell subclasses. Cold Spring Harbor Symp Quant Biol 41:23.

Cantor H, Gershon RK. 1979. Immunological circuits: Cellular compositions. Fed Proc 38:2051.

Cerottini JC. 1980. Clonal analysis of cytolytic T lymphocytes and their precursors. Progress in Immunology 4:622.

Chang TW, Kung PC, Gingras S, Goldstein G. 1981. Does OKT3 monoclonal antibody react with an antigen recognition structure on human T cells? Proc Natl Acad Sci USA 78:1805.

Chien Y, Becker DM, Lindsten T, et al. 1984. A third type of murine T cell receptor gene. Nature 312:31.

Corradin G, Chiller JM. 1979. Lymphocyte specificity to protein antigens: II. Fine specificity of T cell activation with cytochrome c and derived peptides as antigenic probes. J Exp Med 149:436.

Depper JM, Leonard WJ, Robb RJ, Waldmann TA, Greene WC. 1983. Blockade of the interleukin-2 receptor by anti-Tac antibody: Inhibition of human lymphocyte activation. J Immunol 131:690.

Doherty PC. 1980. Surveillance of self: Cell-mediated immunity to virally modified cell surface defined operationally by the major histocompatibility complex. Progress in Immunology 4:563.

Early P, Huang H, Davis M, Calame K, Hood L. 1980. An immunoglobulin heavy chain variable region gene is generated from three segments of DNA: V_H, D and J_H. Cell 19:981.

Fabbi M, Acuto O, Smart JE, Reinherz EL. 1984. Homology of the Ti_α subunit of a T cell antigen-MHC receptor with immunoglobulin. Nature 312:269.

Gershon RK. 1974. T cell control of antibody production. Contemp Top Mol Immunol 3:1.

Gootenberg JE, Ruscetti FW, Mier JW, et al. 1981. Human cutaneous T cell lymphoma and leukemia cell lines produce and respond to T cell growth factor. J Exp Med 154:1403.

Hannum CH, Kappler JW, Trowbridge IA, et al. 1984. Immunoglobulin-like nature of the α chain of a human T cell antigen/MHC receptor. Nature 312:65.

Haskins K, Kubo R, White J, et al. 1983. The major histocompatibility complex restricted antigen receptor on T cells: I. Isolation with a monoclonal antibody. J Exp Med 157:1149.

Hedrick SM, Cohen DI, Nielsen EA, Davis MM. 1984a. Isolation of cDNA clones encoding T cell specific membrane associated proteins. Nature 308:149.

Hedrick SM, Nielsen EA, Kavaler J, et al. 1984b. Sequence relationships between putative T cell receptor polypeptides and immunoglobulins. Nature 308:153.

Hunig T, Bevan M. 1981. Specificity of T cell clones illustrates altered self hypothesis. Nature 294:460.

Kabat EA, Wu TT, Bilofsky H, Reed-Miller M, Perry H. 1983. Sequences of proteins of immunological interest. US Department of Health and Human Services, Bethesda, MD, p. 323.

Krensky AM, Clayberger C, Reiss CS, et al. 1982. Specificity of OKT4+ cytotoxic T lymphocyte clones. J Immunol 129:2001.

Kurnick JT, Gronvik KO, Kimura AK, et al. 1979. Long-term growth in vitro of human T cell blasts with maintenance of specificity and function. J Immunol 122:255.

Kyte J, Doolittle RF. 1983. A simple method for displaying the hydropathic character of a protein. J Mol Biol 157:133.

Leonard WJ, Depper JM, Uchiyama T, et al. 1982. A monoclonal antibody that appears to recognize the receptor for human T cell growth factor: Partial characterization of the receptor. Nature 300:267.

Lipton JM, Reinherz EL, Kudisch M, et al. 1980. Mature bone marrow erythroid burst forming units do not require T cells for induction of erythropoietin-dependent differentiation. J Exp Med 152:350.

Meuer SC, Hussey RE, Hodgdon JC, et al. 1982a. Surface structures involved in target recognition by human cytotoxic T lymphocytes. Science 218:471.

Meuer SC, Schlossman SF, Reinherz EL. 1982b. Differential activation and specificity of human T cell subpopulations. In Vitteta ES, ed., UCLA Symposium on Molecular and Cellular Biology, vol 24. New York, Academic Press p.127.

Meuer SC, Schlossman SF, Reinherz EL. 1982c. Clonal analysis of human cytotoxic T lymphocytes: T4 and T8 effector T cells recognize products of different major histocompatibility regions. Proc Natl Acad Sci USA 79:4395.

Meuer SC, Acuto O, Hussey RE, et al. 1983a. Evidence for the T3-associated 90 kD heterodimer as the T cell antigen receptor. Nature 303:808.

Meuer SC, Cooper DA, Hodgdon JC, et al. 1983b. Identification of the antigen/MHC receptor on human inducer T lymphocytes. Science 222:1239.

Meuer SC, Fitzgerald KA, Hussey RE, et al. 1983c. Clonotypic structures involved in antigen specific human T cell function: Relationship to the T3 molecular complex. J Exp Med 157:705.

Meuer SC, Hodgdon JC, Cooper DA, et al. 1983d. Human cytotoxic T cell clones directed at autologous virus-transformed targets: Further evidence for linkage of genetic restrictions to T4 and T8 surface glycoproteins. J Immunol 131:186.

Meuer SC, Hodgdon JC, Hussey RE, et al. 1983e. Antigen-like effects of monoclonal antibodies directed at receptors on human T cell clones. J Exp Med 158:988.

Meuer SC, Hussey RE, Cantrell DA, et al. 1984. Triggering of the T3-Ti antigen receptor complex results in clonal T cell proliferation via an interleukin 2 dependent autocrine pathway. Proc Natl Acad Sci USA 81:1509.

Morgan DA, Ruscetti RW, Gallo RC. 1976. Selective in vitro growth of T lymphocytes from normal human bone marrow. Science 193:1007.

Pawelec G, Wernet P. 1983. Cyclosporin A inhibits interleukin 2 dependent growth of alloactivated cloned human T lymphocytes. Int J Immunopharmacol 5:315.

Pick E, Cohen S, Oppenheim JJ. 1979. The lymphokine concept. In Cohen S, Pick E, Oppenheim JJ, eds., Biology of the Lymphokines. Academic Press, New York, pp. 1–12.

Quinnan GV, Kirmani N, Rook AH, et al. 1982. Cytotoxic T cells in cytomegalovirus infection: HLA-restricted T-lymphocyte non-T-lymphocyte cytotoxic responses correlate with recovery from cytomegalovirus infection in bone-marrow-transplant recipients. N Engl J Med 307:7.

Reinherz EL, Schlossman SF. 1980a. The differentiation and function of human T lymphocytes. Cell 19:821.

Reinherz EL, Schlossman SF. 1980b. Regulation of the immune response: Inducer

and suppressor T lymphocyte subsets in human beings. N Engl J Med 303:370.
Reinherz EL, Schlossman SF. 1981. The characterization and function of human immunoregulatory T lymphocyte subsets. Immunol Today 2:69.
Reinherz EL, Kung PC, Goldstein G, Schlossman SF. 1979a. Separation of functional subsets of human T cells by a monoclonal antibody. Proc Natl Acad Sci USA 76:4061.
Reinherz EL, Kung PC, Pesando JM, et al. 1979b. Ia determination on human T cell subsets defined by monoclonal antibody: Activation stimuli required for expression. J Exp Med 150:1472.
Reinherz EL, Hussey RE, Schlossman SF. 1980a. A monoclonal antibody blocking human T cell function. Eur J Immunol 10:758.
Reinherz EL, Kung PC, Goldstein G, Schlossman SF. 1980b. A monoclonal antibody reactive with the human cytotoxic/suppressor T cell subset previously defined by a heteroantiserum termed TH$_2$. J Immunol 124:1301.
Reinherz EL, Kung PC, Goldstein G, et al. 1980c. Discrete stages of human intrathymic differentiation: Analysis of normal thymocytes and leukemic lymphoblasts of T lineage. Proc Natl Acad Sci USA 77:1588.
Reinherz EL, Morimoto C, Penta AC, Schlossman SF. 1980d. Regulation of B cell immunoglobulin secretion by functional subsets of T lymphocytes in man. Eur J Immunol 10:570.
Reinherz EL, Cooper MD, Schlossman SF, Rosen FS. 1981a. Abnormalities of T cell maturation and regulation in human beings with immunodeficiency disorders. J Clin Invest 68:699.
Reinherz EL, Geha R, Wohl ME, et al. 1981b. Immunodeficiency associated with loss of T4+ inducer T cell function. N Engl J Med 304:811.
Reinherz EL, Hussey RE, Fitzgerald KA, et al. 1981c. Antibody directed at a surface structure inhibits cytolytic but not suppressor function of human T lymphocytes. Nature 299:168.
Reinherz EL, Meuer SC, Fitzgerald KA, et al. 1982. Antigen recognition by human T lymphocytes is linked to surface expression of the T3 molecular complex. Cell 30:735.
Robb RJ, Munck A, Smith KA. 1981. T cell growth factor receptors: Quantitation, specificity and biological relevance. J Exp Med 154:1455.
Royer HD, Acuto O, Fabbi M, et al. 1984a. Genes encoding the Ti$_\beta$ subunit of the antigen/MHC receptor undergo rearrangement during intrathymic ontogeny prior to surface T3-Ti expression. Cell 39:261.
Royer HD, Bensussan A, Acuto O, Reinherz EL. 1984b. Functional isotypes are not encoded by the constant region genes of the β subunit of the T cell receptor for antigen/major histocompatibility complex. J Exp Med 160:947.
Saito H, Kranz DM, Takagaki D, et al. 1984. A third rearranged and expressed gene in a clone of cytotoxic T lymphocytes. Nature 312:36.
Schlossman SF. 1979. Antigen recognition: The specificity of T cells involved in the cellular immune response. Transplant Rev 10:97.
Siu G, Clark SP, Yoshikai Y, et al. 1984a. The human T cell antigen receptor is encoded by variable, diversity and joining gene segments that rearrange to generate a complete V gene. Cell 37:393.
Siu G, Kronenberg M, Strauss E, Haars R, Mak TW, Hood L. 1984b. The structure, rearrangement and expression of D$_\beta$ gene segments of the murine T cell antigen receptor. Nature 311:562
Smith KA, Baker PE, Gillis S, Ruscetti RW. 1980a. Functional and molecular

characteristics of T cell growth factor. Mol Immunol 17:579.

Smith KA, Lachman LB, Oppenheim JJ, Favata MF. 1980b. The functional relationship of the interleukins. J Exp Med 151:1551.

Spits H, Ijssel H, Thomas A, deVries JE. 1983. Human T4+ and T8+ cytotoxic T lymphocyte clones directed at products of different class II major histocompatibility complex loci. J Immunol 131:678.

Sredni B, Tse HY, Schwartz RH. 1980. Direct cloning and extended culture of antigen-specific, MHC-restricted, proliferating T lymphocytes. Nature 283:581.

Uchiyama T, Broder S, Waldmann TA. 1981. A monoclonal antibody (anti-Tac) reactive with activated and functionally mature human T cells: I. Production of anti-Tac monoclonal antibody and distribution of Tac+ cells. J Immunol 126:1393.

Umiel T, Daley JF, Bhan AK, et al. 1982. Acquisition of immune competence by a subset of human cortical thymocytes expressing mature T cell antigens. J Immunol 129:1054.

van Wauwe FP, DeMay JR, Coosener JG. 1980. OKT3: A monoclonal anti-human T lymphocyte antibody with potent mitogenic properties. J Immunol 124:2708.

Waldmann TA. 1978. Disorders of suppressor immunoregulatory cells in the pathogenesis of immunodeficiency and autoimmunity. Ann Intern Med 88:226.

Wallace LE, Rickinson AB, Rose M, Epstein MA. 1982. Epstein-Barr virus specific cytotoxic T cell clones restricted through a single HLA antigen. Nature 297:413.

Weiss MJ, Daley JF, Hodgdon JC, Reinherz EL. 1984. Calcium dependency of antigen specific (T3-Ti) and alternative (T11) pathways of human T cell activation. Proc Natl Acad Sci USA 81:6836.

Yanagi Y, Yoshikai Y, Legget K, et al. 1984. A human T cell specific cDNA clone encodes a protein having extensive homology to immunoglobulin chains. Nature 308:145.

Yoshikai Y, Anatoniou D, Clark SP, et al. 1984. Sequence and expression of transcripts of the human T cell receptor β chain genes. Nature 312:521.

Zinkernagel RM, Doherty PC. 1975. H-2 compatibility requirement for T cell mediated lysis of target infected with lymphocytic choriomeningitis virus: Different cytotoxic T cell specificities are associated with structures coded in H-2K or H-2D. J Exp Med 141:1427.

Symposium on Fundamental Cancer Research, Vol. 38.

2. Targeting Cells for Attack by Cytotoxic T Lymphocytes Using Heteroconjugates of Monoclonal Antibodies

Uwe D. Staerz and Michael J. Bevan

Department of Immunology, Scripps Clinic and Research Foundation, La Jolla, California 92037

The rationale for the results presented here was our desire to combine the potentially therapeutic advantages of monoclonal antibodies (MAbs) with T cell immunity. Most immunologists would agree that a cell-mediated T cell response is more effective than a humoral, antibody response in rejecting foreign or unwanted cells. In many clinical situations it is apparent, however, that an effective cell-mediated response fails to develop. There are at lease three reasons that make it difficult to conceive of using preimmunized T cells to adoptively transfer effector cell-mediated response into patients who lack it. First, the T cell response to any conventional antigen is major histocompatibility complex (MHC) restricted. This means that the T cells are not specific for the conventional antigen seen in isolation but for the conventional antigen in association with the MHC antigens with which it was presented. Second, T cells express all of the strong histocompatibility antigens and, in most cases, could not be transplanted across such barriers. Third, it is a common finding that T cells grown for prolonged periods as lines or clones in vitro no longer function well when transplanted back to the donor in vivo. They lose the receptors for homing into lymph nodes and, in most cases, also seem unable to enter sites of inflammation.

The great advantages of MAbs are in their known specificity for antigen, their reproducibility, and their availability in large amounts. Thus, having a MAb to a particular antigen allows one to purify that antigen, using affinity chromatographic techniques, to detect that antigen in ELISA tests, for example, and, hopefully, to use it to wipe out cells that express the antigen either alone or when coupled to a toxin molecule. In most cases, it appears that T cell immunity is more effective at rejecting unwanted cells.

The results we present here provide the means whereby the great advantages of MAbs and T cell immunity can be combined. The difficulties of using T cell immunity are overcome. One requirement is having a MAb that recognizes a determinant on the T cell receptor complex. The other is having a MAb that recognizes an antigen of restricted tissue or tumor distribution.

RESULTS AND DISCUSSION

Our work began with the report by Lancki and Fitch (1984) that surprisingly showed that a B cell hybridoma producing a MAb specific for an idiotypic determinant on a cytotoxic T lymphocyte (CTL) clone served as a target for cytolysis by that clone. The B cell hybridoma did not bear the histocompatibility antigens that the CTL clone recognized, and the investigators hypothesized, quite reasonably, that the combining site on the MAb at the surface of the B cell was responsible for focusing the CTL on that cell, which led to its lysis. We decided to investigate whether this interpretation was correct by chemically coupling the surface of various cells with MAbs for anti–T cell receptors and checking whether this rendered them sensitive targets for CTL that expressed receptors that have determinants recognized by such fixed MAbs.

In this work, we used the two CTL clones and four MAbs described below:

1. CTL clone G4 is from a BALB.B (H-2^b) mouse ånd is specific for H-2^d targets (Staerz et al. 1984).

2. CTL clone OE4 is from a B6 (H-2^b) mouse and is specific for H-2^d targets (Kanagawa O unpublished data). Neither clone G4 nor OE4 recognized or lysed H-2^k–bearing target cells.

3. MAb F9 is a clonotypic (idiotype specific) immunoglobulin (Ig) G1 and is prepared from a BALB/c mouse immunized with G4 (Staerz et al. 1984).

4. MAb F23.1 is an IgG2a prepared from C57L/J immunized with BALB.B T cells and is specific for an allotypic determinant expressed on 25% of T cell receptors, including CTL clone OE4 (Staerz et al. 1985).

5. MAb 20.8.4 is an IgG2a prepared from a C3H mouse and is specific for H-2^b (Ozato and Sachs 1981).

6. MAb 19E12 is an IgG2a and is specific for the Thy 1.1 alloantigen (Houston et al. 1980).

S.AKR target cells, derived from AKR/J mice (H-2^k, Thy 1.1) were coupled at their surfaces with various MAbs, using the heterobifunctional cross-linking reagent N-succinimidyl 3-(2-pyridyldithio) propionate (SPDP). Table 2.1 shows that uncoupled S.AKR targets are not lysed by either CTL clone. However, when coupled with the appropriate anti-receptor antibody, they become sensitive targets of the CTL clone recognized by the MAb. Thus, F9-coupled S.AKR targets are lysed by G4 CTL while F23.1 coupled S.AKR cells are lysed by OE4. Interestingly, when these S.AKR cells were coupled with an anti–H-2^b MAb 20.8.4, they were not lysed by either clone. This is despite the fact that this MAb recognizes the H-2^b antigens expressed by the

TABLE 2.1. *Specific Cytolysis of MAb-Coupled Target Cells**

Effector	Specific Lysis of ^{51}Cr Target Cells (%)			
CTL Clone[†]	S.AKR	S.AKR −20.8.4	S.AKR −F9	S.AKR −F23.1
G4(10:1)	6	2	38	3
OE4(3:1)	5	4	3	68

*Protein A Sepharose-purified MAbs were coupled to S.AKR (AKR, H-2^k) tumor cells using the heterobifunctional cross-linker N-succinimidyl 3-(2-pyridyldithio) propionate (SPDP). MAb 20.8.4 is specific for H-2^b; F9 is specific for an idiotypic determinant on G4; F23.1 is specific for an allotypic determinant on OE4.
[†]Both CTL clones derive from H-2^b mice and are specific for H-2^d target antigens.

CTL clones and presumably brings the two cells together. Thus, it appears that there is a requirement that the CTL clone be contacted through its antigen receptor. This may reflect a need to activate the CTL, or it may mean that the killing mechanism is tightly linked to the receptor. Similar results on the chemical coupling of anti-receptor MAbs to cells have recently been reported by Krantz et al. (1984).

Having shown that an anti-receptor antibody can apparently fulfill all of the needs usually provided at the target surface by antigen plus MHC, we then wanted to know whether we could *specifically* target sites for attack by CTL. The most obvious antigen-specific targeting device is another MAb. Heteroconjugates of MAbs (referred to as hybrid antibodies) were constructed using SPDP, in which one site is anti–T cell receptor and the other site is directed against the Thy 1.1 alloantigen. Thy 1.1 was chosen as a target antigen because none of the CTL clones we used expressed this isoantigenic determinant, and there are many AKR/J-derived target cells which do. S.AKR (H-2^k, Thy 1.1) and EL4 (H-2^b, Thy 1.2) cells were ^{51}Cr labeled and incubated with hybrid antibodies constructed as follows: 19E12 (anti–Thy 1.1) linked to F9 and 19E12 linked to F23. After one wash the cells were assayed for lysis by CTL clones G4 and OE4 (Table 2.2). The results showed that the Thy 1.1–positive lymphoma, S.AKR, was specifically targeted for lysis by the hybrid antibodies. Thus, the anti–Thy 1.1 site fixed the hybrid to the surface of the lymphoma, while the anti–T cell receptor site focused the killer cell to act. In other experiments, we have fractionated the cross-linked antibodies by passage through Sephacryl S-400 (Pharmacia, Uppsala, Sweden). This revealed a major peak of targeting activity in the ~300,000 dalton range with no activity in the 7S region or higher than 600,000 daltons. Furthermore,

TABLE 2.2. *Antigen Specific Targeting by Hybrid MAbs*

Target Cell	Hybrid Antibody	Lysis at 6:1 E:T Ratio (%)	
		G4 Effectors (F9$^+$, b anti-d)	OE4 Effectors (F23$^+$, b anti-d)
P815 (H-2^d)	—	82	78
EL4 (H-2^b, Thy 1.2)	—	3	0
S.AKR (H-2^k, Thy 1.1)	—	0	4
EL4	19E12-F9	8	2
EL4	19E12-F23	2	6
S.AKR	19E12-F9	62	2
S.AKR	19E12-F23	0	61

E:T = effector to target.

under some conditions, the CTL can be "armed" with the hybrid antibody and can function against Thy 1.1–positive targets, or the hybrid antibody can be incorporated directly into the mixture of CTL and targets.

We are optimistic that this antigen-specific targeting technique will be able to focus T cell activity to chosen sites in vivo. Our priority is to assess whether we can slow or prevent tumor growth in a murine model system.

REFERENCES

Houston LL, Nowinski RC, Bernstein ID. 1980. Specific in vivo localization of monoclonal antibodies directed against the Thy 1.1 antigen. J Immunol 125: 837–843.

Krantz DM, Tonegawa S, Eisen HN. 1984. Attachment of an anti-receptor antibody to non-target cells renders them susceptible to lysis by a clone of cytotoxic T lymphocytes. Proc Natl Acad Sci USA 81:7922–7926.

Lancki DW, Fitch FW. 1984. A cloned CTL demonstrates different cell interaction requirements for lysis of two distinct target cells (Abstract). Fed Proc 43:1659.

Ozato K, Sachs DH. 1981. Monoclonal antibodies to mouse MHC antigens. J Immunol 126:317–321.

Staerz UD, Pasternack MS, Klein JS, Benedetto JD, Bevan MJ. 1984. Monoclonal antibodies specific for a murine cytotoxic T-lymphocyte clone. Proc Natl Acad Sci USA 81:1799–1803.

Staerz UD, Rammensee H-G, Benedetto JD, Bevan MJ. 1985. Characterization of a murine monoclonal antibody specific for an allotypic determinant on T cell antigen receptor. J Immunol 134:3994–4000.

Symposium on Fundamental Cancer Research, Vol. 38.
© 1986 by The University of Texas System Cancer Center.

3. Lymphokine Regulation of Polyclonal and Antigen-Specific B Cell Responses

Maureen Howard, Peter Stein, and Philippe Dubois

The Laboratory of Microbial Immunity, National Institute of Allergy and Infectious Diseases, National Institutes of Health, Bethesda, Maryland 20205

B lymphocytes respond to antigens via specific clonal expansion and differentiation into immunoglobulin (Ig)-secreting antibody-forming cells (AFC). Recent evidence from many laboratories suggests that this process is controlled by a family of hormonelike glycoproteins with discrete factors regulating the separate activation, proliferation, and differentiation steps involved (reviewed in Howard and Paul 1983, Howard et al. 1984). This concept of lymphokine regulation of B cell responses has emerged from studies where polyclonal activators have been used to initially trigger a large proportion of the "resting" B cell population. Whether or not antigen-driven responses are also governed by the same regulatory stimuli has been more difficult to ascertain. Using affinity-purified hapten-binding B cells or specific hapten antigens, several laboratories have claimed that antigen-driven responses use some, but not all, of the B cell stimulatory factors (BSF) observed in polyclonal systems (Pike et al. 1982, Pike and Nossal 1984, Noelle et al. 1983, Snow et al. 1983a,b, Mond et al. 1983). In each of these studies, however, the responsive cell population has consisted of large B cell blasts obtained either via intentional in vitro stimulation (Noelle et al. 1983) or as the presumed result of environmental stimulation in vivo (Pike et al. 1983, Thompson et al. 1984). Thus, these investigations have not included analysis of the factors involved in the initial events of resting B cell triggering, a fact that might obviously explain the discrepancy between polyclonal and antigen-specific studies. We have now developed a system for analyzing antigen-specific proliferation of affinity-purified small resting B lymphocytes. The following describes the nature of factors regulating such antigen-specific proliferation and compares them to the regulatory stimuli governing polyclonal–B cell responses.

POLYCLONAL–B CELL PROLIFERATION AND DIFFERENTIATION

Factors Involved in Anti–IgM-Induced B Cell Proliferation

To identify factors involved in B cell proliferation, we initially developed a short-term B cell co-stimulator assay where highly purified small B lymphocytes were stimulated with affinity-purified anti-IgM antibodies (Howard et al. 1982). The latter reagent activates approximately 50% of normal splenic B cells (DeFranco et al. 1982) and appears to cross-link membrane Ig in a manner analogous to antigen (Sieckmann et al. 1978). When highly purified resting B lymphocytes were cultured at a sufficiently low cell density, two stimuli, in addition to the anti-IgM antibodies, were required to induce proliferation. The first stimulus was a signal delivered by a T cell–derived factor, originally designated B cell growth factor (Howard et al. 1982) but recently renamed B cell stimulatory factor–p1 (BSF-p1); the second was the macrophage-derived factor interleukin (IL) 1 (Howard et al. 1983). Kinetic studies revealed that BSF-p1 was required in the first few hours of a two-day culture period, whereas the addition of IL 1 could be delayed 18–20 hours after initiation of the cultures, without significant reduction in the final response (Howard and Paul 1983). Recently, several laboratories have provided convincing data that the receptor for BSF-p1 is on "resting" small B lymphocytes (Roehm et al. 1984, Noelle et al. 1984, Rabin et al. 1985, Oliver et al. 1985), a finding that suggests that BSF-p1 may in fact function as an activation signal for unstimulated B lymphocytes.

A Second T Cell–Derived B Cell Proliferation Factor

The existence of a second murine T cell–derived B cell growth factor (BCGF) became apparent when supernatants obtained from different T cell lines were tested in the above anti–IgM B cell co-stimulator assay and in a separate co-stimulator assay utilizing dextran sulfate ($DXSO_4$) rather than anti-IgM as the resting B cell polyclonal activator (Swain et al. 1983). The factor responsive in the latter assay, designated BCGF-II, was additionally distinct from BSF-p1 in terms of its capacity to induce BCL_1 tumor cells to proliferate and to secrete Ig (Dutton et al. 1984). BSF-p1 and BCGF-II have now been separated biochemically; BCGF-II is larger and more acidic than BSF-p1 (Dutton et al. 1984, Howard M unpublished data). The relationship between these two T cell–derived B cell proliferation factors will be discussed further in the following sections.

Factors Required for Induction of Ig Synthesis in Polyclonal B Cell Responses

The preceding sections describe the nature of stimuli required to activate small resting B lymphocytes to polyclonal proliferation. In the anti-IgM induction system, we found that at least two additional T cell–derived factors were required to drive proliferating B cells into Ig-synthesizing cells. These are a factor found in the supernatant from the B151K12 T cell hybridoma (originally designated B15-T cell replacing factor [TRF]) and a factor of isoelectric point 4.5 in phorbol myristic acetate (PMA)–induced supernatant from EL4 thymoma cells (originally designated EL-TRF) (Nakanishi et al. 1983).

Considerable evidence now suggests a possible identity between the differentiation factor in B151K12 T hybridoma supernatant and the BCGF-II proliferation factor described above. This evidence includes similar biochemical properties (e.g., M_r 50,000–60,000; pI 4.5–5.5) and an ability of the B151K12 supernatant to show activity in the various BCGF-II bioassays (e.g., proliferation and secretion of BCL_1 tumor cells, and polyclonal proliferation of $DXSO_4$-activated B cells) (Takatsu et al. 1983, Dutton et al. 1984). Thus BCGF-II and the B151K12 supernatant seem capable of inducing both proliferation and Ig synthesis in certain assays. On this point, others have provided independent evidence for a bifunctional growth and maturation factor with similar biochemical properties to BCGF-II and the differentiation factor in B151K12 supernatant (Pike et al. 1982). These data taken together indicate sufficient similarities between BCGF-II and the B151K12 factor to render their identity a serious consideration.

The second differentiation factor required for induction of Ig synthesis by anti-IgM–activated B cells (e.g., EL-TRF) is a component of PMA-induced EL4 supernatant (Nakanishi et al. 1983). Recent analysis of this material has revealed that both recombinant IL 2 and a separate T cell–derived factor with a molecular weight of 32,000 have the capacity to provide this differentiation stimulus (Nakanishi et al. 1984). Why there should be two separate factors with seemingly identical functions and whether both factors operate in normal B cell responses are not yet known.

Model of Lymphokine Regulation of Polyclonal B Cell Responses

The current working model to emerge from the above studies on polyclonal activation of B cells is depicted in Figure 3.1. Small resting B cells are initially triggered when membrane-bound Ig receptors and BSF-p1 receptors become occupied with their appropriate ligands. This process apparently activates the cells from G_0 to G_1 phase, but does not induce cells to enter S phase

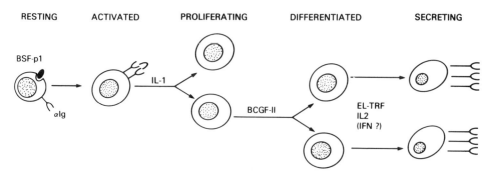

FIGURE 3.1. Model for lymphokine regulation of polyclonal B cell responses.

of the cell cycle. For the latter to ensue, the activated B cells must interact with IL 1. It is not yet clear whether IL 1 and BSF-p1 act beyond this first round of replication. Kinetic studies (Nakanishi et al. 1983) suggest that the differentiation factor in B151K12 supernatant acts either at the end of the first round of replication or the beginning of the second round to sustain proliferation and cause differentiation towards an Ig-secreting cell. As discussed above, this factor in B151K12 supernatant is probably equivalent to BCGF-II. At least one more factor is required before Ig synthesis occurs. This factor may be IL 2 or a separate T cell–derived factor with a molecular weight of 32,000 (i.e., EL-TRF), which is distinct from BSF-p1 and BCGF-II (Nakanishi et al. 1984). Others have also proposed a role for interferon in the induction of Ig secretion from activated B cells (Roehm et al. 1983). Whether interferon is a third factor capable of operating at this final stage of polyclonal B cell responses or whether EL-TRF is interferon is not yet known.

ANTIGEN-SPECIFIC B CELL PROLIFERATION

Enrichment of Antigen-binding Cells

Because the precursor frequency of B cells specific for a single antigenic determinant is extremely low, it is not possible to monitor quantitatively the amount of proliferation a single antigen induces in an unfractionated B cell population. Thus, in order to analyze the nature of factors involved in antigen-specific B cell proliferation, it is necessary to enrich the antigen-reactive population prior to analysis. The enrichment protocol we have used is a modification of the method of Vitetta and colleagues (Snow et al. 1983). The protocol, outlined in Figure 3.2, adds four extra steps to the original method of Snow et al. (1983b).

1. An initial purification of small resting B cells prior to the affinity purification of antigen-binding cells was included. We believe this added step is
critical as: it ensures the subsequent analysis of small unstimulated B lymphocytes rather than the larger activated blasts that have been studied by others; it
eliminates the possibility of antigen-binding T suppressor cells also being enriched during the affinity purification steps; and it removes cells capable of
releasing factors during the affinity purification protocol. Because some of
these steps occur at room temperature, endogenous exposure to factors may
allow activation to proceed at this stage.

2. A different conjugation ratio for joining haptens to the horse erythrocytes used in rosette formation was employed. As this conjugation ratio

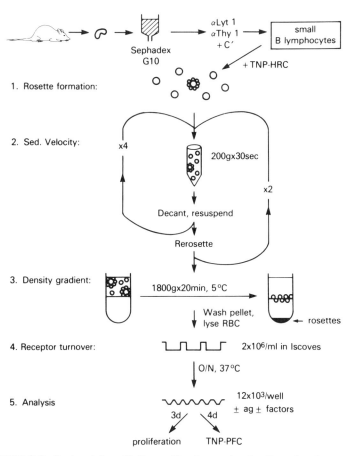

FIGURE 3.2. Protocol for affinity purification and activation of antigen-
binding B lymphocytes.

yielded a lower percentage of rosette-forming cells in the starting B cell population than in the case of Snow et al. (1983b), we believe the conjugation ratio we have used leads to greater specificity of binding.

3. An additional density centrifugation step required to achieve a 100- to 500-fold enrichment of antigen-binding cells using these higher affinity binding hapten-erythrocyte conjugates was employed.

4. The receptor turnover and reexpression step was performed in serum-free Iscove's medium rather than serum-containing medium, in order to minimize enlargement or activation of the cells during this time.

The cells resulting from the enrichment protocol depicted in Figure 3.2 represent approximately 0.03% of the initial spleen cell population. They are more than 95% viable and are approximately 60% capable of forming trinitrophenyl (TNP)-specific rosette-forming cells. This latter number drops to approximately 40% after the 18 hour incubation in Iscove's serum-free medium. This suggests either incomplete turnover and reexpression of receptors or a degree of low affinity or nonspecific binding during the antigen-binding cell-enrichment protocol.

Antigen Activation of Antigen-binding Cells

When TNP-binding B cells, purified as described above, were cultured with the typical type-2 antigen TNP-Ficoll or the typical thymus-dependent antigen TNP-ovalbumin (TNP-OVA), no proliferation was observed (Stein P, Dubois P, Greenblatt D, Howard M unpublished data). If such cultures were supplemented with supernatant obtained from PMA-stimulated EL4 cells, an excellent response was obtained in the case of TNP-Ficoll–stimulated cultures, but not in the case of TNP-OVA–stimulated cultures (Stein P, Dubois P, Greenblatt D, Howard M unpublished data). In such experiments, a small and variable degree of proliferation was obtained with EL4 supernatant alone, suggesting that a variable proportion of B cells had already been partially activated, possibly as the result of the exposure to antigen during the affinity purification. Identical results were obtained if EL4 supernatant was replaced by supernatant obtained from a long-term OVA-reactive helper T cell line stimulated with OVA and antigen-presenting cells, alleviating concern for possible effects of PMA in these experiments. The activation of TNP-binding B cells with TNP-Ficoll and EL4 supernatant was significantly reduced by preexposure of the cells to TNP-OVA, but not to an equivalent concentration of OVA, verifying the hapten specificity of the proliferative response.

To determine exactly which factors in the EL4 supernatant were responsible for reconstitution of TNP-Ficoll responses by TNP-binding B cells, we used partially purified factors prepared by reverse-phase high performance liquid chromatography. An equivalent degree of reconstitution was observed if the EL4 supernatant was replaced with 10 U/ml BSF-p1; in contrast, equivalent concentrations of BCGF-II or IL 2 had no effect. We similarly examined the effects of recombinant IL 1 in these cultures. While IL 1 was unable to reconstitute proliferative responses of TNP-binding cells to TNP-Ficoll, it markedly enhanced the reconstitution obtained in BSF-p1–supplemented cultures. We conclude that the optimum proliferative response of TNP-binding B cells to TNP-Ficoll requires BSF-p1 and IL 1. Thus, the factor regulation of antigen-specific B cell proliferation in the case of type-2 antigens is identical to that of polyclonal anti-IgM–induced B cell proliferation (Figure 3.1).

ACKNOWLEDGMENT

Peter Stein is a medical student research fellow of the American Heart Association; Philippe Dubois is supported by a NATO fellowship.

REFERENCES

DeFranco A, Raveche E, Asofsky R, Paul WE. 1982. Frequency of B lymphocytes responsive to anti-immunoglobulin. J Exp Med 155:1523–1538.

Dutton R, Wetzel G, Swain S. 1984. Partial purification and characterization of a BCGF-II from EL4 culture supernatants. J Immunol 132:2451–2456.

Howard M, Paul WE. 1983. Regulation of B-cell growth and differentiation by soluble factors. Annual Review of Immunology 1:307–333.

Howard M, Farrar J, Hilfiker M, et al. 1982. Identification of a T cell–derived B cell growth factor distinct from interleukin 2. J Exp Med 155:914–923.

Howard M, Mizel S, Lachman L, Ansel J, Johnson B, Paul WE. 1983. Role of interleukin 1 in anti-immunoglobulin–induced B cell proliferation. J Exp Med 157:1529–1543.

Howard M, Nakanishi K, Paul WE. 1984. B cell growth and differentiation factors. Immunol Rev 78:185–210.

Mond J, Farrar J, Paul W, Fuller-Farrar J, Schaefer M, Howard M. 1983. T cell dependence and factor reconstitution of *in vitro* antibody responses to TNP-B Abortus and TNP-Ficoll: Restoration of T depleted responses with chromatographed fractions of a T cell–derived factor. J Immunol 131:633–637.

Nakanishi K, Howard M, Muraguchi A, et al. 1983. Soluble factors involved in B cell differentiation: Identification of two distinct T cell replacing factors (TRF). J Immunol 130:2219–2224.

Nakanishi K, Malek T, Smith K, Hamoaka T, Shevach E, Paul WE. 1984. Both interleukin 2 and a second T cell–derived factor in EL4 supernatant have activity as differentiation factors in IgM synthesis. J Exp Med 160:1605–1621.

Noelle R, Snow C, Uhr J, Vitetta E. 1983. Activation of antigen-specific B cells: Role of T cells, cytokines, and antigen in induction of growth and differentiation. Proc Natl Acad Sci USA 80:6628–6631.

Noelle R, Krammer P, Ohara J, Uhr J, Vitetta E. 1984. Increased expression of Ia antigens on resting B cells: A new role for B cell growth factor. Proc Natl Acad Sci USA 81:6149–6154.

Oliver K, Noelle R, Uhr J, Krammer P, Vitetta E. 1985. B cell growth factor

(BCGF I or BSF-p1) is a differentiation factor for resting B cells and may not induce cell growth. Proc Natl Acad Sci USA 82:2465–2467.

Pike B, Nossal G. 1984. A reappraisal of "T-independent" antigens: Effect of lymphokines on the response of single adult hapten-specific B lymphocytes. J Immunol 132:1687–1695.

Pike B, Vaux D, Clark-Lewis I, Schrader J, Nossal G. 1982. Proliferation and differentiation of single, hapten-specific B lymphocytes promoted by T cell factor(s) distinct from T cell growth factor. Proc Natl Acad Sci USA 79: 6350–6355.

Pike B, Vaux D, Nossal G. 1983. Single cell studies on hapten-specific B lymphocytes: Differential cloning efficiency of cells of various sizes. J Immunol 131:554–560.

Rabin E, Ohara J, Paul WE. 1985. B cell stimulatory factor (BSF-1) activates resting B cells. Proc Natl Acad Sci USA 82:2935–2939.

Roehm N, Marrack P, Kappler J. 1983. Helper signals in the plaque-forming cell response to protein-bound haptens. J Exp Med 158:317–333.

Roehm N, Liebson J, Zlotnick A, Kappler J, Marrack P, Cambier J. 1984. Interleukin-induced increase in Ia expression by normal mouse B cells. J Exp Med 160:679–694.

Sieckmann D, Asofsky R, Mosier D, Zitron I, Paul WE. 1978. Activation of mouse lymphocytes by anti-immunoglobulin: I. Parameters of the response. J Exp Med 147:814.

Snow E, Noelle R, Uhr J, Vitetta E. 1983a. Activation of antigen-enriched B cells: II. Role of linked recognition in B cell proliferation to thymus-dependent antigens. J Immunol 130:614–618.

Snow E, Vitetta E, Uhr J. 1983b. Activation of antigen-enriched B cells: I. Purification and response to thymus-independent antigens. J Immunol 130: 607–613.

Swain S, Howard M, Kappler J, et al. 1983. Evidence for two distinct classes of murine B cell growth factors which have activities in different functional assays. J Exp Med 158:822–837.

Takatsu K, Tomita S, Hara Y, Ishi N, Kanatani T, Hamaoka T. 1983. Role of T cell–replacing factor (TRF) produced by monoclonal T cell hybrid in B cell differentiation. *In* Cohen S, Oppenheim J, eds., Proceedings of the Third International Lymphokine Workshop. Academic Press, New York, pp. 161–168.

Thompson C, Scher I, Schaefer M, Lindstein T, Finkelman F, Mond J. 1984. Size-dependent B lymphocyte subpopulations: Relationship of cell volume to surface phenotype, cell cycle, proliferative response, and requirements for antibody production to TNP-Ficoll and TNP-BA. J Immunol 133:2333–2340.

CELLULAR COMMUNICATION
AND INTERACTION

Symposium on Fundamental Cancer Research, Vol. 38.

4. Cell Interactions in the Immune System: The Role of Self Recognition in the Targeting of Nonspecific Effector Molecules by Helper T Cells

Charles A. Janeway, Jr., John P. Tite, Jay Horowitz, Patricia J. Conrad, Jonathan Kaye,* Barry Jones, and Kim Bottomly

Department of Pathology, Howard Hughes Medical Institute at Yale University School of Medicine, New Haven, Connecticut 06510

The immune system has fascinated biologists and physicians alike because of its ability to destroy foreign microorganisms, grafted normal tissues, and certain types of immunogenic tumors, while generally sparing self tissues. This discrimination between self and nonself has required the development of specific recognition molecules that serve as receptors on lymphocytes. There appear to be three classes of such molecules, and they have solved the problem of linking specificity with function in three distinct fashions (Janeway et al. 1985). B lymphocytes synthesize antibodies, and the progeny of a single B lymphocyte can give rise to antibodies of similar or identical specificity, but of differing biologic function, by the mechanism of isotype switching, the process of replacing one heavy chain constant region with another while maintaining an identical variable region (Honjo 1983). T lymphocytes that mediate helper or cytolytic function recognize antigen on the surfaces of cells. This focusing on cell surfaces results from the fact that T cells of these types only bind antigen when it is associated with self major histocompatibility complex (MHC) gene products (Schwartz 1984). At the present time, there is no known association of particular T cell receptor–constant region gene usage with functional phenotype; rather, function appears to be determined by genes whose expression is independently regulated (see below) (Royer et al. 1984). Finally, T cells involved in immune regulation produce antigen-binding molecules that appear to combine information for specificity with information for function and that are secreted, thus resembling antibody molecules more closely than they do T cell receptors (Cone et al. 1983). Unlike antibody molecules, however, such molecules home to specific cells within the immune system by means of recognition sites specific for polymorphic determinants

*Current address for Dr. Kaye: Department of Biology, University of California at San Diego, La Jolla, CA 92093

encoded either in the MHC or in linkage with the variable region of the immunoglobulin (Ig) heavy chain complex (Green et al. 1983).

In this chapter, we will focus on cell interactions involving T cells that recognize antigen in the context of self MHC gene products. We will ask whether the interaction of the receptor on the T cell with antigen-self MHC itself delivers a signal to its target cell. It has been argued that this must be so in the case of MHC class I recognizing cytolytic T cells, since cytolysis is unidirectional and since the cytolytic T cell is itself a susceptible target for other cytolytic cells (Kuppers and Henny 1976). However, recent studies on the mechanism of cytolysis mediated by such cells has raised doubts about this interpretation (Podack 1985). The situation involving T cells recognizing antigen in the context of self class II MHC gene products has been far more controversial.

Our studies presented here indicate that all the known functions of cloned T cell lines recognizing antigen in the context of self class II MHC gene products, or Ia in the mouse, are mediated by the release of biologically active, antigen-nonspecific mediator molecules, or lymphokines. These lymphokines act over short ranges on cells bearing receptors for them, and thus tend to affect cells closest to the lymphokine-producing cell. Thus, MHC-restricted T cells can combine specificity and function in highly complex ways, since specificity is encoded in genes that specify receptors for antigen-self MHC, while function is encoded in multiple loci that specify lymphokine molecules. Future understanding of T lymphocyte function will thus require an understanding of the mechanisms by which the activity of such genes is regulated.

THE COGNATE-NONCOGNATE DISPUTE AND ITS RESOLUTION

The early studies on helper T cell–B cell interaction in responses to hapten-carrier conjugates in vivo suggested that antigen served as a bridge between the antibody-producing B cell and the helper T cell (Mitchison 1971). However, in certain responses of B cells to antigen, T cells could be replaced with cell-free supernatants, suggesting that direct contact between the helper T cell and the B cell was not necessary for effective B cell activation (Schimpl and Wecker 1973). Over the following years, this argument has taken many forms, with the term "cognate" used to describe direct recognition of antigen by the helper T cell on the B cell surface, and the term "noncognate" to describe B cell activation in the absence of such a recognition event. Of decisive importance was the finding initially reported by Katz et al. (1973) that helper T cells acted exclusively on B cells identical at the I region of the MHC. This finding was hard to reconcile with a noncognate mode of cell interaction. However, it was eventually appreciated that the requirement for self MHC I region matching was a general property of helper T cells in recognizing antigen, and experiments carried out by Singer and Hodes (1983) suggested that B cell activation could be either cognate or noncognate, depending on the B cell being affected.

We have studied three experimental systems involving T cell–B cell interactions, and these led to a general conclusion regarding this question, as well as to an even broader statement about the functional behavior of T cells that recognize antigen in the context of self Ia molecules. In each system, we found that cloned helper T cells produced soluble, antigen-nonspecific effector molecules that mediate function. However, the effect of such cloned T cells on target B cells was cognate in each system, in that not only must the affected cell match the T cell at Ia, but also that the target cells affected most strongly are those bearing the highest density of Ia molecules of the type for which the cloned line is specific.

Cellular Interactions in B Cell Activation

We have analyzed both antigen-specific and polyclonal T cell–dependent B cell responses driven by cloned helper T cell lines (Jones and Janeway 1981a, Bottomly et al. 1983a, Tite et al. 1984). We have analyzed the B cell response to the hapten phosphorylcholine in particular detail. In this response, under all antigen concentrations tested, there was a requirement for the hapten to be linked to the carrier protein for which the cloned helper T cell was specific (Bottomly and Jones 1981), and the activated B cells had to bear the Ia antigen for which the cloned helper T cell line was specific. This is shown most clearly (Table 4.1) by mixing B cells of two different genotypes and determining the genotype of the antibody-producing cells at the end of the culture

TABLE 4.1. *Specificity of T Cell Help in the Anti–PC Antibody Response to PC-OVA*

	Percentage of Antibody-Forming Cells of H-2^b Genotype Helped by	
B Cell Genotype	*H-2^d Cloned Helper T Cell*	*H-2^b Cloned Helper T Cell*
$(H$-$2^b \times H$-$2^d)$F1	100	100
H-$2^b + H$-2^d	0	100

3×10^6 purified B cells from BALB/c (H-2^b), BALB.B (H-2^b), or (BALB/c $\times$ C57BL/6)F1 mice cultured with 10^5 cloned helper T cells plus 0.1 μg phosphocholine-ovalbumin for five days.
Phosphocholine–plaque-forming cells before and after treatment with monoclonal H-2^d anti–H-2^b (anti–H-2.5) antibody plus complement was measured to calculate the percentage of antibody-forming cells of H-2^b genotype.

TABLE 4.2. *B Cell Stimulation by Clone D10.G4.1; Influence of* **xid** *Gene*

Responding B Cells	Stimulus	Proliferation (△CPM)		Ig Secretion (△PFC)	
		Female	Male	Female	Male
(CBA/N × BALB/c̄)F1	Conalbumin	110,000	95,000	42,000	7,000
(CBA/N × BALB.B)F1	I-A^b	82,000	61,000	46,000	11,000
(CBA/N × BALB/c)F1	3D3	177,000	92,000	56,000	5,200

4×10^5 purified B cells plus 3×10^4 mitomycin C-treated D10.G4.1 T cells were mixed with 100 μg/ml conalbumin or 20 ng/ml 3D3 monoclonal anti–T cell receptor antibody and cultured for two days for ^{3}[H]thymidine incorporation or four days for reverse plaque-forming cells. Responses in the absence of antigen, 3D3, or for (CBA/N × BALB.B)F1 B cells, in the absence of D10 cells, subtracted to yield △ values.
CPM = counts per minute; PFC = plaque-forming cells.

(Jones and Janeway 1981a, Bottomly et al. 1983a). Even stronger evidence that the helper T cell is recognizing antigen on the surface of the B cell being activated was the finding that certain cloned T cell lines preferentially helped B cells that had the highest density of Ia antigens, as determined by limited killing of B cells with anti-Ia antibody and complement (Bottomly et al. 1983a). Thus, these studies strongly support the notion that T cell–B cell interactions are cognate, and they suggest that a signal is transduced to the B cell via the Ia molecule itself. However, when the same cloned T cell lines are examined in other assays, we see that they release antigen-nonspecific factors capable of driving B cells to synthesize and secrete antibody without interaction between the T cell receptor and the Ia molecule. Indeed, when various subpopulations of B cells were analyzed for their abilities to be activated in the presence or absence of such an interaction between the B cell's Ia molecules and the T cell's antigen receptor, no differences were observed (Table 4.2).

We are, therefore, left with the paradoxical finding that the same cloned T cell line can activate B cells to secrete antibody without contact with the B cell's Ia molecule and without specific binding of antigen to the B cell's antigen receptor, and can also be shown to help only those B cells that not only bind antigen to their receptors but also bear sufficient quantities of the Ia antigen for which the helper T cell is specific. We will show that this same paradoxical finding can be made in two other experimental systems, and we will then propose a resolution to this paradox, which also serves to resolve the dispute over whether B cell activation is cognate or noncognate.

The Suppression of T Cell–Dependent B Cell Responses by Cloned, Ia-recognizing T Cells

Amongst approximately 100 cloned T cells analyzed for helper function, several have been found that were Ia restricted, antigen specific, and could induce B cell proliferation in an antigen-specific fashion but failed to drive such B cells to antibody formation. One such cell has been analyzed in detail and mediates antigen-specific, Ia-restricted suppression of T cell–dependent antibody responses (Bottomly et al. 1983b). The behavior of this cloned T cell line, C1a, was also tested in the antibody response to phosphorylcholine. The characteristics of suppression mediated by C1a were similar to those outlined above for helper T cells. The suppression required physical linkage of the hapten to the carrier for which C1a was specific, it required that the B cell bear Ia antigens for which C1a was specific, and it preferentially affected those B cells bearing the highest density of Ia molecules. On the other hand, C1a cells were also distinct from cloned helper T cell lines that stimulate B cells to produce antibody in that they secrete lymphotoxin and other molecules that inhibit the proliferation of sensitive target B lymphoma lines in an antigen-nonspecific fashion. Thus, as with helper function, one has the paradox of a cognate effect on the B cell apparently mediated by molecules that are neither antigen specific nor MHC restricted.

Cytolysis of B Lymphoma Cells by Ia-recognizing T Cells

In addition to helper and suppressor function, we have found that many of our cloned Ia-recognizing, antigen-specific T cell lines, as well as freshly isolated antigen-stimulated lymph node cells, will kill antigen-pulsed B lymphoma cells in an Ia-restricted fashion (Tite and Janeway 1984a, Tite et al. 1985). This cytolytic T cell–B cell interaction has many advantages over other experimental systems for analyzing these interactions. It employs only cloned, long-term in vitro cultured lines, making definition of the interacting cells simple; it is rapid, taking four to six hours, thus minimizing secondary changes in the cells that result from the interaction itself; and the target population being transformed can be recovered from the interaction, expanded, and analyzed. To many, the finding that a T cell with the "helper phenotype" can kill B lymphoma cells is heretical. Yet nearly all of our cloned T cell lines that can mediate B cell growth and differentiation into antibody-secreting cells are also able, under different experimental conditions, to kill B lymphoma cells.

The interaction between cloned T cells and B lymphoma cells leading to death of the target B lymphoma cell closely resembles the helper and suppressor interactions described above. First, the B lymphoma cells must match the cloned T cell line at Ia, and antigen must be presented on their surfaces for

TABLE 4.3. *Lysis of B Lymphoma Line Variants*

Cytolytic T Cell Specificity	Target Cell	IA Density	Antigen Concentration	Product ($\times 10^{-4}$)
OVA + I-A^d	Parent	1,200	100	12
	Variant	200	700	14
OVA + I-A^s	Parent	800	100	8
	Variant	1,200	70	8.4

Comparison of parent LS102.9 (H-2^d × H-2^s) B cell hybrid and variant selected for lowered expression of I-A^d. I-A density determined by fluorescence-activated cell sorter analysis with the appropriate monoclonal antibody against restriction element of cytolytic T cell. Antigen concentration is the amount of OVA required to induce lysis equivalent to that induced by 100 μg/ml with parent line. OVA = ovalbumin.

cytolysis to occur. However, because the antigen specificity of such cells is not known, antigen bridge effects have not been analyzed in this system. Second, the B cells that survive the lytic event are reproducibly changed in that they express lower levels of Ia than do the starting cells; under conditions of cytolysis in which the number of B lymphoma cells are limited and antigen is used to activate the cytolytic T cells, most of the cells that survive at limiting B cell number have lowered levels of surface Ia antigens. Such B cells with lowered Ia antigens are resistant to being killed; however, if the concentration of the foreign antigen is adjusted upwards to compensate for the loss of Ia molecules, one finds that the targets are susceptible to these elevated antigen concentrations in exact proportion to the decrease in cell surface Ia antigen expression (Tite and Janeway 1984b). Thus, the product of the concentration of antigen required for half maximal lysis by a given cloned T cell line multiplied by the density of Ia on the target cell is essentially constant (Table 4.3). These data show most clearly that Ia antigen density is a critical determinant of whether a B cell will or will not participate in a functional interaction with an Ia-restricted cloned T cell line or, put differently, that this interaction is cognate.

However, in this case, we have clear evidence that the mechanism of cytolysis is via non–antigen-specific mediator molecules. First, unlike classical cytolytic T cells whose antigen recognition is restricted by class I MHC molecules, these Ia-recognizing cloned T cells readily kill bystander target cells that are added to cultures that contain cloned T cells and Ia antigen-bearing B lymphoma cells that have been pulsed with antigen. Second, only certain target cells can be killed by this mechanism, and the susceptibility to lysis is identical whether they are used in direct contact with the cloned T cell or as bystander targets; these same targets are all susceptible to class I–specific cytolytic effector cells. Third, in testing large panels of cloned T cell lines, there is a direct correlation between direct and bystander killing mediated by a given cloned line, while other functional activities of such cloned lines do not correlate significantly with one another. This finding argues that direct and bystander lysis are mediated by the same mechanism.

An even stronger argument favoring lymphokine-mediated lysis in both direct and bystander cytolysis in this system comes from an analysis of lysis-resistant variants of the B lymphoma lines. These variants were generated by culturing the parent B lymphoma lines with cloned T cells and the T cell activating antibodies found in rabbit anti-mouse brain antisera (RaMBr) (Jones and Janeway 1981b, Norcross and Smith 1979, Jones 1982, 1983). These antibodies must interact with B cell Fc receptors in order to activate T cells. When such antibodies are used in place of antigen, two types of variants arise: B lymphoma lines that appear to have lost cell surface expression of the Fc receptor for rabbit IgG and B lymphoma lines that are resistant to lysis induced by all reagents tested. These latter variants are resistant to direct or bystander lysis mediated by cloned, Ia-recognizing T cells, as well as direct lysis mediated by RaMBr and by concanavalin A. However, they are fully susceptible to lysis by classical class I–specific cytolytic T cells (Table 4.4). Although the mechanism of this resistance is not known, we favor the notion that such cells have lost or modulated surface expression of a receptor for the nonspecific lytic molecules. That these molecules are lymphotoxin and probably interferon γ as well is suggested by the finding that both of these molecules are produced by all of our cloned cytolytic T cell lines, while recombinant inter-

TABLE 4.4. *Selection of A20/2J Variants in Culture*

Ligand			Surface I-A^d Expression	Variant Selection (%)*	
RaMBr	*OVA*	*Con A*		*RaMBr*[†]	*OVA*[‡]
S	R	S	Low	8	91
R	S	S	Normal	17	0
R	R	R	Normal	25	0

*The A20/2J variant type is defined by resistance (R) or susceptibility (S) to cloned T cell cytotoxicity according to the ligand that triggered it.
[†]Twenty-four independent variant lines analyzed.
[‡]Twelve lines analyzed. With both RaMBr and OVA, some lines emerge from selection that are identical to the unselected parental A20/2J line.
RaMBr = Rabbit anti-mouse brain; OVA = ovalbumin; Con A = concanavalin A.

feron γ is without activity, and neither molecule is produced by cloned T cell lines that lack cytolytic activity (Tite et al. 1985).

Thus, this rapid and quantitative bioassay for antigen-specific Ia-restricted T cell–B cell interaction again demonstrates that non–antigen-specific mediator molecules can mediate a cognate T cell–B cell interaction.

Resolution of the Cognate-Noncognate Paradox

Our studies show that, using cloned Ia-restricted T cells, T cell–B cell interactions mediated by the same cloned line can appear to be either cognate or noncognate. The result depends partly on how one sets up the experiment and partly on how one analyzes the result. Thus, if one looks for the release of soluble molecules mediating the effect of the cloned T cell, one, in general, finds them. Likewise, if innocent bystander cells are added to an experimental system, they generally are affected. The one obvious exception occurs in experiments in which the amount of antigen is strictly limited and the response of antigen-specific B cells is analyzed. On the other hand, and under all conditions, the B cell that bears the appropriate Ia antigen at the highest density on its surface is always preferentially affected.

We would resolve this apparent paradox as follows. First, we assume that helper T cell activation requires interaction of the T cell receptor with multiple identical antigen:Ia complexes on the B cell surface, because T cell receptor cross-linking is required for T cell activation (Kaye and Janeway 1984). Second, we would propose that the critical step in any T cell–B cell interaction is activation of the T cell by antigen:Ia complexes on the B cell surface and that the density of such complexes determines the likelihood that T cells will interact with a particular B cell so as to become activated by the interaction (Janeway et al. 1984). Thus, B cells bearing Ig receptors for a particular antigen will have a tremendous advantage over all other B cells under conditions of limiting antigen concentration, as they have a specific binding molecule for the antigen. Likewise, B cells with the highest density of Ia molecules will have the highest density of antigen:Ia complexes, all other conditions being equal. Once the T cell has bound to the antigen:Ia complexes on the B cell surface and become activated by them, it will release certain lymphokines that will preferentially affect the B cell to which the T cell is bound. Whether this preference involves mere proximity or whether the T cell actually releases lymphokines focally, depending upon the area of its surface on which receptor cross-linking is occurring, remains to be determined. This analysis can account for all of our data and, we believe, for the data of other investigators as well.

This model does not propose that T cells transmit signals directly to B cells via the interaction of their receptors with Ia molecules on the B cell nor does it propose that surface Ig on B cells plays an essential role in specific B cell activation. However, the latter is certainly possible and could lead to alterations in both Ia density (Monroe and Cambier 1983) and susceptibility to certain T cell–derived B cell–activating molecules (Howard and Paul 1983), both of which would contribute to the cognate nature of the interaction. Thus, we would argue that there is no biologic difference between cognate and non-cognate T cell–B cell interactions, that the differences result solely from differences in experimental conditions or in the way in which the interaction is analyzed. This resolution has the virtue of clearly delineating what the next step in the analysis of this process should be, namely, to determine what lymphokines are released by helper T cells under various experimental conditions and to delineate the regulation of lymphokine receptor expression on B cells, as well as the mechanism by which B cell–surface Ia density is regulated in normal B cells. We are also examining the extent to which lymphokine release is focused on the area of the T cell membrane over which T cell receptors are cross-linked.

INHIBITION OF IMMUNE RESPONSES BY HELPER T CELLS

T cells that recognize antigen in the context of self Ia molecules and that bear the surface marker L3T4a are usually regarded as being helper T cells. As noted in the previous section, we have observed such cells functioning as helpers in B cell antibody responses, as suppressors of such responses, and as cytolytic T cells. In this section, these functional aspects of T cells of this type will be discussed in more detail. Except where noted, all of these studies have been performed with cloned L3T4a-positive, Ia-restricted T cells that activate B cells in the presence of antigen.

Suppression Mediated by Helper T Cells

We have observed several cloned T cell lines that suppress the responses of B cells to antigen, when the B cells are being helped by other cloned helper T cell lines. All of these cloned lines are also active in killing B lymphoma lines, and some release both lymphotoxin and interferon γ when stimulated with antigen:Ia or with mitogenic lectins. Our initial studies with the clone C1a suggested that the B cell was the target for such suppression. However, another possibility exists that could account for at least some such suppressive phenomena. Cloned helper T cell lines can be highly sensitive to the cytotoxic effects of our cloned, Ia-restricted cytolytic T cells. Indeed, an inverse relationship exists between sensitivity to cytolysis and cytolytic function; the cloned T cell lines that fail to show any cytolytic function are highly sensitive to the cytolytic cloned T cell lines in lectin-dependent killing and are also highly sensitive bystander targets (Table 4.5). Thus, one could account for our findings (Bottomly et al. 1983b), as well as those of Asano and Hodes (1983),

TABLE 4.5. *Sensitivity of Cloned T Cell Lines*

Cloned T Cell Line	Specificity	Cytolytic Capacity[†]	Specific ^{51}Cr Release (%)*	
			With Con A	Without Con A
5.2	I-E^d + OVA	+ + + +	0	0
5.5	I-E^d + OVA	+ + + +	0	0
5.9.24	I-A^d + OVA	+ + + +	0	0
D10.G4.1	I-A^k + CA	−	72.0	5.0
8D3	I-A^d + OVA	−	62.0	4.0
HT-2	None	−	0	0

*Cloned L3T4a$^+$ effector T cells (5.9.24) were used at an effector:target ratio of 5:1 with 2 µg/ml Con A in a six-hour ^{51}Cr release assay with 10^4 ^{51}Cr-labeled target cells. Con A = concanavalin A; OVA = ovalbumin; CA = conalbumin.
[†] As measured in both antigen-specific and lectin-dependent CTL assays.

who have described a similar system, by saying that both helper and suppressor cells tend to interact with the same B cell, namely, one with the highest levels of antigen and Ia on the surface and by saying that the suppressor clones kill or inactivate either the B cell or the helper T cell that is interacting with that B cell.

We have considered whether Ia-restricted cytolytic and suppressor T cells are likely to have an in vivo function. Based on cell and antigen doses required to observe the activity of such cells, we would expect that their primary activity would be to suppress responses to autoantigens, including idiotypic determinants. Only autoantigens are likely to be found on B cell surfaces in large enough quantities and for sufficient periods of time to engage these T cells functionally. Furthermore, resting B cells appear to be relatively resistant to the effects of such cells, at least in cytolysis. In keeping with this postulated role for such cells, we have recently observed a novel form of an MHC-linked Ir gene control in the murine immune response to type IV human collagen (Tite et al. 1985). When T cell proliferative responses to this antigen are measured, only mice having I-A^s respond; mice of nine other common laboratory haplotypes do not. However, when one examines the antibody response, one finds that only mice having I-A^s do *not* respond. In (H-2^d × H-2^s) F1 hybrids, the T cell proliferative response behaves as a dominant trait, while the antibody response behaves as a recessive trait. Although it has not yet been demonstrated experimentally, it seems possible that the proliferating T cells in this system will be primarily suppressive. This is particularly interesting, since the antigen in question is a highly conserved protein and may resemble an autoantigen in mice.

T Cell Regulation of Interleukin 2–dependent T Cell Growth

Many, if not all, T cells require the T cell lymphokine interleukin (IL) 2 for their growth (Smith 1984). IL 2 interacts with a specific cell surface receptor for IL 2 (IL 2R) whose expression can be induced on T cells by encountering antigen, lectins, or anti-receptor antibody (Kaye et al. 1984). We have analyzed this process in detail using a cloned helper T cell line against which we have raised a monoclonal anti-receptor antibody capable of activating the clone in the absence of antigen and accessory cells (Kaye et al. 1983). Activation can be measured as IL 2 secretion; however, no growth occurs unless the monokine IL 1 is also added to the cultures (Table 4.6). The combination of IL 1 and anti-receptor antibody leads to a tenfold increase in IL 2R expression, probably accounting for the stimulation of growth observed in the presence of IL 1. However, this cloned T cell line also responds to IL 2 prepared from T cell hybrids containing no IL 1, as well as to recombinant-derived IL 2 (rIL 2). This paradoxical situation can be explained by postulating the existence of an inhibitory lymphokine produced by the cloned line upon activation, and we have now demonstrated the presence of such a substance in supernatants of this and other cloned T cell lines. This inhibitor can inhibit the rIL 2–induced growth of most cloned T cell lines, although wide differences in sensitivity to the inhibitor exist between such cell lines. An example is shown in Table 4.7. This inhibitory substance is not lymphotoxin or interferon γ nor does it have the characteristics of inhibitor of DNA synthesis (Horowitz J unpublished data). Neither its production nor its effect on indicator cells is altered by IL 1, which must therefore counteract its effects by a different mechanism. We would propose that this inhibitor interferes with the IL 2–IL 2R interaction or its effects and that IL 1 can circumvent this by inducing suf-

TABLE 4.6. *Growth and IL 2 Synthesis of Clone D10*

	Response	
Stimulus	*D10 Growth*	*IL 2 Secretion*
0	450	300
3D3	8,300	62,000
IL 1	830	1,600
3D3 + IL 1	39,000	35,000

2×10^4 D10.G4.1 cloned T cells stimulated for 48 hours with 10 ng/ml monoclonal anti-receptor antibody 3D3, 5% P388.D1 supernatant containing IL 1, or both. D10 growth measured by ^{3}[H]thymidine incorporation in a three-hour pulse treatment. IL 2 production measured as ^{3}[H]thymidine incorporation by HT-2 cells.

TABLE 4.7. *An Inhibitor of IL 2–Dependent T Cell Growth*

Stimulus	Test Cells	Proliferative Response
0	5.5	1,400
3% D10	5.5	1,800
rIL 2	5.5	110,000
3% D10 + rIL 2	5.5	38,000
3% D10	HT-2	406,000

Supernatant of cloned T-cell line D10.G4.1 was induced with monoclonal anti-receptor antibody 3D3 for 24 hours, and tested at 3% final concentration for stimulation or inhibition of growth of the IL 2 indicator line HT-2 or of BALB/c OVA:I-E^d–specific cloned T cell line 5.5. Forty-eight hour proliferative response was measured. rIL 2 was added at 0.5 U/ml final concentration.

ficient IL 2R to bypass the inhibition. This explanation is consistent with our findings and also with the differential sensitivity of various cloned lines to the inhibitor, as this is inversely related to the number of IL 2R per cell on these lines.

The functional significance of this substance is not known, but any molecule that can regulate the effects of such a centrally important molecule as IL 2 seems likely to play a role in vivo and could also be a potent pharmacologic tool. We believe that one role it may play in vivo is to prevent bystander activation of IL 2R–bearing T cells. Thus, if a T cell, upon activation by antigen:Ia on antigen-presenting cell surfaces, also produces an inhibitor of the IL 2 response, T cells in its vicinity will not become activated. However, the T cell producing the IL 2 will itself respond by growing because it has received both signals necessary for growth from the antigen-presenting cell–receptor cross-linking that is mediated by antigen:Ia complexes and IL 1; either a secreted or a membrane molecule on the antigen-presenting cell surface (Kurt-Jones E and Unanue E personal communication 1984, Horowitz J, Kaye J, Janeway C unpublished data).

Inhibition of Helper T Cell Activation via L3T4

Dialynas et al. (1983) suggest that the L3T4 molecule has binding affinity for nonpolymorphic regions of Ia molecules and that it strengthens the interaction of the helper T cell receptor with antigen:Ia on B cell and antigen-presenting cell surfaces. This has been demonstrated in a variety of ways, and it appears highly likely that L3T4 does indeed have Ia binding ability (Greenstein et al. 1984). However, we do not believe that its primary role is to strengthen the interaction of the T cell receptor with antigen:Ia. Instead, we have recent results suggesting that the primary role of L3T4 is to initiate contact between helper T cells and Ia-bearing cells. This is based on two experimental findings. First, anti-L3T4a monoclonal antibody GK1.5 is a potent inhibitor of cloned T cell activation by mitogenic lectins in the complete absence of Ia molecules. This can be measured as inhibition of proliferation, IL 2 release, or rise in intracellular free calcium (Table 4.8). Second, if L3T4 was primarily strengthening already existing interactions between the T cell receptor and antigen:Ia, one would expect the anti-L3T4a antibody to be able to inhibit T cell responses, even when added relatively late in the culture cycle. Instead, such inhibition is seen only very early in the response.

These findings have led us to propose a different role for L3T4 molecules (Tite J, Sloan A, Janeway C unpublished data). We believe that L3T4 molecules initiate contact between L3T4-positive T cells and Ia-bearing cells by means of recognition of invariant portions of the Ia molecule. As there are multiple copies of L3T4 on the T cell and of Ia on the B cell or antigen-presenting cells, we might expect this to lead to an increasingly strong interaction between the two cell types with time, as more such contacts formed. However, if, as our data suggest, the cross-linking of L3T4 molecules sends an "off" signal to the T cell, then this signal might be translated into a mechanism that causes the T cell to release the Ia-bearing cell, possibly by shedding its L3T4 molecules. The situation will be quite different if antigen is also on the surface of the Ia-bearing cell. In this case, the T cell receptor will also become engaged, and the "on" signal generated by the cross-linking of the T cell receptor is dominant over the "off" signal generated by L3T4 cross-

TABLE 4.8. *Inhibition by the GK1.5 Monoclonal Antibody of PHA-stimulated IL 2 Production and of D10.G4.1 T Cell Proliferation*

	Inhibition by GK1.5 (%)*	
Concentration of PHA (μg/ml)	*IL 2 Production*[†]	*T Cell Proliferation*[‡]
100	65.9	66.7
30	65.9	87.5
10	87.8	92.5
3	91.5	98.2
1	96.3	81.7

*Compared to control cultures with PHA alone.
[†]Measured by assay of supernatants on HT-2 cells.
[‡]Measured by incorporation of [3][H]thymidine after co-stimulation with indicated concentration of PHA + IL 1.
PHA = phytohemagglutinin; IL 2 = interleukin 2.

linking, at all levels of stimulation tested (Kaye et al. 1984). We believe that this mode of cell-cell contact could have important implications for the surveillance function of T cells because it allows cell interactions to persist for a finite time, which should allow the Ia-bearing cell to display a large sample of the antigens it has collected to the bound T cell.

DISCUSSION

B lymphocytes make effector molecules that bring together, in a single structure, information for function and specificity for antigen; the progeny of a virgin B cell can give rise to several distinct functional forms of antibody all of identical specificity by the mechanism of isotype switching. These effector molecules then engage secondary, antigen-nonspecific cells and molecules in ridding the organism of the foreign material or cells.

Helper T cells do not appear to be able to secrete their receptors in any form, as molecular analysis of the genes encoding these molecules has not revealed the necessary alternative splice sites at the 3′ end of the genes for the α and β chains (Hood L personal communication 1985). Furthermore, helper T cell receptors only recognize antigen on the surface of an Ia-bearing cell. In our view, the helper T cell receptor serves two, and possibly three, functions. First, the T cell receptor binds the T cell to a target cell–bearing antigen in association with the Ia molecule for which the T cell is specific. Second, this interaction leads to T cell receptor cross-linking, which serves to signal the T cell to release lymphokines and to express lymphokine receptors. Third, the T cell receptor may play a role in a focal delivery of these lymphokines onto the surface of the Ia-bearing cell with which the T cell is interacting. For helper T cells, functional diversity appears to arise not by a mechanism akin to isotype switching but rather through the array of lymphokines secreted by that cell and the types of lymphokine receptors expressed by that cell. Similarly, the result of an interaction between a helper T cell and its Ia antigen–bearing target cell is critically determined by the concentration of antigen:Ia on the target cell surface, by the presence of intermediary molecules such as IL 1, and by the lymphokine receptors the target cell bears. We can model this system using two clonal cell populations, a cloned helper T cell line and a cloned B lymphoma line, as described above.

This analysis suggests that there are three, and perhaps four, distinct modes of regulation of gene expression acting upon lymphokine genes. First, there is the "on-off" signaling of transcription activated when the T cell receptor is cross-linked. Second, there is some more permanent regulation of the lymphokines that an individual cloned line does secrete, as we find cloned lines are quite stable functionally and in their specificity for antigen. Third, there is a form of regulation that determines whether a particular class of cell can or cannot activate a particular gene; thus, B lymphocytes do not make IL 2 or a variety of other lymphokines. Whether there is an additional influence mediated by such ancillary molecules as IL 1 or by the strength of the stimulus on the relative amounts of different lymphokines produced remains to be determined. Given that helper T cells secrete several different lymphokines, it is apparent that T cells with identical receptors could come in a bewildering variety of functional phenotypes, each type determined by the regulation of lymphokine gene expression in that cell.

SUMMARY AND CONCLUSIONS

Helper T cells are activated by cross-linking of their receptors by antigen:Ia complexes on the surface of antigen-presenting cells and B cells. As a result of this cross-linking, the helper T cell releases several lymphokines that in turn affect the Ia-bearing cell with which the helper T cell is in contact. This interaction is cognate when the effect on the target cell is examined, but it operates by a mechanism that is neither antigen specific nor MHC restricted. Whether the cognate nature of this interaction reflects solely the intimate contact of the T cell with the Ia antigen–bearing cell or whether it reflects a receptor-directed focal release of lymphokines remains to be determined. The molecular basis for functional diversity in helper T cells will have to be determined by examining the factors that regulate lymphokine gene expression in such cells, a process that appears to act at several levels.

ACKNOWLEDGMENT

The authors would like to thank Barbara Broughton, Nancy Linberg, Eileen Dunn, and Andrea Wood for their help in carrying out these experiments. We would also like to thank our many colleagues at Yale University, particularly Don Murphy, Nancy Ruddle, Patrick Flood, Mike Iverson, and Al Bothwell for helpful discussion of the ideas in this paper. We also thank Laurie Hauer for preparing this manuscript.

This work was supported in part by National Institutes of Health grant AI-14579, and grants number CA-29606 and CA-38350 awarded by the National Cancer Institute, United States Department of Health and Human Services. Jonathan Kaye was partially supported by National Institutes of Health training grant AI-07019.

REFERENCES

Asano Y, Hodes RJ. 1983. T cell regulation of B cell activation: Cloned Lyt-1 [+],2 [−] T-suppressor cells inhibit the major histocompatibility complex restricted interaction of T-helper cells with B cells and/or accessory cells. J Exp Med 158: 1178–1190.

Bottomly K, Jones F III. 1981. Idiotype dominance manifested during a T-dependent anti-phosphorylcholine response requires a distinct helper T cell. *In* Klinman N, Mosier DE, Scher I, Vitetta FS, eds., B Lymphocytes in the Immune Response: Functional, Developmental, and Interactive Properties. Elsevier-North Holland, Inc., New York, pp. 415–420.

Bottomly K, Jones B, Kaye J, Jones F III. 1983a. Subpopulations of B cells distinguished by cell-surface expression of Ia antigens: Correlation of Ia and idiotype during activation by cloned Ia-restricted T cells. J Exp Med 158:265–279.

Bottomly K, Kaye J, Jones B, Jones F III, Janeway CA Jr. 1983b. A cloned, antigen-specific, Ia-restricted Lyt-1$^+$,2$^-$ T cell with suppressive activity. Journal of Molecular and Cellular Immunology 1:42–49.

Cone RE, Rosenstein RW, Janeway CA Jr, et al. 1983. Affinity-purified antigen-specific products produced by T cells share epitopes recognized by heterologous antisera raised against several different antigen-specific products from T cells. Cell Immunol 82:232–245.

Dialynas DP, Wilde DB, Marrack P, et al. 1983. Characterization of the murine antigenic determinant designated L3T4a, recognized by monoclonal antibody GK1.5: Expression of L3T4a by functional T cell clones appears to correlate with class II MHC antigen-reactivity. Immunol Rev 74:29–56.

Green DR, Flood PM, Gershon RK. 1983. Immunoregulatory T cell pathways. Annual Review of Immunology 1:439–463.

Greenstein JL, Kappler J, Marrack P, Burakoff SJ. 1984. The role of L3T4 in recognition of Ia by a cytotoxic, H-2D^d-specific T cell hybridoma. J Exp Med 159:1213–1224.

Honjo T. 1983. Immunoglobulin genes. Annual Review of Immunology 1:499–528.

Howard M, Paul WE. 1983. Regulation of B cell growth and differentiation by soluble factors. Annual Review of Immunology 1:307–334.

Janeway CA Jr, Bottomly K, Babich J et al. 1984. Quantitative variation in Ia antigen expression plays a central role in immune regulation. Immunology Today 5:99–105.

Janeway CA Jr, Bottomly K, Horowitz J, Kaye J, Jones B, Tite J. 1985. Modes of cell:cell communication in the immune system. J Immunol 135:739s–742s.

Jones B. 1982. Functional activities of antibodies against brain-associated T cell antigens: II. Stimulation of T cell–induced B cell proliferation. Eur J Immunol 12:30–37.

Jones B. 1983. Evidence that the Thy-1 molecule is the target for T cell mitogenic antibody against brain-associated antigens. Eur J Immunol 13:678–684.

Jones B, Janeway CA Jr. 1981a. Cooperative interaction of B lymphocytes with antigen-specific helper T lymphocytes is MHC restricted. Nature 292:547–549.

Jones B, Janeway CA Jr. 1981b. Functional activities of antibodies against brain-associated T cell antigens: I. Induction of T cell proliferation. Eur J Immunol 11:584–592.

Katz DH, Hamaoka T, Dorf ME, Maurer PH, Benacerraf B. 1973. Cell interactions between histoincompatible T and B lymphocytes: IV. Involvement of the immune response (Ir) gene in the control of lymphocyte interactions in responses controlled by the gene. J Exp Med 138:734–739.

Kaye J, Janeway CA Jr. 1984. The Fab fragment of a directly activating monoclonal antibody that precipitates a disulfide-linked heterodimer from a helper T cell clone blocks activation by either allogeneic-Ia or antigen and self-Ia. J Exp Med 159:1397–1412.

Kaye J, Porcelli S, Tite J, Jones B, Janeway CA Jr 1983. Both a monoclonal anti body and antisera specific for determinants unique to individual cloned helper T cell lines can substitute for antigen and antigen presenting cells in the activation of T cells. J Exp Med 158:836–856.

Kaye J, Gills S, Mizel SB, et al. 1984. Growth of a cloned helper T cell line induced by a monoclonal antibody specific for the antigen receptor: Interleukin 1 is required for the expression of receptors for interleukin 2. J Immunol 133:1339–1345.

Kuppers RC, Henney CS. 1976. Evidence for direct linkage between antigen recognition and lytic expression in effector T cells. J Exp Med 143:648–660.

Mitchison NA. 1971. The carrier effect in the secondary response to hapten-protein conjugates: II. Cellular cooperation. Eur J Immunol 1:18–27.

Monroe JG, Cambier JC. 1983. B cell activation: III. B cell plasma membrane depolarization and hyper-Ia expression induced by receptor immunoglobulin cross-linking are coupled. J Exp Med 158:1589–1599.

Norcross MA, Smith RT. 1979. Regulation of T cell mitogen activity of anti-lymphocyte serum by a B-helper cell. J Immunol 122:1620–1628.

Podack ER. 1985. The molecular mechanism of lymphocyte-mediated tumor cell lysis. Immunology Today 6:21–27.

Royer HD, Bensussan A, Acuto O, Reinherz EL. 1984. Functional isotypes are not encoded by the constant region genes of the β subunit of the T cell receptor for antigen/major histocompatibility complex. J Exp Med 160:947–952.

Schimpl A, Wecker A: 1973. Stimulation of IgG antibody response *in vitro* by T cell replacing factor. J Exp Med 137:547–552.

Schwartz RH. 1984. The role of gene products of the major histocompatibility complex in T cell activation and cellular interactions. *In* Paul WE, ed., Fundamental Immunology. Raven Press, New York, pp. 379–438.

Singer A, Hodes R. 1983. Mechanisms of T cell–B cell interaction. Annual Review of Immunology 1:211–241.

Smith KA. 1984. Interleukin 2. Annual Review of Immunology 2:319–333.

Tite JP, Janeway CA Jr. 1984a. Cloned helper cells can kill B lymphoma cells in the presence of specific antigen: Ia restriction and cognate vs. non-cognate interactions in cytolysis. Eur J Immunol 14:878–886.

Tite JP, Janeway CA Jr. 1984b. Antigen-dependent selection of B lymphoma cells varying in Ia density by cloned, antigen-specific L3T4a$^+$ T cells: A possible *in vitro* model for B cell adaptive differentiation. Journal of Molecular and Cellular Immunology 1:255–265.

Tite J, Kaye J, Jones B. 1984. The role of major histocompatibility complex determinant recognition at the B cell surface by T cells in the triggering of B cells: Analysis of the interaction of cloned helper T cells with normal B cells in differing states of activation and with B cells expressing the *xid* defect. Eur J Immunol 14:553–561.

Tite JP, Powell MB, Ruddle NH. 1985. Protein-antigen specific Ia-restricted cytolytic T cells: Analysis of frequency, target cell susceptibility and mechanism of cytolysis. J Immunol 135:25–33.

Symposium on Fundamental Cancer Research, Vol. 38.

5. The Arrangement of Immunoglobulin, T Cell Antigen Receptor, and Interleukin 2 Receptor Genes in Human Lymphoid Neoplasms

Thomas A. Waldmann, Stanley J. Korsmeyer,
and Warner C. Greene

*The Metabolism Branch, National Cancer Institute, National Institutes of Health,
Bethesda, Maryland 20892*

Within recent years, investigators using recombinant DNA technology have provided insights into the processes by which the diversity of antibodies and antigen-specific T cell receptors are generated (Leder 1982, Tonegawa 1983). Furthermore, the analyses of immunoglobulin (Ig), T cell receptor, and interleukin (IL) 2 receptor gene arrangements have proved to be of value in the study of human lymphoid neoplasms (Arnold et al. 1983, Bakhshi et al. 1983, Korsmeyer et al. 1983a, Cleary et al. 1984, Sklar et al. 1984). Ig heavy- and light-chain genes are encoded by discontinuous gene subsegments that are separated from each other in the germ line state. At some point in the development of an antibody-producing cell, there is a somatic recombination that assembles the separated gene segments that encode the variable portion of the molecule. For example, the Ig heavy (H)-chain gene rearranges its germ line DNA to assemble a variable (V_H), diversity (D_H), and joining (J_H) segment into a complete V-D-J region encoding the antigen-binding portion of the peptide. These rearrangements of the heavy-chain gene are followed by rearrangements of the V and J segments of light-chain genes, which themselves proceed in an order of κ (V_κ and J_κ) before λ (V_λ and J_λ). These DNA rearrangements produce a change in the location of restriction endonuclease sites that allows the uniquely rearranged Ig genes in a monoclonal expansion of B cells to be identified by Southern blot analysis. In contrast to B cells, the human T cell malignancies we have studied uniformly retained germ line (unrearranged) light-chain genes and, in most cases (21 of 23), also contained germ line heavy-chain genes (Arnold et al. 1983, Korsmeyer et al. 1983a). Therefore, the detection of both rearranged heavy- and light-chain genes within a lymphoid population served as a marker uniquely associated with malignancies of B cell lineage.

The human antigen-specific T cell receptor is a polymorphic disulfide-linked heterodimer corresponding to a molecular weight (M_r) of about 90 kDa consisting of a 45- to 50-kDa α subunit and a 40- to 45-kDa β subunit (Allison et al. 1982, Haskins et al. 1983, Meuer et al. 1983). This receptor is associated with three 20- to 28-kDa nonpolymorphic peptide chains identified by the T3 monoclonal antibody. cDNA clones encoding the β and α chain of the T cell receptor have been isolated (Chien et al. 1984, Hedrick et al. 1984a,b, Yanagi et al. 1984). The T_β chain genes in their germ line form, like Ig genes, are discontinuous gene subsegments that encode the variable and constant portion of the receptor peptide. This gene locus, found on chromosome 7 q32, comprises multiple germ line variable region gene (V_β) and duplicate sets of diversity ($D_{\beta1}$, $D_{\beta2}$), joining ($J_{\beta1}$, $J_{\beta2}$), and constant ($C_{\beta1}$, $C_{\beta2}$) T_β gene segments. At a point during the differentiation of a pluripotent stem cell into a mature T cell, a process of DNA rearrangements occurs that juxtaposes one of the D_β and J_β segments and then one of the V_β segments to generate the complete T_β variable region gene. In the present study, we have applied recombinant DNA technologies involving analysis of Ig and T cell receptor gene arrangements to classify neoplasms that have been of controversial lineage, to define the clonality of lymphoid proliferations, to assist in the diagnosis of neoplasms of the T cell and B cell series, and to monitor the therapy of lymphoid malignancies.

Ig GENE REARRANGEMENTS THAT GENERATE UNIQUE CLONAL MARKERS IN CELLS OF THE B CELL SERIES

The demonstration that histologically distinct lymphoid neoplasms correspond to stages of B or T cell development has advanced our understanding of these malignancies. Historically, this has often been accomplished using cell surface markers associated with stages of B or T cell maturation. In addition, the demonstration that certain neoplasms are monoclonal proliferations has been of great conceptual importance in understanding their pathogenesis. Often, however, it is impossible to classify a lymphoid neoplasm as B or T cell in origin, despite examining lineage-associated surface markers. This often results from the admixture of large numbers of nonneoplastic cells with tumor cells. Alternatively, some malignancies represent stages of differentiation prior to the expression of lineage-restricted surface markers. These limitations can now be overcome by utilizing DNA rearrangements of receptor genes to reveal clonality, cell lineage, and state of differentiation of such neoplasms. As noted above, DNA rearrangements of Ig genes are mandatory within cells of the B lymphoid lineage. Specifically, sequential assembly of Ig heavy-chain and then light-chain gene subsegments occurs early in B cell development and takes place in a unique fashion within individual B cells to generate a singular antibody specificity. A polyclonal population of normal B cells possesses numerous different Ig gene rearrangements that result in multiple, different size, Ig-containing DNA fragments after restriction enzyme digestion. When this collection of DNA fragments is analyzed on a Southern blot, no single rearranged band is detected because each rearrangement is below the threshold of sensitivity. In contrast, a monoclonal expansion representing a single cell's progeny will have a unique identifying DNA rearrangement pattern specific only for that tumor. In this instance, all cells analyzed are identical and, therefore, contain the same size, rearranged Ig gene–containing fragment. The multiple copies of this unique fragment present in the total DNA from a clonal expansion allow this Ig gene rearrangement to be detected on Southern blot analysis as a distinct band, different in size from the band representing the germ line (unrearranged) form of the gene. We have used such DNA rearrangements detected by Southern blot hybridization to serve as sensitive as well as specific markers capable of identifying even minority populations of clonal cells (2–5%) within tissues of mixed cellularity. Furthermore, rearranged heavy- and light-chain genes within lymphoid populations serve as markers associated specifically with the B cell lineage.

Ig Gene Patterns in B Cell Malignancies

The malignant cells from patients with chronic lymphocytic leukemia and Burkitt's lymphoma all displayed clonal heavy- plus light-chain gene rearrangements. It was of interest that κ-producing B cells displayed at least one κ gene rearrangement, while they usually retained their λ genes in the germ line form. In distinct contrast, λ-producing B cells displayed the obligate λ rearrangement, but in addition had characteristically lost the germ line κ genes. That is, they had deleted or aberrantly rearranged their constant κ genes and, in many cases, the joining κ genes as well, while retaining the variable κ gene subsegments. This reflects an ordered sequence of Ig gene rearrangements in humans in which heavy-chain gene rearrangements precede light-chain genes and κ rearrangements precede λ.

B Cell Precursor Forms of Acute Lymphocytic Leukemia

In order to examine the early events of Ig gene assembly, we examined the leukemic cells from patients with the "non-T, non-B" form of acute lymphoblastic leukemia (Korsmeyer et al. 1983a). These cells lack surface Ig, fail to form rosettes with sheep red blood cells, and do not react with monoclonal antibodies directed at T cells. All 25 cases studied had heavy-chain gene rearrangement, examined utilizing a J_H segment probe. Such rearrangements can be either complete V_H-D_H-J_H junctures or intermediate D_H-J_H forms still missing a V_H segment. Eleven of these leukemia patients had progressed to light-chain gene rearrangements. Once again their pattern of light-chain gene recombination predicted a model in which κ precedes λ rearrangements in humans. Specifically, a series of intermediate light-chain gene rearrangements was observed in which certain patients had aberrantly rearranged or deleted κ

gene subsegments, while retaining their λ genes in the germ line configuration. Although all 25 of the cases showed at least the rearrangement of heavy-chain genes and in 11 cases light-chain genes as well, only 5 cases produced cytoplasmic μ chain, and only a single case produced cytoplasmic light chain, in this case a λ-light chain. In many cases, there may be cells with incomplete D-J intermediates or, alternatively, ineffective aberrant V-D-J rearrangements. Thus, there may be a set of cells trapped in the B cell precursor series because ineffective rearrangements of both alleles encoding the heavy-chain genes have eliminated the necessary germ line gene subsegments required for the assemblage of an effective heavy-chain gene. Such cells may have deleted all available germ line D_H gene subsegments, as well as the signals for rearrangement and thus may be incapable of forming a complete heavy-chain gene. Thus, somatic recombination joining gene subsegments not only provides a dynamic system to generate antibody diversity, but also is very error prone, providing a molecular explanation for some of the cell wastage that accompanies differentiation. Taken as a whole, the examination of acute lymphocytic leukemia cells not reactive with monoclonal antibodies directed at T cells indicates that these cells are within the B cell precursor series. Furthermore, the gene patterns observed reveal a cascade of rearrangements in humans in which heavy-chain gene rearrangements precede light and κ-gene rearrangements precede λ.

Gene Rearrangements that Establish Cell Lineage and Clonality

The molecular genetic analysis with Ig gene probes has proved to be of marked value in determining the cellular lineage of a variety of lymphoid malignancies of controversial origin, including hairy cell leukemia and the lymphoid blast crisis of chronic myelogenous leukemia. Cytogenetic and isoenzyme studies established that chronic myelogenous leukemia is a clonal proliferation arising from a remarkably pluripotent cell (Fialkow et al. 1977). Because of the multipotential capacity of clonal cells in chronic myelogenous leukemia, the cellular origin and exact stage of differentiation of the cells comprising the blast crisis episodes of this disorder have remained uncertain. Occasionally, the lymphoblasts from the acute phase of this disease have been classified as pre–B cells because of the presence of cytoplasmic Ig (LeBien et al. 1979). The granulocytic malignant cells and the myeloid blast crises from such patients did not show rearrangement of Ig genes (Bakhshi et al. 1983). However, rearrangement of heavy-chain genes was demonstrated in eight of the nine lymphoid blast crises cases studied together with light-chain rearrangements in three (Bakhshi et al. 1983). These observations provide important evidence indicating that these lymphoid blast crisis cells are genetically committed B cell precursors.

Furthermore, serial studies of a single patient during several phases of his disease revealed that two separate lymphoid blast crisis episodes were clonal expansions of malignant cells at distinctly different stages of genetic maturation, both crises displayed identical heavy-chain gene rearrangements, but one had progressed to λ light-chain gene recombination, while the other had germ line light-chain genes (Bakhshi et al. 1983). Thus, the clone of cells that bears the Philadelphia chromosomal translocation is capable of clonal progression with differentiation and sequential Ig gene rearrangements. Similar clonal progression or even biclonality has been demonstrated in the malignant lymph nodes of patients with follicular lymphoma (Sklar et al. 1984).

The malignant cells in patients with hairy cell leukemia also have been of controversial lineage. Many investigators have ascribed B cell properties to these cells; however, others have noted monocytic properties and even T cell–associated antigens have been described, especially following activation with the lectin phytohemagglutinin (PHA) (Guglielmi et al. 1980). To help resolve this uncertainty, we asked whether appropriately rearranged and properly expressed Ig genes were present. All cases examined to date had patterns of heavy- and light-chain gene rearrangements characteristic of mature B cell stages of differentiation (Korsmeyer et al. 1983b). In addition, appropriate size mRNA from these rearranged genes was detectable and responsible for the surface Ig. Thus, in those cases examined, hairy cell leukemia appeared to represent a mature B cell stage of differentiation.

Diagnostic dilemmas may arise in lymphomas owing to nondiscriminatory surface marker studies. As noted above, rearrangement of Ig genes serves as a sensitive and specific marker that is capable of identifying even minority populations (2–5%) of clonal B cells within tissues of mixed cellularity (Arnold et al. 1983). This genetic marker of Ig gene rearrangement enabled us to assign a diagnosis of B cell–type lymphoma to a malignancy that could not be classified as a lymphoma (as opposed to an undifferentiated carcinoma) based on histologic surface markers and electron microscopic examination. We also demonstrated the presence of monoclonal B cells in several malignant lymph nodes in which T cells represented over 70% of the cells and in which the mistaken diagnosis of T cell lymphoma may have been made. The T cells in these nodes were polyclonal, as assessed by the techniques discussed below, and they appeared to be T cells reactive to the monoclonal B cell expansion. In addition, a clonal population of cells with Ig gene rearrangements was discovered within the enlarging lymph nodes of a patient with the Wiskott-Aldrich syndrome that was felt to be an atypical hyperplasia (Arnold et al. 1983). These DNA rearrangements in such patients provide the genetic marker unique to clonal cells that will enable us to follow their natural history and determine if such populations of cells are benign and still under regulation or if they represent a malignancy. Furthermore, DNA rearrangements within B cell and B cell precursor malignancies serve as sensitive tumor-specific markers that enhance the ability to identify persistent tumor following therapy and facilitate the early detection of recurrences.

T CELL ANTIGEN RECEPTOR GENE REARRANGEMENTS AS SPECIFIC T CELL LINEAGE AND CLONAL MARKERS IN HUMAN LYMPHOID NEOPLASMS

As noted above, the human antigen-specific T cell receptor is a polymorphic disulfide-linked heterodimer composed of β and α subunits. cDNA clones encoding the β and α chain of a T cell receptor have been isolated (Chien et al. 1984, Hedrick et al. 1984a,b, Saito et al. 1984a, Yanagi et al. 1984). The human T_β chain genes in their germ line form consist of multiple germ line variable region genes (V_β) and duplicate sets of diversity, joining, and constant T_β gene segments. In the present study, we have used a cDNA clone that hybridizes with the $C_{\beta 1}$ and $C_{\beta 2}$ genes to observe the arrangements of these T_β gene subsegments in human lymphoid neoplasms and germ line tissues. The arrangement of the T_β gene in circulating white blood cells of normal individuals was analyzed using a cDNA clone that hybridizes with the $C_{\beta 1}$ and $C_{\beta 2}$ genes to define the germ line arrangement of this gene. In their germ line form, the gene segments encoding the two C_β genes were present on a single 24-kb *Bam*HI fragment, on two *Eco*RI fragments of 4 and 11 kb, and on three *Hin*dIII fragments of 3.5, 6.5, and 8.0 kb. Only in rare cases were polymorphisms observed in this gene pattern. The arrangement of the T_β genes was retained in the germ line form in all nonlymphoid malignancies examined, as well as in polyclonal populations of B cells and Epstein-Barr virus (EBV)–transformed B cell lines. In general, clonal B cell populations derived from patients with Burkitt's lymphoma, B cell precursor, acute lymphoblastic leukemia, or B cell chronic lymphocytic leukemia manifested T_β lines in their germ line configuration.

Normal polyclonal T cells presumably possess numerous different T_β line rearrangements. Collectively, none of these gene rearrangements is detectable as a new band on Southern blot because they are below the threshold of sensitivity of this method. However, such polyclonal T cells have a marked diminution of the intensity of the 11-kb *Eco*RI band when compared to the 4-kb band defined by the T_β probe. The virtual loss of the 11 kb as compared with the 4-kb band in polyclonal T cells reflects the arrangement of the *Eco*RI endonuclease sites. The $C_{\beta 2}$ gene segment present on the 4-kb *Eco*RI fragment is flanked by *Eco*RI sites with an enzyme site between $C_{\beta 2}$ and $J_{\beta 2}$. Thus, the size of the *Eco*RI fragment bearing this gene is not altered by a V-D-J rearrangement of this gene complex, and the intensity of the band reflecting this gene segment is identical in all tissues. In contrast, the size of the *Eco*RI fragment bearing the $C_{\beta 1}$ gene (11 kb in germ line tissues) is altered by virtually all rearrangements affecting V, D_1, or J_1. Thus, the marked diminution of the intensity of the 11-kb *Eco*RI band when compared with the 4-kb band in polyclonal T cells suggests that effective or aberrant rearrangements or deletions at least involving D_β and J_β elements have occurred for both T_β alleles in the majority of polyclonal T cells. A similar diminution of the 11-kb *Eco*RI band on Southern blot analysis was observed with T8-enriched as well as T4-enriched polyclonal T lymphocyte populations. These latter observations concerning T8 lymphocytes suggest that suppressor/cytotoxic T lymphocytes rearrange or delete their T_β genes.

In contrast to the polyclonal T and B lymphocyte populations, each malignant expansion of T cells examined displayed an identifiable DNA rearrangement. The T cells examined included four leukemic populations from patients with the human T cell leukemia/lymphoma virus (HTLV-I)–associated adult T cell leukemia, five with Sézary leukemia, and five with acute lymphoblastic leukemia reactive with monoclonal antibodies to T cells. In 13 of 14 cases, the leukemic cells manifested multiple (2 or even 3) rearrangements with loss of certain germ line bands, as assessed by Southern blot analysis, which supported the view that most T cells manifest an aberrant or effective rearrangement of both T_β alleles. The demonstration of non–germ line bands on Southern blot analysis indicates that these T leukemic populations represent clonal (mono- or, at least, oligoclonal) expansions of T lymphocytes.

In general, clonal B cell populations derived from patients with Burkitt's lymphoma, B cell precursor acute lymphoblastic leukemia, or B cell chronic lymphocytic leukemia retained T_β genes in the germ line configuration. However, in rare cases (3 of 21), there were rearrangements of T_β genes that did not fit this pattern. The three leukemia patients with T_β gene rearrangements were confirmed to have B cell leukemia in that each manifested clonal rearrangements of both heavy- and light-chain Ig genes. Furthermore, fibroblasts cultured from one of the patients retained the T_β gene in the germ line configuration, thus confirming that the T_β gene arrangement in the B cell leukemic population from the patient represents a clonal rearrangement of this gene rather than a genetic polymorphism. Thus, the rearrangement of T_β genes in a small subset of B cells may be analogous to the Ig heavy-chain gene rearrangements observed in 10% of the leukemic T cell populations that we have examined. The DNA sequences that provide signals for the enzymes active in recombining D and J segments in T and B cells are distinct, but have considerable similarities. It is possible that recombinases normally acting in T cells to rearrange T_β genes may occasionally lead to rearrangements of this T_β gene in cells of the B cell series. These rearrangements do not present a major problem in assigning lineage when groups of patients are examined. For example, the leukemic cells of each of the five patients with acute lymphoblastic leukemia whose malignant cells or cell lines derived from these cells that reacted with monoclonal antibodies to T cells demonstrated a rearrangement of the T_β gene, whereas a rearrangement of the Ig heavy-chain genes was not observed. Thus, the leukemic cells of this group of patients could be assigned to the T cell precursor series. The T_β rearrangements observed with certain B cell leukemias can, however, hinder efforts to define the lineage of a particular lymphoid malignancy in an individual patient. A pattern of gene rearrangements has been defined that may allow a more definitive assignment of lineage. Recently, an additional gene complex now termed T_γ was shown to rearrange in T cells and to be expressed in cells of this series (Saito et al. 1984b, Hayday et al. 1985). In preliminary studies performed in collaboration with K. Murre and J. G. Seidman, we have shown that clonal T cells rearrange their T_γ genes, whereas the mature clonal B cells examined did not show rearrangements of this gene complex. Thus, rearrangement of both T_β and T_γ genes appears to occur in cells of the T cell lineage and may provide a molecular arrangement of value in defining cells of this lineage.

Establishment of Clonality in Patients with T Lymphocytosis and Hematocytopenias

There are few techniques available to define clonality in T cell populations. In a number of disorders there is controversy as to whether expansion of T lymphocyte populations reflects clonal expansion of T cells or polyclonal expansion of immunoregulatory cells. For example, there is controversy concerning the clonality of the T8 cell populations in the syndrome characterized by lymphocytosis of large granular lymphocytes expressing the $T3^+$, $T8^+$ phenotype that is associated with granulocytopenia and anemia (Aisenberg et al. 1981, Chan et al. 1984, Reynolds and Foon 1984). The controversy specifically centers around the question of whether this disorder represents an indolent chronic lymphocytic leukemia of T cells or merely an expansion of an immunoregulatory polyclonal population. In conjunction with E. Winton, we have studied three of four such patients with T8 lymphocytosis associated with granulocytopenia and demonstrated that their peripheral blood mononuclear cells had a clonal pattern of T_β gene rearrangement. Thus, the T8 lymphocytosis associated with granulocytopenia frequently represents a clonal expansion of this subset of T lymphocytes.

In summary, the use of Ig gene rearrangements has been of great value in the study of B lymphocytes; however, their application is predominantly restricted to cells of the B cell lineage. We now demonstrate that T cell receptor rearrangements taken in conjuction with studies of Ig gene rearrangements aid in the definition of the lineage (T cell versus B cell) and the clonality of lymphoid populations of all lineages. The application of this molecular genetic approach has great potential for complementing conventional marker analysis, cytogenetics, and histopathology, thereby broadening the scientific basis for the diagnosis, monitoring the therapy, and classifying the lymphoid neoplasias.

IL 2 RECEPTOR GENE EXPRESSION IN HTLV-I–ASSOCIATED ADULT T CELL LEUKEMIA

T cell activation is initiated following the interaction of antigen with the complex, antigen-specific T cell receptor discussed above. Two principal events that are required for T cell proliferation and the development of functionally active effector T cells occur at this point. First, following interaction with antigen and the macrophage-derived IL 1, T cells synthesize and secrete the lymphokine IL 2 (Morgan et al. 1976, Smith 1980). In order to exert its biologic effects, IL 2 must interact with specific high affinity membrane receptors (Robb et al. 1981). Resting T cells do not express IL 2 receptors, but receptors are rapidly expressed on T cells following activation with antigen or mitogen. Thus, both the growth factor IL 2 and its receptor are absent in resting T cells, but following activation, the genes for both proteins are expressed. Thus, both the production of IL 2 and the expression of the IL 2 receptors are pivotal events in the full expression of the human immune response. While the antigen confers specificity for a given immune response, the interaction of IL 2 and IL 2 receptors determines its magnitude and duration.

The specific membrane receptor for IL 2 on human lymphocytes has been identified using a monoclonal antibody (anti-Tac) directed towards this molecule (Uchiyama et al. 1981a, Leonard et al. 1982, 1983a). Utilizing the anti-Tac monoclonal antibody, we have defined a variety of T and B lymphocyte functions that require an interaction of IL 2 with its inducible receptor on activated lymphocytes (Uchiyama 1981b, Depper et al. 1983). The addition of anti-Tac to in vitro culture systems blocked the IL 2–induced DNA synthesis of IL 2–dependent T cell lines and inhibited soluble auto- and alloantigen-induced T cell proliferation. Furthermore, it abrogated the generation of cytotoxic and suppressor-effector T cells, but did not inhibit their action once it was generated. The antireceptor antibody also inhibited the proliferation and Ig synthesis of purified B cells stimulated with staphylococcus Cowan strain I organisms.

The human IL 2 receptor was characterized (Leonard et al. 1983a), and cDNA encoding this receptor has been cloned and expressed. The IL 2 receptor is a 55-kDa glycoprotein composed of a 33-kDa peptide precursor. Mature receptors contain both N-linked and O-linked sugars and are both sulfated and phosphorylated. cDNA encoding the human IL 2 receptor has been molecularly cloned (Leonard et al. 1984a). The deduced amino acid sequence of the IL 2 receptor indicates that this peptide is composed of 272 amino acids, including a 21 amino acid signal peptide. The receptor contains two potential N-linked glycosylation sites, as well as multiple possible O-linked carbohydrate sites. Furthermore, there is a single hydrophobic transmembrane region and a very short (13 amino acid) cytoplasmic domain. The cytoplasmic domain of the IL 2 receptor appears to be too small for enzymatic function. Thus, this receptor differs from other known growth factor receptors, which are tyrosine kinases. Potential phosphate acceptor sites (serine and threonine, but not tyrosine) are present within the intracytoplasmic domain.

In the present study, the anti-Tac monoclonal antibody was used to characterize IL 2 receptor expression in HTLV-I–associated adult T cell leukemia. Furthermore, we report the initial results of a clinical trial to evaluate the efficacy of intravenously administered anti-Tac monoclonal antibody in the treatment of patients with the adult T cell leukemia.

IL 2 Receptor Expression in Adult T Cell Leukemia

We have analyzed the IL 2 receptor expression on three forms of T cell leukemia: acute T cell lymphoblastic leukemia, the Sézary leukemia, and adult T cell leukemia (Waldmann et al. 1984). Acute T cell leukemia is a malignant proliferation of immature T cells that frequently do not express surface antigens, such as the T3 antigen, that are associated with mature T cells. Both the adult T cell leukemia and the Sézary leukemia are malignant proliferations of mature T cells with a propensity to infiltrate the skin. They share similar cell morphology and clinical features. However, certain features aid in distinguishing these leukemias. Cases of adult T cell leukemia, in contrast to those of the Sézary leukemia, are clustered within families and geographically; they occur in the southwest of Japan, the Caribbean basin, and certain areas of the southeastern United States. Furthermore, adult T cell leukemia is caused by HTLV-I, a human type c retrovirus, whereas patients with the Sézary syndrome do not have circulating antibodies to this virus (Poiesz et al. 1980, Gallo and Wong-Staal 1982).

The acute T cell leukemic populations and lines derived from such cells we examined did not express the IL 2 receptor. Furthermore, 9 of the 10 populations of Sézary leukemic T cells not associated with HTLV-I that we examined were Tac antigen negative (Waldmann et al. 1984). In contrast, all of the populations of leukemic cells from patients with the adult T cell leukemia, associated with HTLV-I, expressed the Tac antigen. Thus, the demonstration of IL 2 receptors on leukemic T cells may aid in differentiating leukemias caused by HTLV-I that are Tac antigen positive from other forms of T cell leukemia that are, in general, Tac antigen negative.

The IL 2 receptor expression on adult T cell leukemia cells differs from that on normal T cells. First, unlike normal T cells, adult T cell leukemia cells do not require prior activation to express the IL 2 receptors. Furthermore, using the ^{3}H–anti-Tac receptor assay, HTLV-I–infected leukemic T cell lines characteristically expressed 5- to 10-fold more receptors per cell (270,000 to 640,000) than did maximally PHA-stimulated T lymphoblasts (30,000 to 60,000) (Depper et al. 1984). Since the cell volume of these leukemic cells was only 13% greater than that of PHA lymphoblasts, the density of IL 2 receptors on these leukemic cells increased correspondingly. In addition, while normal human T lymphocytes maintained in long-term culture with IL 2 demonstrate a rapid decline in receptor number, adult T cell leukemia lines do not show a similar decline. Furthermore, we have noted that some, but not all, HTLV-I cell lines display aberrant size IL 2 receptors (Leonard et al. 1983b, 1984b). For example, the receptor on HTLV-I–infected HUT 102-B2 cells is approximately 5 kDa smaller than that on PHA lymphoblasts. Pulse chase, tunicamycin, endoglycosidase, and neuraminidase analyses were used to show that the difference in receptor size was due to differences in posttranslational modification of the 33-kDa protein backbone (Leonard et al. 1983b, 1984b). Furthermore, the receptors on the HUT 102-B2 cells manifested less sulfation than did normal receptors. Finally, in studies by Uchiyama and coworkers (1986), IL 2 receptors on adult T cell leukemia cells, unlike normal, activated T cells, were not modulated (down regulated) by anti-Tac, and IL 2 receptors on adult T cell leukemia cell lines were spontaneously (IL 2 independently) phosphorylated, whereas the phosphorylation of receptors on PHA-stimulated T cells required the addition of IL 2. It is conceivable that the constant presence of high numbers of IL 2 receptors on the adult T cell leukemia cells or the aberrancy of these receptors may play a major role in the pathogenesis of uncontrolled growth of these malignant T cells.

Treatment with the Anti-Tac Monoclonal Antibody of Patients with Adult T Cell Leukemia

We have initiated a clinical trial to evaluate the efficacy of intravenously administered anti-Tac monoclonal antibody in the treatment of patients with the adult T cell leukemia. The scientific basis for these studies is the observation that adult T cell leukemia cells express the Tac antigen, whereas normal resting T cells and their precursors do not (Waldmann et al. 1984). Two patients with adult T cell leukemia have been treated with intravenously administered anti-Tac. Neither patient suffered any untoward reactions nor did they produce antibodies reactive with mouse Ig or the idiotype of the anti-Tac monoclonal. One patient with a very rapidly developing form of adult T cell leukemia had a transient response. However, therapy of the other patient was followed by a six-month remission, as assessed by routine hematologic tests, by immunofluorescence analysis of circulating T cells, and by molecular genetic analysis of the arrangement of T cell β receptor genes. Prior to anti-Tac therapy, the patient had 2,200/mm^3 circulating malignant T cells, as assessed by immunofluorescence analysis using the anti-Tac monoclonal antibody. Furthermore, some (1,200/mm³), but not all, of these circulating leukemic lymphocytes reacted with an antibody to the transferrin receptor, a receptor expressed on malignant T cells, but not on normal circulating cells. Following anti-Tac therapy there was a decline in the number of circulating T cells bearing the Tac antigen from 2,200 to less than 100/mm³ and in transferrin receptor–expressing T cells from 1,200 to less than 100/mm³. During the four-week period following the anti-Tac infusions, there were no cells with free IL 2 receptors, that is, cells with receptors unblocked by the infused anti-Tac monoclonal. Cells with blocked IL 2 receptors were identified as cells that were not reactive with fluorescein isothiocyanate (FITC)–conjugated anti-Tac, but were reactive with FITC-conjugated anti–mouse IgG and with the 7G7 monoclonal antibody, an antibody that identifies an epitope of the IL 2 receptor peptide other than that identified by anti-Tac. The remission of the T cell leukemia in this patient was confirmed utilizing molecular genetic analysis of the arrangement of the gene encoding the β chain of the antigen-specific T cell receptor. Prior to therapy, Southern blot analysis of the arrangement of the T cell β receptor gene, utilizing a radiolabeled probe to the constant region of the T_β chain (Hedrick et al. 1984a), revealed a new band not present in germ line tissues, the hallmark of a clonal expansion of T lymphocytes. This band, reflecting the clonally rearranged T cell receptor gene, was not demonstrable on specimens obtained following anti-Tac therapy when the patient was in remission. Approximately six months following the initial remission, the leukemia recurred with reappearance of circulating leukemic cells identified by immunofluorescence and molecular genetic analysis. The patient also developed large (5 × 7 × 1 cm) malignant skin lesions. A new course of intravenous infusions of anti-Tac was followed by the virtual disappearance of the skin lesions and an over 90% reduction in the number of circulating leukemic cells. Three months later, leukemic cells again were demonstrable in the circulation. At this time the leukemia was no longer responsive to infusions of anti-Tac, and the patient required chemotherapy.

These therapeutic studies have been extended in vitro by examining the efficacy of toxins coupled to anti-Tac in selectively inhibiting protein synthesis and viability of Tac antigen positive adult T cell leukemia cell lines. The addition of anti-Tac antibody coupled to the A chain of the toxin ricin effectively inhibited protein synthesis by the HTLV-I–associated, Tac antigen–positive adult T cell leukemia line HUT 102-B2. In contrast, conjugates of ricin A with a control monoclonal antibody of the same isotype did not inhibit protein synthesis when used in the same concentration (Krönke et al. 1985). The inhibitory action of anti-Tac conjugated with ricin A could be abolished by the addition of excess unlabeled anti-Tac or IL 2. In parallel studies performed in collaboration with David FitzGerald, Mark Willingham, and Ira Pastan (1984), pseudomonas exotoxin conjugates of anti-Tac inhibited the protein synthesis by HUT 102-B2 cells but not that of the Tac antigen negative acute T cell line Molt-4, which does not express the Tac antigen. Again, the toxicity of the anti-Tac toxin conjugates could be inhibited by adding excess unlabeled anti-Tac. Thus, the development of toxin conjugates of the monoclonal anti-Tac that are directed toward the IL 2 receptor expressed on adult T cell leukemia cells may permit the development of a rational approach for the treatment of this almost always fatal form of leukemia.

SUMMARY

Ig and T cell antigen receptor genes in their germ line form are separated DNA segments that are joined by recombinations during lymphocyte development. The analysis of Ig and T cell receptor gene arrangements has been of value in the study of lymphoid neoplasms. The identification of T cell receptor gene rearrangements taken in conjunction with studies of Ig gene rearrangements aids in the elucidation of the lineage (T cell or B cell) and the clonality of lymphoid populations of all series. The application of this molecular genetic approach has great potential for complementing conventional marker analysis, cytogenetics, and histopathology, thus broadening the scientific basis for the classification, diagnosis, and monitoring of the therapy of lymphoid neoplasia.

IL 2 is a lymphokine synthesized by some T cells following activation. Resting T cells do not express IL 2 receptors, but receptors are rapidly expressed on T cells following the interaction of antigens, mitogens, or monoclonal antibodies with the antigen-specific T cell receptor complex. Normal resting T cells and most leukemic T cell populations do not express IL 2 receptors; however, the leukemic cells of all patients with HTLV-I–associated adult T cell leukemia examined expressed the Tac antigen. The constant display of large numbers of IL 2 receptors that may be aberrant may play a role in the uncontrolled growth of these leukemic T cells. Patients with the Tac antigen positive adult T cell leukemia are being treated with the anti-Tac monoclonal antibody directed toward this growth factor receptor.

REFERENCES

Aisenberg A, Wilkes B, Harris N, Ault K, Carey R. 1981. Chronic T-cell lymphocytosis with neutropenia: Report of a case studied with monoclonal antibody. Blood 58:818–822.

Allison JP, McIntyre BW, Bloch D. 1982. Tumor-specific antigen of murine T lymphoma defined with monoclonal antibody. J Immunol 129:2293–2300.

Arnold A, Cossman J, Bakhshi A, Jaffe ES, Waldmann TA, Korsmeyer SJ. 1983. Immunoglobulin gene rearrangements as unique clonal markers in human lymphoid neoplasms. N Engl J Med 309:1593–1599.

Bakhshi A, Minowada J, Arnold A, et al. 1983. Lymphoid blast crises of chronic myelogenous leukemia represent stages in the development of B cell precursors. N Engl J Med 309:826–831.

Chan W, Check I, Schick C, Brynes R, Kateley J, Winton E. 1984. A morphologic and immunologic study of the large granular lymphocyte in neutropenia with T lymphocytosis. Blood 63:1133–1140.

Chien YH, Becker DM, Lindsten T, Okamuras M, Cohen DI, Davis MM. 1984. A third type of murine T-cell receptor gene. Nature 312:31–35.

Cleary MI, Warnke R, Sklar J. 1984. Monoclonality of lymphoproliferative lesions in cardiac transplant recipients. N Engl J Med 310:477–482.

Depper JM, Leonard WJ, Waldmann TA, Greene WC. 1983. Blockade of the interleukin-2 receptor by anti-Tac antibody: Inhibition of human lymphocyte activation. J Immunol 131:690–696.

Depper JM, Leonard WJ, Krönke M, Waldmann TA, Greene WC. 1984. Augmentation of T-cell growth factor expression in HTLV-I-infected human leukemic T cells. J Immunol 133:1691–1695.

Fialkow PJ, Jacobson RJ, Papayannopoulou T. 1977. Chronic myelocytic leukemia: Clonal origin in a stem cell common to the granulocyte, erythrocyte, platelet, and monocyte/macrophage. Am J Med 63:125–130.

FitzGerald DJP, Waldmann TA, Willingham MC, Pastan I. 1984. Pseudomonas exotoxin-anti-Tac: Cell-specific immunotoxin active against cells expressing the human T-cell growth factor receptor. J Clin Invest 74:966–971.

Gallo RC, Wong-Staal F. 1982. Retroviruses as etiologic agents of some animal and human leukemias and lymphomas and as tools for elucidating the molecular mechanism of leukemogenesis. Blood 60:545–557.

Guglielmi P, Preud'homme JL, Flandrin G. 1980. Phenotypic changes of phytohaemagglutinin-stimulated hairy cells. Nature 286:166–168.

Haskins K, Kubo R, White J, Pigeon M, Kappler J, Marrack P. 1983. The major histocompatibility complex-restricted antigen receptor on T cells: Isolation with a monoclonal antibody. J Exp Med 157:1149–1169.

Hayday AC, Saito H, Gillies SD, et al. 1985. Structure, organization, and somatic rearrangement of T-cell gamma genes. Cell 40:259–281.

Hedrick SM, Cohen DI, Nielsen EA, Davis MM. 1984a. Isolation of cDNA clones encoding T cell specific membrane-associated proteins. Nature 308:149–153.

Hedrick SM, Nielsen EA, Kavaler J, Cohen DI, Davis MM. 1984b. Sequence relationships between putative T-cell receptor polypeptides and immunoglobulins. Nature 308:153–158.

Korsmeyer SJ, Arnold A, Bakhshi A, et al. 1983a. Immunoglobulin gene rearrangement and cell surface antigen expression of acute lymphocytic leukemia of T-cell and B-cell precursor origin. J Clin Invest 71:301–313.

Korsmeyer SJ, Greene WC, Cossman J, et al. 1983b. Rearrangement and expression of immunoglobulin genes and expression of Tac antigen in hairy cell leukemia. Proc Natl Acad Sci USA 80:4522–4526.

Krönke M, Depper JM, Leonard WJ, Vitetta ES, Waldmann TA, Greene WC. 1985. Anti-Tac-ricin A conjugates selectively inhibit protein synthesis in human T-cell leukemia/lymphoma virus infected leukemic T cells. Blood 65:1416–1421.

LeBien TW, Hozier J, Minowada J, Kersey JH. 1979. Origin of chronic myelocytic leukemia in a precursor of pre-B lymphocytes. N Engl J Med 301: 144–147.

Leder P. 1982. The genetics of antibody diversity. Sci Am 246:102–115.

Leonard WJ, Depper JM, Uchiyama T, Smith KA, Waldmann TA, Greene WC. 1982. A monoclonal antibody that appears to recognize the receptor for human T-cell growth factor; partial characterization of the receptor. Nature 300: 267–269.

Leonard WJ, Depper JM, Robb RJ, Waldmann TA, Greene WC. 1983a. Characterization of the human receptor for T cell growth factor. Proc Natl Acad Sci USA 80:6957–6961.

Leonard WJ, Depper JM, Roth JS, Rudikoff S, Waldmann TA, Greene WC. 1983b. Aberrant T cell growth factor (TCGF) receptors on human T-cell leukemia virus (HTLV) infected leukemic cells (Abstract). Clinical Research 31:348.

Leonard WJ, Depper JM, Crabtree GR, et al. 1984a. Molecular cloning and expression of cDNAs for the human interleukin 2 receptor. Nature 311:626–631.

Leonard WJ, Depper JM, Waldmann TA, Greene WC. 1984b. A monoclonal antibody to the human receptor for T cell growth factor. *In* Greaves MF, ed., Monoclonal Antibodies to Receptors: Probes for Receptor Structure and Function. Receptor and Recognition Series B, vol. 17. Chapman and Hall, London, pp. 45–46.

Meuer SC, Fitzgerald KA, Hussey RE, Hodgdon JC, Schlossman SF, Reinherz EL. 1983. Clonotypic structures involved in antigen-specific human T cell function. J Exp Med 157:705–719.

Morgan DA, Ruscetti FW, Gallo RC. 1976. Selective in vitro growth of T lymphocytes from normal human bone marrows. Science 193:1007–1008.

Poiesz BJ, Ruscetti FW, Gazdar AF, Bunn PA, Minna JD, Gallo RC. 1980. Detection and isolation of type-C retrovirus particles from fresh and cultured lymphocytes of a patient with cutaneous T-cell lymphoma. Proc Natl Acad Sci USA 77:7415–7419.

Reynolds C, Foon K. 1984. T_γ-lymphoproliferative disease and related disorders in humans and experimental animals: A review of the clinical, cellular, and functional characteristics. Blood 64:1146–1158.

Robb RJ, Munck A, Smith KA. 1981. T-cell growth factor receptors. J Exp Med 154:1455–1474.

Saito H, Kranz DM, Takagaki Y, Hayday AC, Eisen HN, Tonegawa S. 1984a. A third rearranged and expressed gene in a clone of cytotoxic T lymphocytes. Nature 312:36–40.

Saito H, Kranz DM, Takagaki Y, Hayday AC, Eisen HN, Tonegawa S. 1984b. Complete primary structure of a heterodimeric T cell receptor deduced from cDNA sequences. Nature 309:757–762.

Sklar J, Cleary ML, Thielman K, Gralow J, Warnke R, Levy R. 1984. Biclonal B cell lymphoma. N Engl J Med 311:20–27.

Smith KA. 1980. T-cell growth factor. Immunol Rev 51:337–357.

Tonegawa S. 1983. Somatic generation of antibody diversity. Nature 302:575–581.

Uchiyama T, Broder S, Waldmann TA. 1981a. A monoclonal antibody (anti-Tac) reactive with activated and functionally mature human T cells: I. Production of anti-Tac monoclonal antibody and distribution of Tac ($^+$) cells. J Immunol

126:1393–1397.

Uchiyama T, Nelson DL, Fleisher TA, Waldmann TA. 1981b. A monoclonal antibody (anti-Tac) reactive with activated and functionally mature human T cells: II. Expression of Tac antigen on activated cytotoxic killer T cells, suppressor cells, and on one of two types of helper T cells. J Immunol 126:1398–1403.

Uchiyama T, Wano Y, Tsudo M, et al. 1986. Abnormal expression of Tac antigen (IL-2 receptor) in adult T-cell leukemia. *In* Miwa M, ed., Retroviruses in Human Lymphoma/Leukemia: The Fifteenth International Symposium of the Princess Takamatsu Cancer Research Fund. Japan Sci Soc Press (In press).

Waldmann TA, Greene WC, Sarin PS, et al. 1984. Functional and phenotypic comparison of human T cell leukemia/lymphoma virus positive adult T cell leukemia with human T cell leukemia/lymphoma virus negative Sézary leukemia, and their distinction using anti-Tac: Monoclonal antibody identifying the human receptor for T cell growth factor. J Clin Invest 73:1711–1718.

Yanagi Y, Yoshikai Y, Leggett R, Clark SP, Aleksander I, Mak TW. 1984. A human T-cell specific cDNA clone encodes a protein having extensive homology to immunoglobulin chains. Nature 308:145–149.

Symposium on Fundamental Cancer Research, Vol. 38.
© 1986 by The University of Texas System Cancer Center.

6. Molecular Genetics of Human B Cell Neoplasia

Yoshihide Tsujimoto, Jan Erikson, Peter C. Nowell,*
and Carlo M. Croce

*The Wistar Institute of Anatomy and Biology and the *Department of Pathology and Laboratory Medicine, University of Pennsylvania School of Medicine, Philadelphia, Pennsylvania 19104*

Most malignancies of the hematopoietic system carry nonrandom chromosome alterations, predominantly chromosome translocations and inversions (Rowley 1973, 1982, Nowell and Hungerford 1960, Yunis 1983). During the past three years, it has been possible to link two specific human genes, which represent the human homologues of the v-*myc* and of the v-*abl* retroviral oncogene, with two malignant diseases, Burkitt's lymphoma (Dalla-Favera et al. 1982, Erikson et al. 1983, Taub et al. 1982) and chronic myelogenous leukemia (CML), respectively (de Klein et al. 1982).

In Burkitt's lymphoma with the t(8;14) chromosome translocation, the c-*myc* oncogene that is normally located at band q24 of human chromosome 8 translocates to the immunoglobulin (Ig) heavy-chain locus at band q32 of human chromosome 14 (Dalla-Favera et al. 1982). On the contrary, in Burkitt's lymphoma with the variant t(8;22) and t(2;8) chromosome translocations, the c-*myc* oncogene remains on human chromosome 8, and the Igλ or Igκ locus translocates to a chromosome 8 region distal to the c-*myc* site (Croce et al. 1983, Erikson et al. 1983b). The consequences of these different chromosomal rearrangements are a deregulation of transcription of the c-*myc* oncogene involved in the translocations, usually resulting in its being transcribed constitutively at elevated levels (Croce et al. 1983, Erikson et al. 1983b, Nishikura et al. 1983) while the c-*myc* oncogene on the uninvolved chromosome 8 responds normally to regulatory mechanisms (Croce et al. 1983, Erikson et al. 1983b, Nishikura et al. 1983).

In CML, the c-*abl* oncogene translocates to region q11 of chromosome 22 (de Klein et al. 1982). As a result, the c-*abl* oncogene rearranges with a gene on chromosome 22, leading to the formation of a hybrid gene (Heisterkamp et al. 1983). This hybrid gene seems to be transcribed into a hybrid (8.5 kb) mRNA that is expressed in Ph[1] chromosome-positive CML cells (Collins et al. 1984). While the c-*abl* normal product is a 150-kDa protein, CML cells express an additional 210-kDa protein that has protein kinase activity (Konopka et al. 1984).

In addition to these two diseases with chromosome changes that involve known oncogenes, there are other human hematopoietic tumors in which cytogenetic data may provide clues to important gene loci. For instance, many human B cell lymphomas of adults also carry nonrandom chromosome alterations, predominantly translocations (Yunis 1983, Yunis et al. 1982) Interestingly, band q32 of chromosome 14 at the Ig heavy-chain locus is often involved in these chromosome rearrangements. We speculated that it should be possible to clone gene loci involved in adult B cell neoplasms by taking advantage of their proximity to the heavy-chain locus, which results from the chromosomal translocations. Our results to date are summarized in the following sections, along with preliminary data that may be relevant to T cell neoplasms.

CLUSTERING OF BREAKPOINTS ON CHROMOSOME 11 IN HUMAN B CELL TUMORS WITH THE t(11;14) CHROMOSOME TRANSLOCATION

A translocation between chromosomes 11 and 14, t(11;14) (q13;q32), has been described in chronic lymphocytic leukemias of the B cell type (B-CLL), in diffuse small and large B cell lymphomas (Yunis 1983, Yunis et al. 1982), and in multiple myeloma (Van den Berghe et al. 1984). By examining somatic cell hybrids between mouse myeloma cells and CLL cells (CLL 271) carrying the t(11;14) chromosome translocation, we discovered that the Ig heavy-chain constant region genes (C_H) remained on the 14q$^+$ chromosome, while the variable region genes (V_H) translocated to the 11q$^-$ chromosome in these leukemic cells. We concluded that in neoplastic B cells carrying the t(11;14) translocation, the chromosome breakpoint directly involved the heavy-chain locus on chromosome 14 (Erikson et al. 1984). We cloned the joining region between chromosomes 11 and 14 on the 14q$^+$ chromosome and found that the

---

FIGURE 6.1. Southern blot hybridization of CLL 271, CLL 1386, and LN87 DNA with human chromosome 11–derived probes (A) and the maps of chromosome 14q$^+$ in CLL 271, CLL 1386, and LN87 (C) and of normal chromosome 11 (B). (A) DNA derived from neoplastic cells of CLL 271, CLL 1386, and LN87 were cut with the restriction enzymes shown, run on 0.7% agarose gels, and transferred to nitrocellulose filters. The filtrates were hybridized with a nick-translated probe (a) (pRc8SmR) (Tsujimoto et al. 1984b) or (b) (shown in B). Hybridizations were carried out in 50% formamide/4 × standard saline citrate at 37°C and finally washed with 0.2 × standard saline citrate at 65°C. DNA 1104 and 1412 were obtained from T cell lymphomas and used as germ

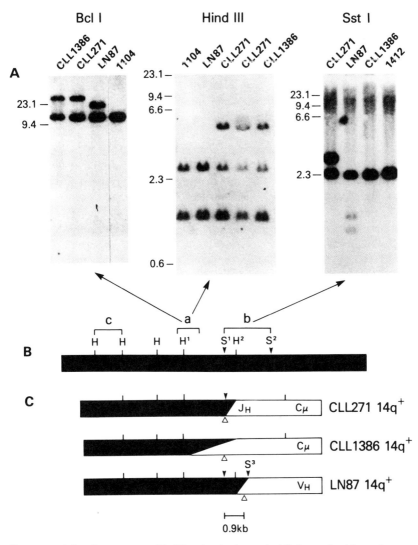

line control for chromosome 11. The size is shown in kilobases beside each panel. (B) and (C): Structure of normal chromosome 11 in B is deduced by analyzing the chromosome 11 sequence-containing recombinant clones in Figure 2 obtained from CLL 271 and CLL 1386 genomic phage libraries. Filled and open portions of boxes show chromosomes 11 and 14, respectively. The cleavage sites by restriction enzymes: *Sst*I ($\blacktriangledown$, S^1 or S^2) and *Hind*III ($|$, H^1 or H^2). Not all restriction sites are shown. Open triangles represent the joining sites between chromosome 11 and 14 on chromosome $14q^+$, which are determined as described in the text.

breakpoint occurred within the joining (J_H) region of the heavy-chain locus (Tsujimoto et al. 1984b). We used chromosome 11–derived DNA probes flanking the chromosomal breakpoint to detect rearrangements in B cell neoplasms that carry the t(11;14) chromosome translocation (Tsujimoto et al. 1984b.) As shown in Figure 6.1, a single DNA probe could detect rearrangements in all three cases of B cell malignancies that carry the t(11;14) chromosome translocation. Interestingly, the breakpoints in all three cases involved a 0.9-kb DNA region.

We then cloned the breakpoint from an additional case of B-CLL carrying the t(11;14) chromosome translocation (CLL 1386) (Tsujimoto et al. 1985b). The restriction maps of the regions flanking the joining region between chromosomes 11 and 14 in the leukemic cells of CLL 271 and CLL 1386 and of the corresponding normal chromosome 11 are shown in Figure 6.2. Comparison of the DNA sequences of the regions surrounding the breakpoints in the leukemic cells and of the corresponding segment of normal chromosome 11 from CLL 271 cells indicates that the first 31 bases following the common *Sst*I site (S^1 shown in Figure 6.2) are identical between normal chromosome 11 and the joining regions on the $14q^+$ chromosomes of the two leukemias. Then the DNA of CLL 1386 diverges. Eight bases further along the gene, the DNA sequences of normal chromosome 11 and that of the joining segment of CLL 271 diverge. The DNA sequence beyond the breakpoints indicates that the rearrangements involved the J_4 segment of the heavy-chain locus in both cases. At the joining sites, we noticed sequences between the breakpoints on chromosomes 11 and 14 that did not derive from these chromosomes. Addition of a few nucleotides (N regions) during V-D-J joining has been previously described (Desiderio et al. 1984).

These findings suggest that the chromosomal translocation might have occurred during V-D-J joining at the pre–B cell stage of differentiation. In fact, the breakpoints on chromosome 14 in both cases of CLL are in the region where the D segment is rearranged with the J_H segment during physiological V-D-J joining. These results suggest that the putative recombinase involved in Ig V-D-J joining might have a role in the development of the chromosomal translocations. This enzyme is thought to recognize signal sequences, heptamer-nonamer, that are close to the Ig V, D, and J segments in germ line DNA (Tonegawa 1983). Then the heptamer-nonamer sequence with a 12 base–long spacer is paired with a heptamer-nonamer sequence with 23 ± 1 base–long spacer during V-D-J joining (Tonegawa 1983). As shown in Figure 6.3, we found in the DNA of normal chromosome 11 a sequence very similar to the heptamer-nonamer signal sequence (Tonegawa 1983). Interestingly, the signal sequence on chromosome 11 is separated by a 12 base–long spacer, whereas the signal sequence of the J_4 segment is separated by a 23 base–long spacer (Figure 6.4). These results suggest that the t(11;14) chromosome translocations in B cell neoplasms are sequence specific and may involve the en-

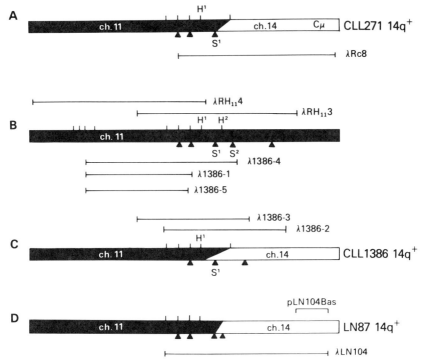

FIGURE 6.2. Restriction maps of the regions surrounding the breakpoints on chromosome 14q$^+$ in CLL 271 (A), CLL 1386 (C), LN87 (D), and of normal chromosome 11 (B). Filled and open portions of boxes represent chromosomes 11 and 14, respectively. Horizontal lines represent the insert DNAs of representative recombinant clones. λRc8 was described previously (Tsujimoto et al. 1984b). λRH11-3 and -4 were obtained by screening the CLL 271 library with chromosome 11 sequences. The λ1386s were obtained from the CLL 1386 library, as described in the text. The λ1386-1, -4, and -5 all contain only DNA sequences of chromosome 11. The cleavage sites of restriction enzymes: *Sst*I (▼,S^1 or S^2) and *Hin*dIII (|, H^1 or H^2).

```
            J4
ch. 14    GGTTTTTGTGCACCCCTTAATGGGGCCTCCCCACAATGTGACTACTTTGACTACTGGGGCCAAGGAACCCTGGTCACCGTCTCCTCAGG
CLL 1386  GAGCTCCCTGAACACCTGGCGCTGCCATTGGTGTTGGAGGGAACCCGCATCTGACTACTGGGGCCAGGGAACCCTGGTCACCGTCTCCTCAGG
ch. 11    GAGCTCCCTGAACACCTGGCGCTGCCATTGGCGTGAACGAGGGGAAGCCCCTCCTGACAGCTGGATGGTAGGACAAAGCCTCTAA
CLL 271   GAGCTCCCTGAACACCTGGCGCTGCCATTGGCGTGAACTACCAGACTTGACTACTGGGGCCAGGGAACCCTGGTCACCGTCTCCTCAGG
ch. 14    GGTTTTTGTGCACCCCTTAATGGGGCCTCCCACAATGTGACTACTTTGACTACTGGGGCCAAGGAACCCTGGTCACCGTCTCCTCAGG
            J4

CLL 1386  TGAGTCCTCACAACCTCTCTCCTGCTTTAACTCTGAAGGGTTTTGCTGCATTTTTGGGGGAAAATAAG
CLL 271   TGAGTCCTCACAACCTCTCTCCTGCTTTAACTCTGAAGGGTTTTGCTGCATTTTTGGGGGAAAATAAAGGGTGCTGGGTCTCCTGCC
ch. 14    TGAGTCCTCACAACCX3TCTCCTCCGTTAACTCCG AGG TTTG TG ACTTTTGGGG  AATAAGGGTGCTGGG GGCCTGCC
```

FIGURE 6.3. DNA sequences of the joining sites between chromosome 11 and 14 in CLL 271, CLL 1386, and of corresponding normal chromosome 11. The identical nucleotide sequences are shown by vertical lines. The boxed region indicates the J$_4$ coding segment of the Ig heavy-chain gene (Ravetch et al. 1981). The DNA sequences shown by brackets on chromosome 14 indicate that the conserved sequence heptamer-nonamer DNA sequences were obtained from *Sst*I (S^1) site shown in Figure 2 toward chromosome 14 sequence by using chemical degradation method of Maxam and Gilbert (1980) with a modification of the A reaction (Som and Tomizawa 1982).

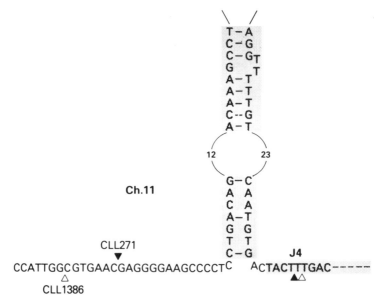

FIGURE 6.4. A possible secondary structure between chromosome 11 and the J_4 segment of the Ig gene.

zyme system for V-D-J joining. Thus, translocations would occur when the recombinase, by mistake, joins two different human chromosomes carrying signal sequences for V-D-J segment joining (Figure 6.4).

The fact that the different breakpoints in tumor cells that carry the t(11;14) chromosome translocation cluster within a very short segment of DNA implies that we can now use the Southern blot procedure to establish the presence of a t(11;14) chromosome translocation in human neoplastic specimens.

Cloning the Joining Region Between Chromosomes 14 and 18 in B Cell Neoplasms that Carry the t(14;18) Chromosome Translocation

A t(14;18) (q32;q21) chromosome translocation also occurs nonrandomly in human B cell tumors, particularly follicular lymphomas (Yunis 1983, Yunis et al. 1982). We have taken advantage of a pre–B cell leukemia line (380) that carries both a t(8;14) (q24;q32) and a t(14;18) (q32;q21) translocation (Pegoraro et al. 1984) to clone the joining regions between chromosomes 14 and 18 on one of the two 14q⁺ chromosomes of the 380 cell line (Tsujimoto et al. 1984a). As shown in Figure 6.5, two classes of recombinant clones were obtained from a library of the 380 cell line DNA. One class represented the unproductively rearranged μ gene on the 14q⁺ chromosome derived from the t(14;18) chromosome translocation, while the other class represented the unproductively rearranged μ gene on the 14q$^+$ derived from the t(8;14) chromosome translocation (Figure 6.5). We then determined a restriction map of normal chromosome 18 in both directions by using overlapping DNA clones and used different DNA probes (a, b, c, and d in Figure 6.6) to examine the DNA of several cases of follicular lymphoma (Tsujimoto et al. 1985a). We detected rearrangements of chromosome 18 in approximately 60% of such cases (Tsujimoto et al. 1985a). Figure 6.7 shows that most of the breakpoints occurred in two small regions of chromosome 18 separated by approximately 13 kb. Interestingly, we have detected signal sequences for V-D-J joining in the proximity of the breakpoints on chromosome 18 (Tsujimoto Y and Croce CM unpublished data).

We have also used probe b (Figure 6.6) from the t(14;18) translocation to determine whether we could detect transcripts in B cells. We have hybridized polyA$^+$ RNA derived from the 380 cell line and from cells of another pre–B cell leukemia line (697), which contains a t(1;19) chromosome translocation instead of a t(14;18) translocation, with probe b. We detected 6 kb transcripts

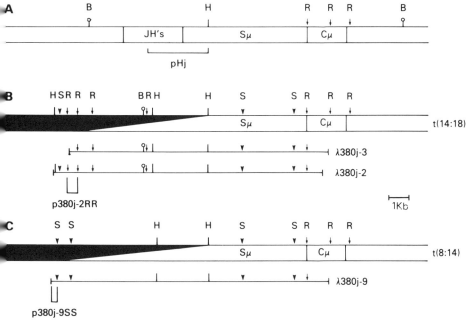

FIGURE 6.5. Restriction maps of the germ line Cμ gene (A) and of the two classes of recombinant clones from the 14q$^+$ chromosomes resulting from the t(14;18) (B) and the t(8;14) (C) translocations. The filled portion of the boxes represents the chromosome 18–derived sequences in (B) and the chromosome 8–derived sequences in (C). The open portion of the boxes represents the chromosome 14–derived sequences. H–*Hind*III; R–*Eco*RI; B–*Bam*HI; S–*Sst*I.

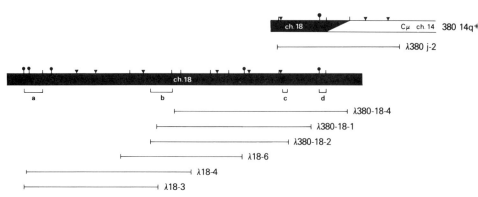

FIGURE 6.6. The restriction map of the region surrounding the breakpoint on the 14q⁺ chromosome of t(14;18) in the 380 cell line and of normal chromosome 18 are shown. The restriction map of the 14q⁺ chromosome has been shown previously. The structure of normal chromosome 18 was deduced by analyzing the overlapping recombinant clones isolated from a 380 phage library screened with the chromosome 18–specific probes. Each horizontal line indicates DNA inserts of representative recombinant clones. DNA probes used in this study are shown by a, b, c, and d with brackets. The cleavage sites of restriction enzymes: *Sst*I, (▼) *Bam*HI (↑), and *Hin*dIII (|).

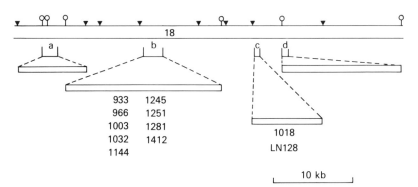

FIGURE 6.7. Clustering of the breakpoints of t(14;18) on chromosome 18 in follicular lymphomas. The top bar represents normal chromosome 18. The restriction sites: *Sst*I (▼) and *Bam*HI (↑). The open bar below chromosome 18 indicates the germ line restriction fragment detected by each probe. *Sst*I cleavage was used for probes a and c and *Bam*HI digestion was used for probes b and d (Figure 6.6). The numbers below open bars indicate follicular lymphoma DNA that showed rearrangement of the germ line restriction fragment shown by open bar.

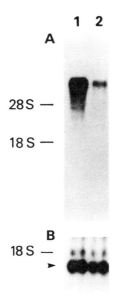

FIGURE 6.8. RNA blot hybridization. Total cytoplasmic RNA was extracted from cell lines shown and polyA$^+$ RNA was selected by oligo(dT)-cellulose column chromatography. About 5 μg of polyA$^+$ RNA from each cell line was glyoxalated, separated on a 1% agarose gel, and transferred to nitrocellulose filters (Thomas 1980). The filter was hybridized with a nick-translated probe in 50% formamide/4 × standard saline citrate at 37°C and washed finally in 0.5 × standard saline citrate at 55°C. (A) Lane 1, 380 RNA; lane 2, 697 RNA. The filtrate was hybridized with probe b (Figure 6.6). In (B), the same filtrate as in (A) was rehybridized with a human phosphoglycerokinase cDNA probe, pHPGK-7e (Michelson 1983). The transcript is shown by the arrow.

hybridizing with probe b in both 380 and 697 cell lines (Figure 6.8). This result indicated that the gene on chromosome 18 that is directly involved in follicular lymphoma, for which we have proposed the name *bcl*-2, is transcribed into a 6-kb message (Tsujimoto et al. 1985a). As shown in Figure 6.8A, the levels of *bcl*-2 transcripts in the 380 cells are at least tenfold higher than in the 697 cells, indicating that the t(14;18) translocation enhanced the expression of the *bcl*-2 gene. The northern blot shown in Figure 6.8A was rehybridized with a cDNA clone of the enzyme phosphoglycerate kinase (PGK). We detected the same levels of PGK transcripts in both the 380 and 697 cells, supporting the view that the *bcl*-2 gene has been specifically deregulated by the t(14;18) chromosome translocation (Figure 6.8B).

Since the rearrangements on chromosome 14 in the t(14;18) translocation involve the J$_H$ segment of the heavy-chain locus, the enhancer located between

TABLE 6.1. *Assignment of the Gene for the α Chain of the T Cell Receptor to Human Chromosome 14*

Hybrids	Human Chromosomes																							Tα Chain Gene
	1	2	3	4	5	6	7	8	9	10	11	12	13	14	15	16	17	18	19	20	21	22	X	
PXBIV-Cl 5	−	+	−	−	+	−	−	+	−	−	−	+	−	−	−	−	−	−	+	−	−	−	−	−
77 B10 Cl 28	+	−	+	−	+	−	−	−	−	−	−	−	−	+	−	−	−	+	−	−	+	+	+	+
DSK Cl 20-C	−	−	−	−	−	−	−	−	−	−	−	−	−	−	+	−	−	+	−	−	+	+	+	−
106 2B4 4C4	−	−	−	−	−	−	−	−	−	−	−	−	−	−	−	−	−	−	−	−	−	−	−	+
5263 Cl 7 S17*	−	−	−	−	−	+	−	−	−	−	−	−	+	+	−	−	−	−	−	−	−	+	−	+
D69 Cl 4S7	−	−	−	−	−	+	−	+	−	−	−	−	−	+	−	−	−	−	−	+	−	−	−	+
M44 Cl 2S5†	−	−	−	−	−	+	+	+	−	−	−	−	−	+	−	−	−	−	−	−	−	−	−	+
Nu9	−	−	−	−	−	+	−	−	−	−	−	−	−	−	+	−	−	−	−	−	−	−	−	−
D2 Cl 6SS	−	−	+	+	−	−	+	−	−	−	+	−	−	+	+	−	+	−	+	−	+	+	+	+
401 AD5 EF 3-1	−	−	+	+	−	−	−	+	−	−	−	−	−	−	−	+	−	−	−	−	−	−	−	−
77 B10 Cl 30	−	−	+	+	+	−	−	+	+	+	−	−	+	−	+	+	−	+	+	+	−	−	+	+
77 B10 Cl 31	+	−	+	+	+	−	−	+	+	+	−	−	+	−	+	+	−	−	+	+	−	−	+	+
53-87-3 Cl 10	−	−	−	−	−	−	+	+	−	−	−	−	−	−	−	−	+	−	−	−	−	−	−	−
GM54VA Cl 31	−	−	−	+	−	−	−	+	−	−	−	−	−	+	+	+	+	−	+	−	−	−	+	−
GM x LM Cl 5	−	−	−	+	−	+	−	+	−	−	+	−	−	+	+	+	−	−	+	−	−	−	+	−
D2 Cl 6S3	−	−	−	−	−	−	−	−	−	−	−	−	−	−	−	−	−	−	−	−	−	−	−	−
77 B10 Cl 5	+	−	+	+	+	−	+	+	−	+	+	−	+	+	+	+	+	−	+	−	−	−	+	+
1P1	−	−	−	−	−	−	−	−	+	−	+	−	−	−	−	−	−	−	−	−	−	−	−	−
PT47 Cl 5	−	−	−	−	−	−	−	−	−	+	+	+	−	−	−	−	+	+	−	−	+	+	−	−
5468 F1 Cl 1-11	−	−	−	−	−	−	−	+	+	−	−	−	−	+	−	+	−	−	−	−	+	+	−	−
5468 F2 Cl 5	−	−	−	−	−	−	−	+	−	−	−	−	−	−	+	−	+	−	−	−	+	+	+	+
DSK Cl 2	−	+	−	−	−	−	−	+	−	−	−	−	+	+	+	−	+	−	−	−	+	+	−	−
706B6-40 Cl 17	−	−	−	−	−	−	−	−	+	−	−	−	+	+	−	+	−	−	−	−	−	−	−	−
640-63	−	+	−	−	−	−	−	−	−	−	−	−	−	−	−	−	−	−	−	−	+	−	−	−
706-D1	−	+	−	−	+	+	−	−	−	−	−	−	−	−	−	+	−	+	−	−	−	+	−	−

*Hybrid 52-63 Cl 7S17 carries the $14q^+$ chromosome of KOP-2 cells which have a t(14;X) chromosome translocation.
†Hybrid M44 Cl 2S5 contains only the $14q^+$ chromosome of P 3HR-1 Burkitt's lymphoma with the t(8;14) chromosome translocation.

J_H and S_μ is close to the translocated *bcl*-2 gene (Tsujimoto et al. 1985a) and may be responsible for its deregulation.

LOCATION OF THE ALPHA-CHAIN GENE OF THE T CELL RECEPTOR

Chromosome 14 is often involved in translocations and inversions in T cell neoplasms (Williams et al. 1984, Ueshima et al. 1984, Zech et al. 1983, 1984, Hecht 1984). By using a cDNA clone specific for the α chain of the T cell receptor to analyze, by Southern blot techniques, the DNA of somatic cell hybrids between mouse and human cells, we found that the gene for the α chain of the T cell receptor is on chromosome 14 (Table 6.1) (Croce et al. 1985). In situ hybridization to metaphase chromosomes further indicated that the gene is located at band 14q11.2, the precise region involved in translocations and inversions in T cell neoplasia (Figure 6.9) (Croce et al. 1985). Thus,

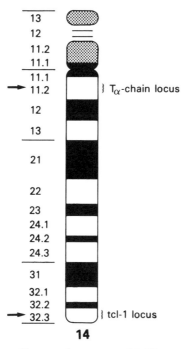

FIGURE 6.9. Diagram of human chromosome 14. The arrows indicate the breakpoints observed in neoplastic T cells with an inversion of chromosome 14. The brackets indicate the positions of the locus for the alpha chain of the T cell receptor (upper) and of a putative oncogene (*tcl*-1) (lower). We hypothesize that this chromosomal inversion, as well as the t(14;14) (q11;q32) translocation seen in other T cell tumors could result in juxtaposition of the T alpha-chain locus and the *tcl*-1 oncogene, thereby activating *tcl*-1.

these results suggest a role for the α chain gene of the T cell receptor in the pathogenesis of T cell neoplasms. Preliminary results with neoplastic T cells suggest that the locus for the α chain of the T cell receptor is split by chromosome translocation.

CONCLUSIONS

Two major approaches have been used recently to isolate and characterize genes that may be involved in the pathogenesis of human cancer. In one case, retrovirus oncogenes have been used as probes to clone and characterize their human homologues. While in most cases it is not yet clear what role the human homologues of retrovirus oncogenes play in the pathogenesis of human cancer, at least in the case of Burkitt's lymphoma, it is evident that the c-*myc* gene is directly involved as a result of its deregulation by proximity to one of the three Ig loci (Dalla-Favera et al. 1982, Erikson et al. 1983a,b, Taub 1982, Croce 1983, Nishikura et al. 1983). Similarly the human homologue of the v-*abl* oncogene may be involved in the pathogenesis of chronic myelogenous leukemia because of its rearrangement with the so-called bcr region of band q11 on chromosome 22 (de Klein et al. 1982, Croce 1985).

The second approach involves the use of a transfection assay to transform 3T3 cells or other phenotypically untransformed cell lines to rescue human oncogenes from neoplastic tissue (for review, see Weinberg 1981). While this second approach may provide useful and important information concerning the mechanisms of cell transformation, it does not indicate the role of the rescued oncogene in the tumors from which they derive. Such oncogenes can be rescued from only 10–20% of human tumors; there is no correlation between a specific rescued oncogene and a specific type of human tumor, and the target cells may have a strong bias, at the level of expression, in favor of certain oncogenes, such as those within the *ras* family (Der et al. 1982, Hall et al. 1983, Parada et al. 1982, Pulciani et al. 1982, Shimizu et al. 1983, Santos et al. 1982).

In this study, we describe a third approach to identify genes that are involved in the pathogenesis of human cancer. Previously, we took advantage of the knowledge that highly specific chromosome rearrangements occur in many human hematopoietic malignancies (Rowley 1973, 1982, Nowell 1960, Yunis 1983) and of the fact that the Ig heavy-chain locus on chromosome 14 is the frequent target of rearrangements occurring in B cell neoplasms (Yunis 1983) to clone the chromosomal breakpoints involved in the t(11;14) and t(14;18) chromosome translocations in B cell neoplasms (Tsujimoto 1984a,b). Using a DNA probe thus obtained, we were able to show in tumor cells with the t(14;18) translocation elevated transcription levels of a 6 kb RNA apparently derived from the postulated *bcl*-2 gene involved in the translocation. Since most of the chromosome breakpoints observed in cases of fol- licular lymphomas directly involve the transcription unit of the *bcl*-2 gene (Tsujimoto et al. 1985a), it seems likely that in most such lymphomas, like c-*myc* in some Burkitt's lymphomas, the involved oncogene may be struc- tually altered, as well as deregulated.

Thus, it is possible to take advantage of specific chromosomal alterations occurring in particular human neoplasms to isolate and to characterize the genes that are directly involved in the neoplastic process. A logical extension of this approach is to use these DNA probes to detect specific chromosomal alterations in human tumors. It is reasonable to predict that within a relatively short time, the classification and the diagnosis of human B and T cell malig- nancies will be significantly aided by the knowledge of the genomic re- arrangements of the genes involved in their pathogenesis.

REFERENCES

Collins SJ, Kubonishi I, Miyoshi I, Groudine MT. 1984. Altered transcription of the c-*abl* oncogene in K-562 and other chronic myelogenous leukemia cells. Science 225:72–74.

Croce CM, Isobe M, Palumbo A, et al. 1985. Gene for alpha-chain of human T- cell receptor: Location on chromosome 14 region involved in T-cell neoplasms. Science 227:1044–1047.

Croce CM, Thierfelder W, Erikson J, et al. 1983. Transcriptional activation of an unrearranged and untranslocated c-myc oncogene by translocation of a C lambda locus in Burkitt. Proc Natl Acad Sci USA 80:6922–6926.

Dalla-Favera R, Bregni M, Erikson J, Patterson D, Gallo RC, Croce CM. 1982. Human c-*myc* onc gene is located on the region of chromosome 8 that is trans- located in Burkitt lymphoma cells. Proc Natl Acad Sci USA 79:7824–7827.

de Klein A, van Kessel AG, Grosveld G, et al. 1982. A cellular oncogene is trans- located to the Philadelphia chromosome in chronic myelocytic leukaemia. Nature 300:765–767.

Der CJ, Krontiris TG, Cooper GM. 1982. Transforming genes of human bladder and lung carcinoma cell lines are homologous to the *ras* genes of Harvey and Kirsten sarcoma viruses. Proc Natl Acad Sci USA 79:3637–3640.

Desiderio SV, Yancopoulos GD, Paskind M, et al. 1984. Insertion of *N* regions into heavy-chain genes is correlated with expression of terminal deoxytrans- ferase in B cells. Nature 311:752–755.

Erikson J, Finan J, Tsujimoto Y, Nowell PC, Croce CM. 1984. The chromosome 14 breakpoint in neoplastic B cells with the t(11;14) translocation involves the immunoglobulin heavy chain locus. Proc Natl Acad Sci USA 81:4144–4148.

Erikson J, ar-Rushdi A, Drwinga HL, Nowell PC, Croce CM. 1983a. Transcrip- tional activation of the translocated c-myc oncogene in burkitt lymphoma. Proc Natl Acad Sci USA 80:820–824.

Erikson J, Nishikura K, ar-Rushdi A, et al. 1983b. Translocation of an immu- noglobulin kappa locus to a region 3′ of an unrearranged c-*myc* oncogene en- hances c-*myc* transcription. Proc Natl Acad Sci USA 80:7581–7585.

Groffen J, Stephenson JR, Heisterkamp N, de Klein A, Bartram CR, Grosveld G.

1984. Philadelphia chromosomal breakpoints are clustered within a limited region, bcr, on chromosome 22. Cell 36:93–99.

Hall A, Marshall CJ, Spurr NK, Weiss RA. 1983. Identification of transforming gene in two human sarcoma cell lines as a new member of the *ras* gene family located on chromosome 1. Nature 303:396–400.

Hecht F, Morgan R, Kaiser-McCaw B, Smith SD. 1984. Common region on chromosome 14 in T-cell leukemia and lymphoma. Science 226:1445–1446.

Heisterkamp N, Stephenson JR, Groffen J, et al. 1983. Localization of the c-abl oncogene adjacent to a translocation break point in chronic myelocytic leukaemia. Nature 306:239–242.

Konopka JB, Watanabe SM, Witte ON. 1984. An alteration of the human c-abl protein in K562 leukemia cells unmasks associated tyrosine kinase activity. Cell 37:1035–1042.

Maxam AM, Gilbert W. 1980. Sequencing end-labeled DNA with base-specific chemical cleavages. Methods Enzymol 65:499–560.

Michelson AM, Markham AF, Orkin SH. 1983. Isolation and DNA sequence of a full-length cDNA clone for human × chromosome-encoded phosphoglycerate kinase. Proc Natl Acad Sci USA 80:472–476.

Nishikura K, ar-Rushdi A, Erikson J, Watt R, Rovera G, Croce CM. 1983. Differential expression of the normal and of the translocated human c-*myc* oncogenes in B cells. Proc Natl Acad Sci USA 80:4822–4826.

Nowell PC, Hungerford DA. 1960. A minute chromosome in chronic granulocyte leukemia. Science 132:1497.

Parada LF, Tabin CJ, Shih C, Weinberg RA. 1982. Human EJ bladder carcinoma oncogene is homologue of Harvey sarcoma virus *ras* gene. Nature 297:474–478.

Pegoraro L, Palumbo A, Erikson J, et al. 1984. A 14;18 and an 8;14 chromosome translocation in a cell line derived from an acute B-cell leukemia. Proc Natl Acad Sci USA 81:7166–7170.

Pulciani S, Santos E, Lauver AV, Long LK, Robbins KC, Barbacid M. 1982. Oncogenes in human tumor cell lines: Molecular cloning of a transforming gene from human bladder carcinoma cells. Proc Natl Acad Sci USA 79:2845–2849.

Ravetch JV, Siebenlist U, Korsmeyer S, Waldmann T, Leder P. 1981. Structure of the human immunoglobulin mu locus: Characterization of embryonic and rearranged J and D genes. Cell 27:583–591.

Rowley JD. 1973. A new consistent chromosomal abnormality in chronic myelogenous leukaemia identified by quinacrine fluorescence and Giemsa staining. Nature 243:290–293.

Rowley JD. 1982. Identification of the constant chromosome regions involved in human hematologic malignant disease. Science 216:749–751.

Santos E, Tronick SR, Aaronson SA, Pulciani S, Barbacid M. 1982. T24 human bladder carcinoma oncogene is an activated form of the normal human homologue of BALB- and Harvey-MSV transformimg genes. Nature 298:343–347.

Shimizu K, Goldfarb M, Suard Y, et al. 1983. Three human transforming genes are related to the viral ras oncogenes. Proc Natl Acad Sci USA 80:2112–2116.

Som T, Tomizawa J. 1982. Origin of replication of *Escherichia coli* plasmid RSF 1030. MGG 187:375–383.

Taub R, Kirsch I, Morton C, et al. 1982. Translocation of the c-*myc* gene into the immunoglobulin heavy chain locus in human Burkitt lymphoma and murine plasmacytoma cells. Proc Natl Acad Sci USA 79:7837–7841.

Thomas PS. 1980. Hybridization of denatured RNA and small DNA fragments transferred to nitrocellulose. Proc Natl Acad Sci USA 77:5201–5205.
Tonegawa S. 1983. Somatic generation of antibody diversity. Nature 302:575–581.
Tsujimoto Y, Cossman J, Jaffe E, Croce CM. 1985a. Involvement of *bcl-2* gene in human follicular lymphoma. Science 228:1440–1443.
Tsujimoto Y, Jaffe E, Cossman J, Gorham J, Nowell PC, Croce CM. 1985b. Clustering of breakpoints on chromosome 11 in human B-cell neoplasms with the t(11;14) chromosome translocation. Nature 315:340–345.
Tsujimoto Y, Finger LR, Yunis J, Nowell PC, Croce CM. 1984a. Cloning of the chromosome breakpoint of neoplastic B cells with the t(14;18) chromosome translocation. Science 226:1097–1099.
Tsujimoto Y, Yunis J, Onorato-Showe L, Erikson J, Nowell PC, Croce CM. 1984b. Molecular cloning of the chromosomal breakpoint of B-cell lymphomas and leukemias with the t(11;14) chromosome translocation. Science 224:1403–1406.
Ueshima Y, Rowley JD, Variakojis D, Winter J, Gordon L. 1984. Cytogenetic studies on patients with chronic T cell leukemia/lymphoma. Blood 63:1028–1038.
Van den Berghe H, Vermaelen K, Louwagie A, Criel A, Mecucci C, Vaerman JP. 1984. High incidence of chromosome abnormalities in IgG3 myeloma. Cancer Genet Cytogenet 11:381–387.
Weinberg RA. 1981. Use of transfection to analyze genetic information and malignant transformation. Biochim Biophys Acta 651:25–35.
Williams DL, Look AT, Melvin SL, et al. 1984. New chromosomal translocations correlate with specific immunophenotypes of childhood acute lymphoblastic leukemia. Cell 36:101–109.
Yunis JJ. 1983. The chromosomal basis of human neoplasia. Science 221:227–236.
Yunis JJ, Oken MM, Kaplan ME, Ensrud BS, Howe RR, Theologides A. 1982. Distinctive chromosomal abnormalities in histologic subtype of non-Hodgkin's lymphoma. N Engl J Med 307:1231–1236.
Zech L, Gahrton G, Hammarstrom L, et al. 1984. Inversion of chromosome 14 marks human T-cell chronic lymphocytic leukaemia. Nature 308:858–860.
Zech L, Hammarstrom L, Smith CIE. 1983. Chromosomal aberrations in a case of T-cell CLL with concomitant IgA myeloma. Int J Cancer 32:431–435.

IMMUNE RESPONSES TO CANCER

Symposium on Fundamental Cancer Research, Vol. 38.
© 1986 by The University of Texas System Cancer Center.

7. Leporine Acquired Immune Deficiency Disease

Stewart Sell, David Strayer,* Eileen Skaletsky,† Lynette Corbeil,‡
Gary Cabirac, and Julian Leibowitz

*Department of Pathology and Laboratory Medicine, The University of Texas Health
Science Center at Houston, Houston, Texas 77030; *Department of Pathology,
Yale University, New Haven, Connecticut, 06510; †Department of Pathology,
University of California at San Diego, La Jolla, California 92093; and ‡Department
of Veterinary Microbiology and Pathology, Washington State University,
Pullman, Washington 99164*

In 1895, Professor Giuseppe Santarelli moved his laboratory from the University of Sienna, Italy to Montevideo, Uruguay. The next year a rapidly fatal, highly contagious disease characterized by severe conjunctivitis and multiple myxomatous skin tumors devastated his colony of domestic European rabbits, imported for the purpose of producing antisera (Santarelli 1898). In 1911, Moses demonstrated that the transmissable agent was a filterable virus (Moses 1911). Epidemiologic studies later showed that this myxoma virus is endemic in native South American rabbits (*Sylvilagus brasiliensis*), in which it produces a chronic localized skin tumor (Aragao 1920). The lesions are reservoirs for viruses that are transmitted by mosquitoes (Aragao 1943). A similar situation exists in the western United States, where fatal myxoma in domestic rabbits is transmitted from wild rabbits (*Sylvilagus bachmani*) (Marshall and Regnery 1963). The virus can survive for up to 30 days in the mouth parts of mosquitoes but does not multiply in the mosquito (Fenner et al. 1952).

In 1918, Aragao (see Fenner 1959) suggested the use of the myxoma virus for biologic control of the European wild rabbit, which had become established in Australia. The European rabbit in Australia was a major pest, causing crop and foliage damage amounting to hundreds of millions of pounds each year. The myxoma virus was successfully introduced in 1950 (Fenner 1959) and rapidly spread over southern Australia. Over 99% of the wild European rabbits infected with the myxoma virus died. Over the following 10 years, the grade of virulence of the virus declined and the resistance of the rabbits increased so that a natural balance between a less virulent virus and a more resistant host has been established (Fenner 1959).

A similar situation developed in Europe where the indigenous rabbit, *Oryctolagus cuniculus*, is highly susceptible to the virus. In 1953, Dr. A. Delille introduced the myxoma virus into two rabbits on his estate, and it quickly spread throughout Europe, decimating the rabbit population. This result did not produce the same favorable public response as it did in Australia because the rabbit is a traditionally prized game animal in France.

The European rabbit flea, *Spilopsyllus cuniculi*, is a more effective vector for the myxoma virus particularly in areas that are not hospitable to mosquitoes. The flea has been introduced to enhance infective rates in an area of Australia where mosquitoes are relatively ineffective (Shepard and Edwards 1977).

In November 1931, Richard E. Shope transferred pieces of fibrous subcutaneous tumor tissue from a wild cottontail rabbit captured in New Jersey into laboratory rabbits, and the rabbits grew tumors now known as Shope fibroma (Shope 1932a). Transmission was possible using filtrates. The filterable agent produced a local tumor that regressed, in contrast to the rapidly fatal systemic disease produced by myxoma virus. Rabbits that recovered from the fibroma were resistant to challenge with myxoma, but their sera did not contain neutralizing antibodies to myxoma. On the other hand, one rabbit that survived myxoma did develop neutralizing antibodies to fibroma (Shope 1932b). Shope later showed that rabbits that recovered from Shope fibroma harbored viable myxoma virus in local lesions when infected, but they developed less severe systemic disease. After 7–14 days, these rabbits produced neutralizing antibodies to the myxoma virus and cleared the myxoma virus infection, whereas rabbits not previously inoculated with fibroma virus did not develop neutralizing antibodies and died from the rapidly progressing myxomatosis (Shope 1936).

CLASSIFICATION OF POXVIRUSES

Myxoma viruses and Shope fibroma viruses (SFV) belong to the poxvirus family. Members of this group of viruses share common physicochemical properties, are generally dermatotropic, and often induce characteristic ulcerated lesions, termed pocks, when grown on chicken chorioallantoic membranes. Many of these viruses also contain a common antigen. The poxviruses can be further divided into subgroups on the basis of their host range, antigenic relationships, and nucleic acid homology. A classification developed by Fenner (1976) on the basis of their susceptible hosts is presented in Table 7.1. The SFV and the myxoma viruses are leporipoxviruses. These two closely related viruses were classically differentiated from one another by their effects in different species of rabbit (Table 7.2) (Gross 1970).

Myxoma and fibroma viruses are indistinguishable from most other poxviruses, including vaccinia, when viewed under the electron microscope. Early studies showed that these viruses contain approximately 6% DNA, 6% lipid, and no RNA (Fenner 1979). The DNA is a single double-stranded, base-paired, linear molecule with covalently closed ends, containing approximately 160 kb of DNA (Willis et al. 1983, Delange et al. 1984). Other common char-

TABLE 7.1. Host Classification of Poxviruses

Orthopoxvirus (Conventional)	Avipoxvirus (Birds)	Capripoxvirus (Goats)	Leporipoxvirus (Rabbits)	Parapoxvirus (Different)	Entomopoxvirus (Insects)
Ectromelia	Fowl pox	Sheep pox	Hare fibroma	Bovine Pustular Stomatitis	Melolontha
Cow pox	Canary pox	Goat pox	Myxoma	Milker's node	Amsacta
Monkey pox	Pigeon pox	Lumpy-skin disease	Rabbit fibroma	Orf	Chironomus
Rabbit pox	Turkey pox		Squirrel fibroma	Camel Contagious Ecthyma	
Vaccinia					
Variola					
Buffalo pox					
Camel pox					

Not allocated: Molluscum contagiosum, swine pox, tana pox, Yaba monkey tumor virus.
Adapted from Fenner 1976.

TABLE 7.2. *Pathologic Features of Myxoma and Fibroma*

Rabbit Family	Myxoma	Fibroma
Oryctolagus cuniculus	Rapidly fatal	Local lesion
(Europe, Australia) (Bunny rabbit)	Disseminated lesion	
Sylvilagus floridanus	Resistant	Natural host
(Eastern North America) (Cotton tail)	Local lesion	Local lesion
Sylvilagus brasiliensis	Natural host	Resistant
(South America) (Tapeti)	Local lesion	Local lesion
Sylvilagus bachmani	Natural host	Resistant
(Western North America) (Bush rabbit)	Local lesion	Local lesion
Lepus	Resistant	Resistant
(Hares, Jackrabbits)		

TABLE 7.3. *Common Characteristics of Myxoma and Fibroma Virus*

No Hemagglutinin
Acidophilic cytoplasmic inclusions
Infective for chorioallantoic membrane and tissue culture lines
175 μm diameter by filtration
230–280 μm diameter by electron microscopy
Cross immunity
One-way serologic cross-reactivity

acteristics of myxoma and fibroma viruses are presented in Table 7.3. Because of their large size and propensity to form large inclusions in infected cells, these viruses were among the earliest recognized. Studies on other poxviruses, such as bird epithelioma, molluscum contagiosum, and Yaba monkey pox, provided early evidence that viruses could cause tumors. However, unlike most cancers, actual viable virus could be recovered from lesions produced by oncogenic poxviruses. The focus on the role of viruses in cancer shifted away from poxviruses with the discovery of the oncogenic properties of the polyoma virus (Stewart et al. 1957), with an increasing emphasis on retroviruses and oncogenes (Heubner and Todaro 1968).

IMMUNOPATHOLOGY OF THE SHOPE FIBROMA

We began our studies on the SFV during a time of great interest in tumor immunity. We hypothesized that tumors induced by the SFV are rejected by immune responses. Immunofluorescence localization of virus antigen, T cells, and immunoglobulin (Ig) during growth and rejection of SFV-induced tumors in adult laboratory rabbits revealed large amounts of viral antigen in the tumor cells, followed by infiltration of the tumor by T cells and finally, rejection of the tumor (Sell and Scott 1981). Associated with rejection was marked T cell hyperplasia of draining lymph nodes and spleen and production of killer T cells to virus-infected RK-13 tissue culture cells (Scott et al. 1981). T and B cell mitogen responses were not depressed during growth or rejection of the tumor, and the response to anti-Ig was increased, indicating that there was B cell as well as T cell hyperplasia (see below). Antibody-dependent and cell-mediated cytotoxicity and natural killer activity to SFV were also detected, but we could not identify how or if they contributed to tumor rejection. We concluded that SFV induces proliferation of host cells and a humoral and cellular immune response to viral antigens and that the tumor is mainly rejected by cellular mechanisms (delayed hypersensitivity).

In neonatal rabbits, in contrast to adult rabbits, SFV inoculation often produced disseminated tumors and fatal disease (for review, see Strayer et al. 1984). On immunofluorescence, SFV antigen is seen systemically in the reticuloendothelial cells. In most neonates, prolonged healing of lesions is accomplished by granuloma formation. SFV-infected neonates develop cytotoxic T cells and antibody (Scott CB, Sell S unpublished data), but prolonged disease occurs presumably because of inadequate mobilization of immunity or because of malignant fibroma syndrome development (see below). Neonatal rabbits with maternal antibody to myxoma virus are not protected from the lethal effects of myxoma infection (Sobey and Conolly 1975).

THE MALIGNANT FIBROMA SYNDROME

The virus we used for our initial studies of Shope fibroma was grown as a large batch in cell culture. Subsequently, we attempted to obtain larger amounts of virus by rabbit-to-rabbit passage of tumor homogenates. Unexpectedly, the recipient rabbits developed a rapidly fatal syndrome with disseminated tumors, more similar to myxoma than fibroma (Strayer et al. 1983a). In vitro, it was noted that virus suspensions from the tumors of these rabbits produced clear plaques as well as the proliferative foci that were seen with fibroma virus when cultured on RK-13 rabbit kidney cells (Strayer et al. 1983a). Fibroma virus was purified by double focus cloning and the new virus by double plaque cloning. The clonally purified viruses reproduced their respective diseases. The fibroma virus produced self-limited lesions; the other, disseminated lesions and death. We named the new virus malignant rabbit fibroma virus (MV) (Strayer et al. 1983c).

The malignant fibroma syndrome is characterized by secondary infections with *Pasteurella multocida* and other nosocomial organisms, primarily in the nasal cavity (Corbeil et al. 1983). The nasal cavity is also involved with submucosal fibromas and marked hyperplasia of the overlying mucosa. (A role for growth factors produced by poxviruses must be considered in view of the

TABLE 7.4. *Cross-Reactivity of SFV and MV Neutralizing Antisera*

Virus Target	Neutralizing Titers	
	Anti-SFV	*Anti-MV*
Shope fibroma (SFV)	1/334	1/4096
Malignant rabbit fibroma (MV)	1/143	1/3681

Antisera obtained 10 days after infection with MV. The endpoint is the dilution of serum that reduces the number of plaques or foci by 50% compared with normal rabbit serum.

homology among the transforming growth factor I, epidermal growth factor, and a 19-kDa protein coded by a portion of the terminal repeat of vaccinia virus DNA; Blomquist et al. 1985.) This, combined with systemic immuno-suppression (see below), sets the stage for severe conjunctivitis and rhinitis. Rabbits are obligate nose breathers, and death is caused by asphyxiation. Immunization of rabbits with heat-killed *Pasteurella* will slow the course of the secondary infections, but does not prevent eventual death (Corbeil et al. 1983). Previous infection with SFV protects against MV and produces cross-reacting neutralizing antibody (Table 7.4).

THE GENETIC RELATIONSHIP OF SFV, MV, AND MYXOMA

Restriction endonuclease digestion of SFV, MV, and myxoma DNAs reveal that MV has many fragments in common with myxoma and only a few in common with SFV (Strayer et al. 1983a). Digests of the original SFV stock, when compared to clonally purified SFV and MV, indicate that the original stock of SFV contained a trace amount of MV (Strayer et al. 1983c). Apparently, passage from animal to animal permitted selection for the MV.

Restriction endonuclease analysis of the genomes of five strains of SFV, the Moses strain of myxoma virus, and vaccinia virus reveals that, as expected, the leporipoxvirus genomes have several structural features in common with the prototypic member of the poxvirus family, vaccinia. These viral genomes contain inverted terminal repetitions approximately 12 kb in length with cross-linked ends (Wills et al. 1983, Cabirac et al. 1985). However, neither SFV nor myxoma virus appear to have any significant homology with vaccinia, a result supported by cross-hybridization data. The five different strains of SFV demonstrate a high degree of conservation of restriction sites amongst one another, whereas the SFV and myxoma genomes are quite different. The Boerlage strain of SFV contains a deletion of approximately 300 base pairs in the terminal region of the genome relative to the other strains of SFV. A comparison of MV, SFV, and myxoma restriction digests clearly demonstrates that

MV is a recombinant between myxoma and SFV. Restriction mapping and blot hybridization experiments in our laboratory have shown that in the malignant variant, approximately 5.5 kb of myxoma virus DNA within each of the inverted terminal repeats is replaced by a similar amount of DNA derived from the corresponding region of the SFV genome (also see Block et al. 1985). Thus, MV contains approximately 149 kb of myxoma sequences and 11 kb of SFV sequences. The lack of comigrating fragments of SFV and myxoma DNA indicate that these viruses do not share a highly conserved internal region of their genome and thus are clearly two different viruses.

Transcriptional mapping studies have determined that the region of the SFV genome, which is present in MV, is expressed early in the infectious cycle. These experiments have shown that at least five genes from SFV are active in MV and that one gene is a fusion of an SFV gene and a myxoma gene. The functions of these genes are not yet known, but presumably they are responsible for the differences in biologic activity between MV and myxoma virus.

The origin of the recombinant MV that we have identified remains conjectural. We know that it was present in trace amounts in the stock of SFV that we prepared from the sample obtained from W. A. F. Tomkins, University of Illinois. Recombination could have occurred naturally or in the laboratory. The relationship of the demonstrated recombinational capacity of these viruses to the Berry-Dedrick phenomenon is fascinating. Selected recombinants are now being used to determine the relationship of genomic structure to biologic and immunologic properties of the viruses.

The Berry-Dedrick Phenomenon

In 1936, Berry and Dedrick issued a report entitled, "A method for changing the virus of rabbit fibroma (Shope) into that of infectious myxoma (Santarelli)." In this experiment, the heat-killed myxoma virus was mixed with active fibroma virus and recovery of myxoma virus achieved. They concluded that the heat-killed myxoma virus was "transformed" and that it acquired infectivity. Later, Fenner and Woodroofe (1960) demonstrated that this was a general phenomenon among poxviruses and that a poxvirus killed by methods involving damage to its proteins rather than to its nucleic acids could be restored by adding intact proteins from another poxvirus. However, if the DNA of the poxvirus was lethally damaged, it could not be restored (Joklik et al. 1960).

Effects of SFV, MV, and Myxoma Virus In Vivo

A comparison of the biologic effects of SFV, MV, and myxoma is given in Table 7.5 (see Strayer and Sell 1983, Strayer et al. 1983b). Both myxoma and

TABLE 7.5. Comparison of SFV, MV, and Myxoma in Domestic Rabbits

Shope Fibroma Virus (SFV)	Malignant Rabbit Fibroma Virus (MV)	Myxoma
Benign, local, small regresses	Large local nodule	Local flat plaque
	Disseminates, discrete nodule	Diffuse flat disseminated lesions
	Gram infection	Gram infection
Myxoid fibroma	Myxosarcoma	Myxosarcoma
		Virus inclusions in cytoplasm
Normal	Squamous metaplasia	Squamous metaplasia*
	Atypia	Atypia
		Virus inclusions
Hyperplasia (T Cell)	Hyperplasia	Hyperplasia
	Sinus histiocytosis	Sinus histiocytosis
Virus antigen in tumor cells only	Virus antigen in tumor, in epithelium over-lying tumor, and in macrophages in liver, lung, and lymphoid tissue	Virus antigen in tumor, mucous glands, skin, kidney tubules, hepatocytes, bronchial epithelium, and in macrophages in liver, lung and lymphoid tissue
Foci	Plaques	Plaques
5×10^6/culture	5×10^7/culture	5×10^7/culture

*In myxoma seen in bronchial epithelium as well. In MV epithelial metaplasia overlying tumors only.

MV produce disseminated tumors, marked immune suppression, and epithelial hyperplasia overlying the tumors, but there are also subtle differences between myxoma and MV. The hyperplastic epithelium overlying myxoma-induced lesions contains much more viral antigen than MV lesions do. Acidophilic inclusions are found in epithelial cells in myxoma but not in MV (Strayer and Sell 1983, Strayer et al. 1983b). Other epithelial cells in liver, kidney, and lung of myxoma-infected rabbits contain viral antigen, whereas in MV-infected rabbits, these cells do not contain viral antigens. Systemic dissemination of viral antigens in the reticuloendothelial system and large amounts of viral antigen in hyperplastic nasal mucosa is seen with both viruses (Strayer and Sell 1983).

MV and Immunosuppression

Both specific and nonspecific immune responses are severely depressed during MV tumor induction (Table 7.6). MV added to lymphocyte cultures stimulated by T or B cell mitogens or by specific antigen (sheep red blood cells (SRBC) added to lymphocytes from SRBC-primed rabbits) markedly suppresses the proliferative response. This effect is noted two days following the addition of MV to the cultures. MV also inhibits generation of SRBC-stimulated plaque-forming cells (PFC) but does not affect an ongoing antibody response in vivo (Strayer et al. 1983b). There is evidence that MV actually infects lymphocytes as titers of infective virus increase in lymphocyte

TABLE 7.6. *Comparison of Blastogenesis in Shope Fibroma and Malignant Rabbit Fibroma Virus–Infected Rabbits (% of control)*

Virus Injected	Day 3			Day 6			Day 10		
	Spleen	Lymph node	PBL	Spleen	Lymph node	PBL	Spleen	Lymph node	PBL
				Concanavalin A					
SFV	110	94	98	60	100	120	108	94	80
MV	102	90	100	16	31	87	6	12	13
				Anti-Ig					
SFV	116	150	140	80	140	105	106	140	160
MV	100	125	118	40	34	89	20	110	18

Representative Control Values (i.e., normal uninfected rabbits assayed the same day as infected rabbits): Concanavalin A = 22,000; Anti-Ig = 2,500.
PBL = peripheral blood lymphocytes.

cultures (Strayer D, Skaletsky E, Leibowitz J unpublished data). A similar effect is seen when measles or influenza virus is added to human lymphocytes in vitro (Casali et al. 1984). In addition, splenic lymphocytes and lysates of spleen cells from MV tumor-bearing rabbits inhibit PFC and proliferative responses of normal rabbit lymphocytes in vitro (Table 7.7). This suggests that there are multiple suppressive mechanisms, including direct infection of responding cells and production of suppressor cells and soluble suppressor factors (Strayer et al. 1983b). Inhibition of early viral DNA polymerases by addition of doses of phosphonoacetic acid (PAA) to lymphocyte cultures, which blocks MV proliferation by 99%, does not affect the ability of MV to inhibit lymphocyte proliferation or initiation of antibody production (Strayer E, Skletsky E, Leibowitz J unpublished data). Thus, the immunosuppressive effects of MV appear to be associated with early MV gene functions.

Lymphoid cells from rabbits injected with SFV are stimulated by SFV, ultraviolet (UV) radiation–inactivated SFV, or radiation-inactivated MV to proliferate in vitro (Skaletsky et al. 1984). On the other hand, lymphoid cells from MV-infected rabbits do not respond to SFV or to MV in any form used. In addition, MV added to cultures of lymphoid cells from SFV-infected rabbits suppress the response to SFV (Table 7.8). As with inhibition of mitogen-stimulated lymphocyte cultures, inhibition of the response occurs two days after addition of MV to the cultures (Skaletsky et al. 1984). The profound specific and nonspecific immunosuppressive effects of MV and myxoma have not been duplicated by any other infection or treatment in the rabbit. Cortisone treatment, which inhibits induction of specific immunity, neither suppresses mitogen responses nor results in nosocomial infections (Lukehart et

TABLE 7.7. *Effect of Spleen Cells and Lysates from MV-Infected Rabbits on In Vitro Proliferation and PFC Response to SRBC Using Spleen Cells From Primed Rabbits*

| | Ratio to Controls | |
	PFC	CPM (Day 6)
MV cells	0.36 ± 0.12	0.20 ± 0.10
SFV cells	1.23 ± 0.08	1.35 ± 0.30
MV lysates	0.19 ± 0.12	0.20 ± 0.08
SFV lysates	0.92 ± 0.01	0.33 ± 0.05

Responses of SRBC-primed cultures (controls) = 1.00.
All additions at 2:1 (5:1 gives similar result).
MV = malignant rabbit fibroma virus; PFC = plaque-forming cells;
SRBC = sheep red blood cells; SFV = Shope fibroma virus; CPM = counts per minute (per culture).

TABLE 7.8. *Effect of MV on Proliferation of Lymphoid Cells from SFV Immunized Rabbits**

	^{125}I *IUdR Incorporation (CPM/culture)*		
Culture Addition	*Lymph node*	*Spleen*	*PBL*
SFV	6,000	7,100	240
SFV + MV	800	0	0
SFV + heat inactivated MV	7,400	6,100	310

Adapted from Skaletsky et al. 1984.
*Cells obtained 6 days after inoculation of SFV.
(See Table 7.7 for abbreviations.)

al. 1981), and even after lethal irradiation, rabbits are able to respond to immunization (Taliaferro et al. 1964).

Strain Differences in SFV

Most strains of SFV tested produce similar effects. However, the Boerlage strain, which has slight differences in endonuclease fragments of DNA when compared to the other strains (Cabirac et al. 1985), produces a different pathologic effect when compared to the Patuxent strain (Strayer et al. 1984). The Boerlage strain results in larger tumors than those produced by the Patuxent strain. The epithelium overlying Boerlage tumors contains viral antigen, whereas the epithelium over Patuxent tumors does not. Foci of hepatocyte necrosis, persistent extramedullarly hematopoiesis, necrosis in thymic lobules, and systematic localization of viral antigen in the reticuloendothelial system and in the thymus, liver, and kidney cells are associated with the Boerlage but not with the Patuxent strain infections. The relationship of these biologic differences to the slight difference in endonuclease fragments is under study. It is notable that this difference maps in the terminal region of the genome, a genetically unstable region in orthopoxviruses and the region that has been acquired from SFV by the myxoma virus to become the MV.

SFV in Immunocompromised Rabbits

It has long been noted that SFV may produce systemic dissemination of virus, metastatic tumors, and death in neonatal rabbits or in adult rabbits treated with cortisone, irradiation, or carcinogens (Strayer et al. 1984). Earlier studies in our laboratory using the nonpurified SFV resulted in prolonged infection, metastatic lesions, and granulomas in neonatal rabbits (Sell and Scott

1981). We became interested in determining if the clonally purified SFV strains would produce systemic lesions in immunocompromised rabbits. The clonally purified Patuxent strain of SFV produced only local tumors without systemic dissemination in neonatal rabbits or in cortisone-treated adult rabbits (Strayer et al. 1984). The Boerlage strain of SFV did disseminate in neonatal rabbits but did not produce progressive tumor growth or death. This suggests that the fatal effects induced in immunosuppressed rabbits by nonpurified SFV in the past may have been caused by contamination with a more virulent form of the virus (MV).

SUMMARY

We have identified a recombinant leporipoxvirus that produces disseminated fibromas and a severe combined immune deficiency disease of sudden onset. The virus is recombinant between the SFV and the MV. MV was identified as a trace contaminant in stocks of SFV (Patuxent strain). Rabbits inoculated with the original uncloned stock of SFV prepared in vitro develop local tumors that subsequently regress. However, tumor extracts prepared from these animals, when injected into a second group of rabbits, produced MV syndrome. Rabbits with MV syndrome develop severe, usually lethal, *Pasteurella* or *Bordetella* infections and have disseminated fibroxanthosarcomas more similar to those produced by myxoma virus. The virus that induces this syndrome has been isolated by two cycles of plaque purification. This virus is indistinguishable from SFV using cross-neutralization and electron microscopy. Analyses of restriction enzyme digests of MV and plaque-purified SFV show them to be quite dissimilar and indicate that MV is recombinant between SFV and myxoma virus. This recombinational event resulted in approximately 5.5 kb of myxoma virus DNA within each of the inverted terminal repeats being replaced by a similar amount of DNA derived from the corresponding region of the SFV genome. Thus, MV contains approximately 149 kb of myxoma sequences and 11 kb of SFV sequences. Immunofluorescent studies of spleen and lymph nodes from MV-infected rabbits demonstrate that viral antigens are present predominantly in the sinusoidal lining cells in lymph nodes and in phagocytes in the splenic cords. This contrasts with the distribution of antigen observed in myxoma virus-infected rabbits where myxoma-specific antigens are present in large amounts in hyperplastic epithelium overlying tumors, particularly in the nasal mucosa and in spleen and lymph node cells. MV-infected rabbits essentially lose their lymphocyte proliferative response to T and B cell mitogens and are unable to initiate an antibody response to SRBC, as determined by a modified Jerne plaque assay. In vitro MV severely depresses the mitogen responses of normal B and T lymphocytes after two days of culture. Lymphoid cells and lysates of lymphoid cells from MV-infected rabbits will suppress mitogen- and antigen-induced responses in vitro. MV can grow in lymphocytes, but replication of MV is less efficient in lymphocytes than in RK-13 cells. Thus, MV produces a disseminated viral infection, systemic myxofibromas, and a severe combined immune deficiency in rabbits. The molecular and immunologic basis for these effects is now under study.

REFERENCES

Aragao HB. 1920. Transmissao do virus do myxoma dos coelhos pelos pulgas. Brasil-Medico 34:753–754.

Aragao HB. 1943. O virus do mixoma no coelho do mato (Sylvilagus minenses), Sua transmissao pelos Aedes scapularis e aegypti. Mem Inst Oswaldo Cruz 38:93–99.

Berry CP, Dedrick HM. 1936. A method for changing the virus of rabbit fibroma (Shope) into that of infectious myxomatosis (Santarelli). J Bacteriol 31: 50–51.

Block W, Upton C, McFadden G. 1985. Tumorigenic poxviruses: Genomic organization of malignant rabbit virus, a recombinant between Shope fibroma virus and myxoma virus. Virology 140:113–124.

Blomquist MC, Hunt LT, Barker WC. 1985. Vaccinia virus 19-kilodalton protein: Relationship to several mammalian proteins, including two growth factors. Proc Natl Acad Sci USA 81:7363–7367.

Cabirac GF, Strayer DS, Sell S, Leibowitz JL. 1985. Characterization, molecular cloning and physical mapping of the Shope fibroma virus genome. Virology 143:663–670.

Casali P, Rice GPA, Oldstone MBA. 1984. Viruses disrupt functions of human lymphocytes: Effect of measles virus and influenza virus on lymphocyte mediated killing and antibody production. J Exp Med 159:1322–1337.

Corbeil LB, Strayer DS, Skaletsky E, Wunderlich A, Sell S. 1983. Immunity to pasteurellosis in compromised rabbits. Am J Vet Res 44:845–850.

Delange AM, Macavly C, Block W, McFadden G. 1984. Tumorigenic poxviruses: Construction of the composite physical map of the Shope fibroma genome. J Virol 50:408–416.

Fenner F. 1959. Myxomatosis. Br Med Bull 15:240–245.

Fenner F. 1976. Classification and nomenclature of viruses. Second report of the International Committee on Taxonomy of Viruses. Intervirology 7:1–16.

Fenner F. 1979. Portraits of viruses: The poxviruses. Intervirology 11:137–157.

Fenner F, Day MF, Woodroofe GM. 1952. The mechanisms of the transmission of myxomatosis in the European rabbit (Oryctolagus cuniculus) by the mosquito Aedes aegypti. Aust J Exp Biol Med Sci 30:139–152.

Fenner F, Woodroofe GM. 1960. Reactivation of poxviruses: II. Range of reactivating viruses. Virology 11:185–201.

Gross L. 1970. Oncogenic Viruses. Pergamon Press, London, pp. 17–48.

Heubner RJ, Todaro GJ. 1968. Oncogenes of RNA tumor viruses as determinants of cancer. Proc Natl Acad Sci USA 64:1087–1091.

Joklik WK, Abel P, Holmes IH. 1960. Reactivation of poxvirus by a non-genetic mechanism. Nature 186:992–993.

Lukehart SA, Baker-Zander SA, Lloyd RMC, Sell S. 1981. Effect of cortisone on host parasite relationships in early experimental syphilis. J Immunol 127: 1361–1368.

Marshall ID, Regnery DC. 1963. Studies in the epidemiology of myxomatosis in California: III. The response of bush rabbits (Sylvilagus bachmani) to infection with exotic and enzootic strains of myxoma virus and the relative infectivity of the tumors for mosquitoes. American Journal of Hygiene 77:213–219.

Moses A. 1911. O virus do mixoma des coelhos: Untersuchungen ueber das Virus Myxomatosum der Kaninchen. Mem Inst Oswaldo Cruz 3:46–53.

Santarelli G. 1898. Das myxomatogene Virus: Beitrag zum Studium der Krankheit-serreger auberhalb des Sichtbaren. Centralblatt für Bakteriologie, Parasiten-kunde u. Infektionskrankheiten, Erste Abteilung. Medizinisch-Hygienische Bakteriologie und Tierische Parasitenkunde 23:865–873.

Scott CB, Holdbrook R, Sell S. 1981. Cell mediated immunity to Shope fibroma virus induced tumors in adult rabbits. JNCI 66:681–689.

Sell S, Scott CB. 1981. An immunologic study of Shope fibroma in rabbits: Tumor rejection by cellular reaction in adult and progressive systemic reticuloen-dothelial infection in neonates. JNCI 66:363–373.

Shepard RC, Edwards JW. 1977. Myxomatoses: The transmission of a highly virulent strain of myxoma virus by the European rabbit flea Spilopsyllus cuniculi (Dale) in the Mallee region of Australia. J Hyg 79:405–409.

Shope RE. 1932a. A transmissable tumor-like condition in rabbits. J Exp Med 56:793–802.

Shope RE. 1932b. A filterable virus causing a tumor-like condition in rabbits and its relationship to virus myxomatosum. J Exp Med 56:803–822.

Shope RE. 1936. Infectious fibroma of rabbits: IV. The infection with virus myxo-matosum of rabbits recovered from fibroma. J Exp Med 63:43–57.

Skaletsky E, Sharp PA, Sell S, Strayer DS. 1984. Immunologic dysfunction during viral oncogenesis: II. Inhibition of cellular immunity to viral antigens by malignant rabbit fibroma virus. Cell Immunol 86:64–74.

Sobey WR, Conolly D. 1975. Myxomatosis: Passive immunity in the offspring of immune rabbits (Oryctolagus cuniculus) infested with fleas (Spilopsyllus cuniculi Dale) and exposed to myxoma virus. J Hyg 74:43–55.

Stewart SE, Eddy BE, Gochenour AM, Borgese MG, Grubbs GE. 1957. The induction of neoplasms with a substance released from mouse tumors by tissue culture. Virology 3:380–400.

Strayer DS, Sell S. 1983. Immunohistology of malignant rabbit fibroma virus: A comparative study with rabbit myxoma virus. JNCI 71:105–116.

Strayer DS, Cabirac G, Sell S, Leibowitz JL. 1983a. Malignant rabbit fibroma virus: Observations on the culture and histopathologic characteristics of a new virus induced tumor. JNCI 71:91–104.

Strayer DS, Sell S, Skaletsky E, Leibowitz JL. 1983b. Immunologic dysfunction during viral oncogenesis: I. Nonspecific immunosuppression caused by malignant rabbit fibroma virus. J Immunol 131:2595–2602.

Strayer DS, Skaletsky E, Cabirac G, et al. 1983c. Malignant rabbit fibroma virus causes secondary immunosuppression in rabbits. J Immunol 130:399–404.

Strayer DS, Skaletsky E, Sell S. 1984. Strain differences in Shope fibroma virus: An immunopathologic study. Am J Pathol 116:342–358.

Taliaferro WH, Taliaferro LG, Jaroslow BN. 1964. Radiation and Immune Mechanisms. Academic Press, New York, pp. 1–152.

Wills A, Delange AM, Gregson C, Macauley C, McFadden G. 1983. Physical characterization and molecular cloning of the Shope fibroma virus DNA genome. Virology 130:403–414.

Symposium on Fundamental Cancer Research, Vol. 38.

8. The Immunology of Skin Cancer

Margaret L. Kripke

Department of Immunology, The University of Texas M. D. Anderson Hospital and Tumor Institute at Houston, Houston, Texas 77030

It has been known for almost 30 years that cancers induced by chemical carcinogens are immunogenic and can be recognized under appropriate circumstances as foreign by syngeneic hosts. In spite of numerous demonstrations of this phenomenon, there is still little evidence that the immune system plays a definitive role in the development of such tumors in the primary host. In nearly every instance in which the immune system can be implicated as a participant in the carcinogenic process, the tumors have been associated with an oncogenic virus. It has been very difficult to provide convincing evidence that the immune system plays a surveillance role against cancers that are not associated with viruses.

The one exception to this pattern that has been identified to date is the system of skin cancers induced in inbred mice by ultraviolet (UV) radiation. It is important to study this unusual system for two reasons: first, by studying the exceptional, we may learn something about the unexceptional; second, UV radiation is an environmental agent that is carcinogenic for humans, and what we learn from the mouse system may be applicable to the prevention or treatment of human skin cancers.

IMMUNOLOGY OF UV CARCINOGENESIS

The feature of this tumor system that makes it interesting from an immunologic point of view is that when most skin cancers induced by chronic UV irradiation are transplanted into normal syngeneic recipients, they are immunologically rejected (Kripke 1974). The lack of growth is immunologically mediated because the tumors grow progressively in immunosuppressed mice. In addition, tumor regression is associated with the development of an immune response that can be detected by adoptive transfer of T lymphocytes (Kripke 1974) and by in vitro cytotoxicity tests (Fortner and Kripke 1977,

Thorn 1978); the immune response generated by such transplantation is specific for the particular tumor transplanted (Kripke 1974, Pasternak et al. 1964).

This rejection by the immune system is unusual because most carcinogen-induced murine tumors are readily transplantable among members of the same inbred strain. It led us to ask how primary skin cancers survive immunologic destruction in the primary host. We discovered that exposure of the mice to UV radiation caused a systemic alteration that interfered with tumor rejection. This conclusion was based on the following type of experiment (Kripke and Fisher 1976): C3H mice were shaved once per week and exposed to FS40 sunlamps for one hour, three times per week. After about 20 weeks, primary skin cancers began to appear, and in about one year, all mice had developed skin cancer. We wanted to determine at what point during the course of carcinogenesis the mice lost their ability to reject the antigenic skin cancers. Therefore, we transplanted primary tumors into groups of normal and immunosuppressed mice and into animals exposed for increasing periods of time to UV radiation. We found that quite early in the course of irradiation, the mice lost their ability to reject UV-induced skin cancers. The systemic nature of this UV-induced alteration is illustrated in experiments in which suspensions of tumor cells are injected intravenously and the lungs are examined several weeks later (Kripke and Fidler 1980). Under identical conditions, mice whose skin is exposed to UV radiation develop many more lung metastases than animals who were not irradiated. These studies demonstrated that exposing the skin to UV light produced a systemic alteration that interfered with tumor rejection.

We and others have studied the immunologic capabilities of UV-irradiated mice and have found that most immune responses are unaffected by exposure to UV radiation (Kripke et al. 1977, Norbury et al. 1977, Spellman et al. 1977). For example, antibody formation and allogeneic responses appear to be unperturbed in UV-irradiated mice. However, contact hypersensitivity reactions and the rejection of UV-induced skin cancers are impaired. Therefore, the UV-induced alteration is highly selective.

The UV-induced alteration is also immunologically mediated because it can be transferred with lymphoid cells. We used the following protocol to demonstrate this conclusion (Fisher and Kripke 1977): mice were lethally x irradiated and their lymphoid system was replaced with cells from normal or UV-irradiated donors. When UV-induced tumors were implanted into these mice, they were rejected by animals whose immune system came from normal donors, but they grew progressively in mice whose immune system came from UV-irradiated donors. This indicated that the systemic alteration induced by UV radiation is immunologic because it can be transferred with lymphoid cells. It is also selective because the animals can reject allogeneic tumors even though they cannot reject syngeneic UV-induced tumors.

Using this approach, we asked a second question (Fisher and Kripke 1977), whether the failure of lymphoid cells from UV-irradiated animals to reject tumors results from the absence of effector cells or from the presence of suppressor cells. When these lymphoid cells are mixed with normal cells prior to injection into x-irradiated mice, the recipients are still susceptible to tumor challenge, indicating that a suppressor mechanism is involved. Daynes and Spellman (1977) were the first to show that injection of T lymphocytes from UV-irradiated mice directly into normal animals renders them unable to reject UV-induced tumors. Recently, we reported that the suppressive activity can be abolished by treating the cell population with anti–Lyt-1 antiserum and complement but not anti–Lyt-2 antiserum (Ullrich and Kripke 1984).

To summarize, the effect of UV radiation has three characteristics: it is systemic, it is selective, and it is suppressive.

SPECIFICITY OF THE SUPPRESSOR CELLS

As mentioned above, UV-induced tumors resemble chemically induced tumors in that each tumor is individually specific in tests of transplantation immunity (Kripke 1974, Pasternak et al. 1964). However, the UV-induced suppressor cells appear to interfere with the rejection of all UV-induced tumors (Fisher and Kripke 1977, Daynes and Spellman 1977). This observation raises the question of how there can be immunologic recognition of a set of apparently non–cross-reacting antigens. To examine this point in more detail, tests of the specificity of the UV-induced alteration were carried out (Fisher and Kripke 1977, Kripke et al. 1979). Mice that were injected with UV-induced suppressor cells could reject allogeneic UV-induced tumors and syngeneic methylcholanthrene-induced tumors, even though they could not reject syngeneic UV-induced tumors. A more interesting example is provided by tumors induced by 8-methoxypsoralen and longwave, UVA, radiation. This compound is a chemical photosensitizer that intercalates into DNA and absorbs UVA radiation. The absorbed energy forms chemical bonds between the psoralen molecule and DNA, resulting in the formation of monofunctional adducts and DNA crosslinks. This treatment mimics the effects of sunlamp, or UVB, irradiation: it produces sunburn and tanning reactions in skin, and it activates the same DNA repair pathways. It also induces, in mice, skin cancers that are indistinguishable histologically from sunlamp-induced tumors (Kripke et al. 1982). Unlike the sunlamp-induced tumors, these tumors are not highly antigenic. However, it is possible with some tumors to find a dose of cells that grows preferentially in immunosuppressed mice, relative to normal animals. Under these conditions, it is possible to ask whether the tumors also exhibit preferential growth in UV-irradiated mice, as do the tumors induced by sunlamp irradiation. We found that even these tumors are not affected by the UV-induced alteration (Kripke et al. 1982). Therefore, the UV-induced suppressor cells appear to be able to distinguish UV-induced tumors from syngeneic tumors induced by other carcinogens.

It is possible that the suppressor cells are directed against a differentiation antigen that occurs in the skin on a cell that is particularly susceptible to transformation by UVB radiation. To test this hypothesis, tumor cell lines derived by in vitro transformation of a cloned 10T1/2 C3H fibroblast line were obtained. We tested the growth of cells transformed in vitro by UV radiation, 3-methylcholanthrene, and x-rays in normal, immunosuppressed, and UV-irradiated mice. At doses of cells that exhibited preferential growth in immunosuppressed animals, only the UV-induced transformants grew preferentially in UV-irradiated hosts (Fisher et al. 1984). We demonstrated, in addition, that the increased susceptibility of UV-irradiated mice was mediated by suppressor lymphocytes. Because all cell lines were derived from the same cloned population, this result demonstrated that the antigen recognized by the suppressor cells was not related to the cell of origin, but to the UV radiation. Recent studies by Hostetler et al. (1985) suggest, in addition, that the antigen does not result from the transformation event, but may simply be a by-product of the exposure of cells to UV radiation.

One model for explaining the unusual specificity of the UV-induced suppressor T cells is that the suppressor cells are directed against a common, UV-associated determinant, whereas the effector cells are directed against the individually specific determinant. This model is reminiscent of the studies of Sercarz and colleagues (Turkin and Sercarz 1977) on the lysozyme molecule, which show that there are suppressor determinants that control the formation of antibodies directed against different determinants on the same molecule. Direct evidence supporting this model was presented in a poster session* by Lee Roberts of the University of Utah, Salt Lake City (personal communication 1985), who has now cloned the suppressor cells and shown that the cloned cells still recognize all UV-induced tumors as a group. This provides evidence that the suppressor cells recognize a common determinant that is shared among tumors of a particular etiology. This finding raises the question of whether there are common regulatory determinants on other types of tumors that appear to be non–cross-reacting and whether such common determinants could be used to identify the etiology of a tumor or to regulate the immune response against individual tumor antigens.

ORIGIN OF THE SUPPRESSOR CELLS

One of the most interesting questions raised by this system is, how exposing the skin to UV rays induces suppressor T lymphocytes that interfere with tu-

---

*Symposium on Fundamental Cancer Research. UT M.D. Anderson Hospital and Tumor Institute at Houston, Houston, Texas, Feb. 26–March 1, 1986

mor rejection. The answer is not yet certain, but there are two hypotheses that come from studies of the suppression of contact hypersensitivity by UV radiation.

Bergstresser, Streilein, and colleagues (Toews et al. 1980, Elmets et al. 1983) demonstrated that exposing mouse skin to very small doses of UV radiation (just a few minutes of exposure) prevented the development of a contact hypersensitivity reaction to haptens painted on the irradiated skin. Instead, the mice developed hapten-specific suppressor T lymphocytes. Recent studies by this group (Sullivan et al. 1984) and by Granstein et al. (1984) suggest that suppressor cells are induced because UV radiation changes the manner in which the sensitizer is presented to the central immune system. According to these current models, ordinarily, a hapten is presented by Langerhans cells, which are cutaneous macrophages that present antigens to stimulate the effector pathway of the immune response. The Langerhans cells are inactivated by UV radiation, which blocks activation of the effector cell pathway. Instead, the hapten is presented by a different antigen-presenting cell, which is UV resistant, and activates the suppressor cell pathway of the immune system. By analogy, we can speculate that the suppressor cells that inhibit tumor rejection may arise by the same mechanism.

A second model comes from the finding that UV radiation can also suppress contact hypersensitivity at a distant site. Studies by Noonan et al. (1981) show that exposing mice to higher doses of UV radiation (a single, three-hour exposure), followed by painting unexposed skin with a hapten, fails to induce contact hypersensitivity, which is measured by painting hapten on the unexposed ears. Instead, hapten-specific suppressor T lymphocytes are induced. How the suppressor cell pathway is activated in this case is not yet known, but it appears to be due to a change in the central lymphoid organs, rather than to a change in cutaneous Langerhans cells (Morison et al. 1984). Again, the suppressor cells for tumor rejection may also be induced by this second pathway.

ROLE OF THE SUPPRESSOR CELLS IN CARCINOGENESIS

What do these suppressor cells have to do with carcinogenesis? So far, we have considered only the effects of these cells on transplanted, UV-induced tumors. A more important issue is whether the cells play a role in carcinogenesis in the primary host. To address this issue, we separated the immunologic effects of UV radiation from the carcinogenic effects, by means of the following experiment (Fisher and Kripke 1982): the immune system of lethally x-irradiated mice was reconstituted with lymphoid cells from normal or UV-irradiated mice, or the mixed population, as described above. However, instead of challenging the mice with tumor transplants, we grafted each group with UV-irradiated skin, and we monitored the development of primary tumors in the grafts. Even though the skin grafted onto animals in each treatment group had received the same carcinogenic insult, many more tumors developed in skin grafted onto mice that were given suppressor cells than in those given normal lymphocytes. This demonstrates that the suppressor cells permit the outgrowth of nascent transformed cells and that the presence of these suppressor cells is a determining factor in the development of primary skin cancers.

In a second experiment (Fisher and Kripke 1982), normal mice were injected with T cells from UV-irradiated or normal animals and then primary skin cancers were induced in the recipients by chronic UV irradiation. The objective of this experiment was to determine whether the presence of suppressor cells early in carcinogenesis would affect the rate of development of primary skin cancers. We found that injection of suppressor cells three times, beginning at the time of the first UV irradiation, significantly reduced the latent period of the primary tumors. These results also indicate that the UV-induced suppressor cells are a determining factor in the development of primary skin cancers. Furthermore, they suggest that one reason for the long latency period in UV carcinogenesis is that tumors that occur early in the course of UV irradiation are eliminated or held in check by an immunologic mechanism.

CONCLUSIONS

We see from these studies that immune surveillance exists for some tumors that are not virus induced. In this case, it is probably due to two factors. First, the tumors are very highly antigenic and therefore are capable of being recognized by the immune system. Second, these tumors may be particularly vulnerable to immunologic detection because they arise in the skin—an organ specifically designed for immune surveillance against foreign intruders.

What conclusions can we draw about tumor immunology in general from studies of this exceptional tumor system? Many arguments have been made that "spontaneous" tumors in rodents are not antigenic and that there is little evidence for the antigenicity of human tumors (Hewitt et al. 1976). What we learn from this system is that first, antigenicity is related to etiology. Whether or not a tumor will be antigenic may depend entirely on what induced it. If a human cancer was induced by a virus or by UV radiation, it is likely to be highly antigenic. If, however, a tumor occurs late in life from no apparent external causative agent, it may not be antigenic at all. The key issue in antigenicity is not histologic type, but the identity of the etiologic agent.

Second, we learn from this system that the primary host is not necessarily a very good indicator of whether a tumor is antigenic or not. UV-induced tumors are among the most antigenic tumors described, yet, the primary host does not appear to make effector responses against these tumors. In human cancer, where we have only the primary host as an indicator, it is possible that many cancers that appear to be nonantigenic may in fact be highly antigenic under different circumstances and may appear nonantigenic because they have induced a negative response, rather than a positive one.

Finally, we have learned that to manipulate the immune response against cancer will require a more sophisticated understanding of how the immune system is regulated than we now have.

REFERENCES

Daynes RA, Spellman CW. 1977. Evidence for the generation of suppressor cells by ultraviolet radiation. Cell Immunol 31:182–187.

Elmets CA, Bergstresser PR, Tigelaar RE, Wood PJ, Streilein JW. 1983. Analysis of the mechanism of unresponsiveness produced by haptens painted on skin exposed to low-dose ultraviolet radiation. J Exp Med 158:781–794.

Fisher MS, Kripke ML. 1977. Systemic alteration induced in mice by ultraviolet light irradiation and its relationship to ultraviolet carcinogenesis. Proc Natl Acad Sci USA 74:1688–1692.

Fisher MS, Kripke ML. 1982. Suppressor T lymphocytes control the development of primary skin cancers in UV-irradiated mice. Science 216:1133–1134.

Fisher MS, Kripke ML, Chan GL. 1984. Antigenic similarity between cells transformed by ultraviolet radiation in vitro and in vivo. Science 223:593–594.

Fortner GW, Kripke ML. 1977. In vitro reactivity of splenic lymphocytes from normal and UV-irradiated mice against syngeneic UV-induced tumors. J Immunol 118:1483–1487.

Granstein RD, Lowy A, Greene MI. 1984. Epidermal antigen-presenting cells in activation of suppression: Identification of a new functional type of ultraviolet radiation-resistant epidermal cell. J Immunol 132:563–565.

Hewitt HB, Blake ER, Walder AS. 1976. A critique of the evidence for the host defense against cancer based on personal studies of 27 murine tumors of spontaneous origin. Br J Cancer 33:241–259.

Hostetler LW, Ananthaswamy HN, Kripke ML. 1985. Induction of antigenic variants exhibiting UV-associated antigens from a spontaneous murine fibrosarcoma by in vitro UV-irradiation (Abstract). Proceedings of the American Association for Cancer Research 26:312.

Kripke ML. 1974. Antigenicity of murine skin tumors induced by ultraviolet light. JNCI 53:1333–1336.

Kripke ML, Fidler IJ. 1980. Enhanced experimental metastasis of ultraviolet light-induced fibrosarcomas in ultraviolet light-irradiated syngeneic mice. Cancer Res 40:625–629.

Kripke ML, Fisher MS. 1976. Immunologic parameters of ultraviolet carcinogenesis. JNCI 57:211–215.

Kripke ML, Lofgreen JS, Beard J, Jessup JM, Fisher MS. 1977. In vivo immune responses of mice during carcinogenesis by ultraviolet radiation. JNCI 59:1227–1230.

Kripke ML, Thorn RM, Lill PH, Civin CI, Fisher MS. 1979. Further characterization of immunologic unresponsiveness induced in mice by UV radiation: Growth and induction of non–UV-induced tumors in UV-irradiated mice. Transplantation 28:212–217.

Kripke ML, Morison WL, Parrish JA. 1982. Induction and transplantation of murine skin cancers induced by methoxsalen plus ultraviolet (320-400nm) radiation. JNCI 68:685–690.

Morison WL, Bucana CB, Kripke ML. 1984. Systemic suppression of contact hypersensitivity by UVB radiation is unrelated to the UVB-induced alterations in the morphology and number of Langerhans cells. Immunology 52:299–306.

Noonan FP, DeFabo EC, Kripke ML. 1981. Suppression of contact hypersensitivity in mice by UV radiation and its relationship to UV-induced suppression of tumor immunity. Photochem Photobiol 34:683–689.

Norbury KC, Kripke ML, Budmen MB. 1977. In vitro reactivity of macrophages and lymphocytes from UV-irradiated mice. JNCI 59:1231–1235.

Pasternak G, Graffi A, Horn KH. 1964. Der Nachweis individual-spezifischer Antigenitat bei UV-induzierten Sarkomen der Maus. Acta Biol Med Ger 13:276–279.

Spellman CW, Woodward JG, Daynes RA. 1977. Modification of immunologic potential by ultraviolet radiation: I. Immune status of short-term UV-irradiated mice. Transplantation 24:112–119.

Sullivan S, Streilein JW, Bergstresser PR, Tigelaar RE. 1984. Hapten-derivatized, purified epidermal Langerhans cells induce contact hypersensitivity without down-regulation (Abstract). J Invest Dermatol 82:440.

Thorn RT. 1978. Specific inhibition of cytotoxic memory cells produced against UV-induced tumors in UV-irradiated mice. J Immunol 121:1920–1926.

Toews GB, Bergstresser PR, Streilein JW. 1980. Epidermal Langerhans cell density determines whether contact hypersensitivity or unresponsiveness follows skin painting with DNFB. J Immunol 124:445–453.

Turkin D, Sercarz E. 1977. Key antigenic determinants in regulation of the immune response. Proc Natl Acad Sci USA 74:3984–3987.

Ullrich SE, Kripke ML. 1984. Mechanisms in the suppression of tumor rejection produced in mice by repeated UV irradiation. J Immunol 133:2786–2790.

Symposium on Fundamental Cancer Research, Vol. 38.
© 1986 by The University of Texas System Cancer Center.

9. A Monoclonal Antibody against a Methylcholanthrene-induced Fibrosarcoma That Defines an Important T cell–Activation Antigen

Patrick M. Flood

Department of Pathology, Howard Hughes Medical Institute at Yale University School of Medicine, New Haven, Connecticut 06510

Malignantly transformed cells express cell surface antigens that are not found on nontransformed cells of the identical cell type. These antigens, known as tumor-associated surface antigens (TASA), are identified with antisera or monoclonal antibodies raised against individual tumor cell lines. These antibodies divide the antigens into two subclasses, (1) those that appear to be unique for that particular tumor, since the antibodies used to identify that antigen do not react with normal cells or other malignantly transformed cells, and (2) those that are found on a number of different malignantly transformed cells or on both malignant and normal tissue types, since these antibodies serologically cross-react with other cell types. Despite the identification of a large number of antigens in both categories, the absence of functional, molecular, and genetic data on these antigens leaves the nature of TASA largely a mystery.

An intense search has been carried out in recent years to discover the molecular nature of TASA, their function on malignantly transformed cells, and their relationship to cross-reactive antigens on normal tissue. Recent evidence has suggested that a number of TASA are related to highly polymorphic antigens used by cells of the immune system to communicate biologically active signals. Tumor antigens related to major histocompatibility complex (MHC)–linked class I antigens (Invernizzi and Parmiani 1975, Festenstein and Schmidt 1981), immunoglobulin (Ig) h–linked antigens (DeLeo et al. 1977, Flood et al. 1983a, Henderson et al. 1984), and minor histocompatibility antigens (Henderson et al. 1984) have been described. These antigens can act as targets of the immune system or can serologically mimic many important immunoregulatory determinants. However, the exact relationship of these tumor antigens to the immunoregulatory molecules remains to be determined.

Our laboratories have been involved in studies on the nature of TASA on the BALB/c methylcholanthrene (MCA)-induced fibrosarcoma Meth A (DeLeo et al. 1977, Flood et al. 1983a,b,c, Flood 1985). In this chapter, we describe serologic and functional analysis of a cell surface antigen expressed on the Meth A sarcoma and lymphoid cells of BALB/c origin, as defined by the monoclonal antibody (MAb) HD-42. This antibody appears to define an antigen on lymphoid cells that is important in the generation of functional T cell subsets.

SEROLOGIC ANALYSIS OF HD-42–DEFINED ANTIGEN

Antigen That Appears Tumor Specific for Meth A Fibrosarcoma

The HD-42 hybridoma was generated by fusion of NS/1 myeloma cells with spleen cells from Meth A hyperimmunized C57B1/6 mice. HD-42 MAb was originally detected in a complement (C')-dependent cytotoxicity assay and cloned three times by limiting dilution. The reactivity of HD-42 MAb on positive Meth A cells or negative CMS 4 (another BALB/c MCA-induced fibrosarcoma line) and a large panel of BALB/c, C3H, and B6 tumor lines were then tested for reactivity with HD-42 MAb using a direct cytotoxicity test or quantitative absorption analysis (Table 9.1). The expression of the HD-42–defined antigen was restricted to the Meth A sarcoma and appeared to represent a tumor-specific transplantation antigen.

Expression of HD-42 Antigen on Normal Lymphoid Cells

When tested on normal tissue from BALB/c and B6 mice, we found that HD-42 MAb did not react in direct cytotoxicity tests with BALB/c or B6 spleen, thymus, bone marrow, brain, or fibroblast tissue or B6 lymph node cells (Table 9.2). However, HD-42 MAb did kill 20–30% of normal BALB/c lymph node cells in a microcytotoxicity assay. In absorption analysis, the antigen was expressed on BALB/c thymus, spleen, lymph node, and bone marrow cells, as well as BALB/c embryo cells but not on the same cells from B6 mice. In both direct cytotoxocity tests and absorption analysis, the antigen was expressed on both BALB/c concanavalin A (Con A)–induced T cells and lipopolysaccharide (LPS)-induced B cells. Direct cytotoxicity tests and fluorescence-activated cell sorter analysis revealed that nearly 100% of Con A–induced T cells expressed the HD-42 MAb–defined antigen, while 30–40% of LPS-activated B cells expressed the antigen.

This differential expression of the antigen by BALB/c but not B6, T, and B cells suggested that the antigen exhibits a limited polymorphism and that the HD-42 antibody recognized one allelic determinant of this polymorphic antigen. Therefore, an absorption analysis was done on a large panel of indepen-

TABLE 9.1. *Expression of HD-42 Antigen on Tumor Cell Lines*

Tumors	Strain	Tumor Designation	Direct Test	Absorption Assay*
Chemically induced sarcomas	BALB/c	CMS1, 3, 4, 5, 7, 8	−	−
	BALB/c	Meth A	+	+
	B6	B6MS2,5	−	−
Leukemias	BALB/c	BALBRVC, BALBRVD, BALBRV ♀80, 81, 82, 83, RL♂1, RL♀7	−	−
	B6	B5RV ♀50, 52, 54, B6RV ♂60, 61, ERLD	−	−
Myelomas	BALB/c	MOPC−70A, −245, −21, −104E	−	−

*Antibody was absorbed and residual activity assayed on Meth A.

TABLE 9.2. *Serological Analysis of MAb HD-42*

Strain	Normal Tissue	Direct Test	Absorption Assay*
BALB/c	Adult lung fibroblasts	−	−
	Bone marrow	−	+
	Brain	−	−
	Lymph node	+	+
	Spleen	−	+
	Thymus	−	+
	Con A–activated spleen	+	+
	LPS-activated spleen	+	+
B6	Adult lung fibroblasts	−	−
	Bone marrow	−	−
	Brain	−	−
	Lymph node	−	−
	Spleen	−	−
	Thymus	−	−
	Con A–activated spleen	−	−
	LPS-activated spleen	−	−
CB6F₁	Helper T cell line	+	+

*Antibody was absorbed and residual activity assayed on Meth A.

TABLE 9.3. *Strain Expression of HD-42 Identified Antigen Expression on Normal Lymph Node Cells*

Group Number	Strains Positive for HD-42 Antigen Expression*	Strains Negative for HD-42 Antigen Expression*
I	BALB/cJ	C57B1/6J
	A/HeSn	
	C3H/HeJ	C57B1/10J
	C3H/HeN	SJL/J
	A/J	AKR/J
	CBA/J	C57L/J
	CE/J	
	NZB	DBA/2J
II	BALB/cJ	C57B1/6J
	C.B20	B.C9
	BAB.14	
III	BALB/cJ	C57B1/10J
	BALB.B	B10.D3
	BALB.K	B10.BR
IV	CB6F$_1$	CXB-D
	CXB-G	CXB-E
	CXB-H	CXB-I
	CXB-J	CXB-K
V	C3H/HeJ	C3H.Ly-6^b

*Inbred, congenic, or recombinant inbred strains of mice were determined to be positive for the HD-42–identified antigen by absorption of HD-42 MAb with lymph node cells.

dent strains and genetic cross-bred strains, in order to determine if the polymorphism exhibited by this antigen was identical to other antigens that are also expressed in different allelic forms (Table 9.3). In addition to BALB/c, the determinant recognized by HD-42 MAb was expressed on a wide variety of strains, including C3H/HeJ, C3H/HeN, A/J, A/HeSn, CBA/J, CE, and NZB mice. Strains negative for HD-42 antigen expression were C57B1/6J, C57B1/10J, C57L/J, DBA/2J, AKR/J, and SJL/J. Our results with BALB/c and B6 congenic and cross-bred mice showed that (1) the expression of this polymorphic determinant was not linked to Igh (group II)- or MHC (group III)-linked genes, (2) the antigen is codominantly expressed on (BALB/c × B6) F$_1$ mice, and (3) the pattern of expression using BALB/c × B6 inbred mice matches two gene polymorphisms, a minor histocompatibility antigen H-30, and a lymphocyte differentiation antigen Ly-6. We therefore tested Ly-6 congenic mice in order to determine if the expression of the antigen identified by HD-42 was linked to the Ly-6 gene locus, and we found that the expression of this antigen was identical to that found for the Ly-6.1 gene loci. We have provisionally designated it as Ly-6.1 and therefore refer to the HD-42 MAb as a-Ly-6.1.

FUNCTIONAL ANALYSIS OF Ly-6.1 ANTIGEN

a-Ly-6.1 MAb and Lymphokine-dependent Proliferation of Lectin-Activated Lymphocytes

While Ly-6.1 antigen expression was found on spleen, thymus, bone marrow, and lymph node cells from naive BALB/c mice, the activation of lymphocytes with lectin clearly enhances the expression of this antigen. Therefore, we attempted to determine if the Ly-6.1 antigen played any role in the activation process of either Con A–stimulated T cells or LPS-stimulated B cells. Spleen cells from naive BALB/c mice were treated with a-Ly-6.1 plus C' and tested for their proliferative response to the mitogens Con A or LPS. We found that pretreating spleen cells with a-Ly-6.1 did not appreciably affect the viability of spleen cells nor did it affect their ability to respond to either Con A or LPS. In contrast, posttreatment of both Con A–activated and LPS-activated spleen cells with a-Ly-6.1 plus C' resulted in significant cell death and diminished or eliminated their ability to respond to a restimulation with the same mitogen.

Since the Ly-6.1 antigen is expressed as a result of activation by mitogen, we asked whether adding a-Ly-6.1 MAb during the activation by lectins would appreciably affect the mitogen-induced proliferation of these cells (Table 9.4). Addition of a-Ly-6.1 MAb at dilutions of 1:100 to cultures of spleen cells and Con A did appear to marginally affect the proliferative response of BALB/c but not of B6 cells. When the MAb was diluted further, no effect was seen on either BALB/c or B6 spleen cells. Surprisingly, the addition of a-Ly-6.1 MAb to cultures of spleen cells and LPS had absolutely no effect on proliferation by either BALB/c or B6 cells.

The seemingly restricted effects of a-Ly-6.1 MAb on Con A–activated T cells but not LPS-activated B cells, led us to determine if the a-Ly-6.1 MAb also blocked the proliferative response of Con A–activated T cells to interleukin (IL) 2. Therefore, a-Ly-6.1 MAb was added to gradient-purified blast cells activated 72 hours earlier with Con A (Table 9.5). The addition of a-Ly-6.1 MAb significantly inhibited the IL 2–dependent growth of T cells in the absence of Con A. This inhibition could be seen at antibody dilutions of 1:2500 and was seen with BALB/c but not B6 T cell blasts.

TABLE 9.4. *Con A – Induced versus LPS-Induced Proliferation of BALB/c Spleen Cells*

Assay Cells*	Mitogen Added	a-Ly-6.1 MAb Added to Culture	Incorporation of [³H]-TdR (cpm) ± SEM†
BALB/c	—	—	800 ± 150
BALB/c	Con A	—	98,100 ± 7,800
BALB/c	Con A	1:100	31,000 ± 5,100
BALB/c	Con A	1:500	84,000 ± 9,000
BALB/c	Con A	1:2,500	110,900 ± 12,200
BALB/c	Con A	1:10,000	94,600 ± 9,100
BALB/c	LPS	—	68,500 ± 7,400
BALB/c	LPS	1:100	72,400 ± 6,000
BALB/c	LPS	1:500	63,300 ± 5,200
BALB/c	LPS	1:2,500	69,400 ± 9,000
BALB/c	LPS	1:10,000	67,200 ± 5,100
B6	—	—	700 ± 100
B6	Con A	—	124,800 ± 16,300
B6	Con A	1:100	141,500 ± 14,300
B6	Con A	1:500	132,400 ± 18,200
B6	Con A	1:2,500	121,300 ± 16,100
B6	Con A	1:10,000	130,400 ± 11,700
B6	LPS	—	89,500 ± 7,900
B6	LPS	1:100	85,700 ± 8,800
B6	LPS	1:500	87,400 ± 10,300
B6	LPS	1:2,500	93,500 ± 7,600
B6	LPS	1:10,000	82,400 ± 6,800

*Assay cells were 10^6 spleen cells/well from BALB/c or B6 mice in 200 μl of culture medium in 96-well tissue culture plate. Cells were incubated for 48 hours before being pulse treated with [³H]-TdR and harvested three hours later. Con A was added at 1.5 μg/ml; LPS was added at 50 μg/ml final concentration at the beginning of culture.

Source of a-Ly-6.1 MAb was ascites fluid from $CB6F_1$ mice bearing the HD-42 hybridoma.

a-Ly-6.1 MAb was added to cultures of spleen cells at the beginning of the culture period.

†Results are the average of three independent culture conditions indicated above.

a-Ly-6.1 MAb in Meth A Tumor Cell Proliferation Blocking

The fact that a-Ly-6.1 MAb blocks the IL 2–dependent proliferation of T cells prompted us to test if a-Ly-6.1 MAb could block the proliferation of the Meth A fibrosarcoma in vitro. a-Ly-6.1 MAb was added to Meth A cells or to T cells plus IL 2, and the proliferation was measured by [³H]-TdR uptake (Table 9.6). As seen before, a-Ly-6.1 MAb blocks the IL 2–dependent T cell

TABLE 9.5. *IL 2–Dependent Proliferation of Con A–Activated Spleen Cells*

Assay Cells*	Lympho-kine Added[†]	a-Ly-6.1 MAb Added to Culture[‡]	Incorporation of [³H]-TdR (cpm) ± SEM
BALB/c Con A Spleen	None	—	800 ± 200
	IL 2	—	75,200 ± 6,300
	IL 2	1:100	2,700 ± 1,100
	IL 2	1:500	20,500 ± 2,300
	IL 2	1:2,500	58,700 ± 6,400
	IL 2	1:10,000	71,800 ± 8,500
	IL 2	1:50,000	83,600 ± 7,100
B6 Con A Spleen	None	—	300 ± 50
	IL 2	—	89,300 ± 7,600
	IL 2	1:100	78,600 ± 8,400
	IL 2	1:500	83,400 ± 9,200
	IL 2	1:2,500	110,500 ± 9,000
	IL 2	1:10,000	114,800 ± 12,200
	IL 2	1:50,000	95,100 ± 8,200

*Assay cells were spleen cells from BALB/c or B6 spleen cells activated for 48 hours with 1.5 μg/ml Con A. Blast cells were purified by equilibrium density gradient centrifugation, and 10^5 cells were added to each culture in 100 μl of medium to a 96-well tissue culture plate.

[†]IL 2 was obtained from the supernatant of rat spleen cells incubated for 48 hours with Con A. α methyl mannoside was added to the IL 2–containing supernatant to neutralize residual Con A. IL 2–containing supernatant was added at a final concentration of 10% to Con A–activated spleen cells.

[‡]See Footnote *, Table 9.4.

proliferation of Con A–activated T cells (Table 9.6). However, the addition of a-Ly-6.1 has no effect on the proliferation of the Meth A fibrosarcoma cells. Therefore, it appears that whatever the function of the Ly-6.1 antigen on Meth A cells, it is not identical to the Ly-6.1 antigen on Con A–activated T cells.

Definition of IL 2 Receptor on T Cells

A number of explanations for the above results can be advanced to account for the observations made on T cells after the addition of a-Ly-6.1 MAb. One possibility is that the presence of a-Ly-6.1 MAb in culture results in lysis of cells bearing the Ly-6.1 marker. There are a number of reasons why this explanation is unlikely: (1) cultures of Con A–activated T cells that show, in some cases, greater than 80% inhibition of proliferation by the a-Ly-6.1 MAb show less than 10% cell death when compared to the original number of cells

TABLE 9.6. *Proliferation of Meth A Sarcoma Cells In Vitro*

Assay Cells*	Lymphokine Added[†]	a-Ly-6.1 MAb Added to Culture[‡]	Incorporation of [^{3}H]-TdR (cpm)±SEM
BALB/c Con A T	None	—	500 ± 100
	IL 2	—	84,000 ± 7,200
	IL 2	1:100	2,700 ± 600
	IL 2	1:500	5,800 ± 1,100
	IL 2	1:2,500	54,300 ± 6,800
	IL 2	1:10,000	86,800 ± 6,800
Meth A	None	—	171,300 ± 10,200
	IL 2	1:100	179,600 ± 12,400
	IL 2	1:500	190,200 ± 15,300
	IL 2	1:2,500	182,600 ± 17,100
	IL 2	1:10,000	164,500 ± 11,200

*Assay cells are either 10^5 BALB/c spleen cells activated 48 hours previously with Con A and separated into blast cells by equilibrium density gradient separation or 10^5 Meth A tumor cells adhered for 24 hours to a tissue culture dish. Assay cells were incubated for 48 hours then pulse treated with [^{3}H]-TdR for 3 hours before being harvested.
[†]See Footnote[†], Table 9.5.
[‡]See Footnote*, Table 9.4.

added to culture, (2) addition of anti–H-2L^d MAb to cultures of the same Ig isotype and subclass as the a-Ly-6.1 MAb had no effect on the response of those cells to Con A, (3) cells that are removed from a-Ly-6.1 MAb, placed back into culture and then given the same stimulus again responded normally, and (4) the effects of a-Ly-6.1 MAb in culture could be overcome with the addition of high concentrations of di-butyl cyclic guanosine monophosphate (cGMP) (Table 9.7). While it is clear from our studies that a-Ly-6.1 MAb can act as a lytic agent under the appropriate circumstances, it seems that the mechanism of suppression that we see in vitro is unrelated to a-Ly-6.1 MAb–mediated cell lysis. On the contrary, these results suggest that the effects of a-Ly-6.1 MAb in culture are transient and can be overcome simply by removing the suppressive agent. In this sense, the a-Ly-6.1 MAb may behave much like a hormone, signaling the cell with a positive transmembrane signal to reverse or terminate functional programming (Gordon et al. 1981).

An alternative to the above explanation is that the a-Ly-6.1 MAb is blocking the receptor cells' need to maintain an activated state. In the case of T cells, one possibility is that the antigen recognized by HD-42 antibody is the T cell receptor for IL 2 (Miyawaki et al. 1982). What makes a-Ly-6.1 MAb an unlikely candidate for a mouse anti–IL 2 receptor antibody are the following results: (1) the fact that (BALB/c $\times$ B6) F_1 T cells are at least as sensitive if not more sensitive to the effects of a-Ly-6.1 MAb and the fact that the effective dose of a-Ly-6.1 MAb on F_1 cells is even lower than for parental BALB/c cells (suggesting that it is not simply due to the number of receptors on the cell surface) make it unlikely that the a-Ly-6.1 MAb suppresses by blocking a receptor for IL 2, (2) saturation of the cell surface Ly-6.1 antigens on T cell blasts with a-Ly-6.1 MAb does not affect the ability of these cells to absorb IL 2 activity while saturation of cell surface determinants on the same T cell blasts with monoclonal anti–IL 2 receptor antibody (3C7) (Malek et al. 1983) significantly inhibits their ability to absorb IL 2 (Table 9.8), and (3) there have been no previous reports of a polymorphism detected on the IL 2 receptor; molecular genetic data have confirmed this for the human IL 2 receptor. Therefore, it appears that a-Ly-6.1 MAb identifies a very important, but as yet undefined, antigen on the surface of activated lymphocytes that, in addition to receptors for known lymphokines, plays a critical role in the proliferation and maturation of functional T cells.

TABLE 9.7. *Suppressive Effects of a-Ly-6.1 MAb*

Assay Cells	Lympho-kine Added	a-Ly 6.1 MAb Added to Culture	dib-cGMP Added*	Incorporation of [³H]-TdR (cpm)±SEM
BALB/c Con A T	None			800 ± 200
BALB/c Con A T	IL 2			78,000 ± 6,300
BALB/c Con A T	IL 2	1:100		1,200 ± 200
BALB/c Con A T	IL 2	1:500		3,800 ± 600
BALB/c Con A T	IL 2	1:2,500		42,700 ± 3,800
BALB/c Con A T	IL 2	1:10,000		82,500 ± 9,100
BALB/c Con A T	IL 2	1:50,000		74,350 ± 2,500
BALB/c Con A T	IL 2	1:100	10^{-3}M	61,300 ± 5,800
BALB/c Con A T	IL 2	1:500	10^{-3}M	79,400 ± 8,300
BALB/c Con A T	IL 2	1:2,500	10^{-3}M	81,500 ± 6,300
BALB/c Con A T	IL 2	1:10,000	10^{-3}M	74,900 ± 8,100
BALB/c Con A T	IL 2	1:50,000	10^{-3}M	78,700 ± 4,500
BALB/c Con A T	IL 2	1:100	10^{-4}M	9,600 ± 800
BALB/c Con A T	IL 2	1:500	10^{-4}M	11,800 ± 900
BALB/c Con A T	IL 2	1:2,500	10^{-4}M	45,300 ± 4,000
BALB/c Con A T	IL 2	1:10,000	10^{-4}M	75,300 ± 3,600
BALB/c Con A T	IL 2	1:50,000	10^{-4}M	82,400 ± 2,600

*Di-butyl cyclic guanosine monophosphate (cGMP) was added at the given concentrations at the beginning of culture. Cells were incubated for 48 hours then harvested 3 hours after pulse treating with [³H]-TdR.
Results are given as the average ± the SEM for three individual cultures.

TABLE 9.8. *Absorption of IL 2 Activity by Con A–Activated T Cells*

Assay Cells*	Lympho- kine Added[†]	Absorption of Lymphokine[‡]	Cell Number	Incorporation of [³H]-TdR (cpm) ± SEM
HT-2	None			500 ± 150
HT-2	IL 2			89,500 ± 7,200
HT-2	IL 2	BALB/c Con A T	10^7	21,500 ± 3,100
HT-2	IL 2	" " "	3×10^6	49,800 ± 5,700
HT-2	IL 2	" " "	10^6	91,600 ± 8,400
HT-2	IL 2	" " "	3×10^5	98,800 ± 11,200
HT-2	IL 2	a-Ly-6.1-Treated	10^7	16,400 ± 2,100
HT-2	IL 2	BALB/c Con A T	3×10^6	31,500 ± 2,700
HT-2	IL 2	" " "	10^6	80,900 ± 7,400
HT-2	IL 2	" " "	3×10^5	85,600 ± 9,100
HT-2	IL 2	3C7-Treated	10^7	74,300 ± 6,200
HT-2	IL 2	BALB/c Con A T	3×10^6	81,400 ± 8,200
HT-2	IL 2	" " "	10^6	79,800 ± 5,300
HT-2	IL 2	" " "	3×10^5	87,300 ± 5,300

* 10^5 IL 2–dependent HT-2 T cells were added to the 100 μl of tissue culture medium in one well of a 96-well tissue culture plate. Cells were incubated for 48 hours then harvested three hours after being pulse treated with [³H]-TdR.
† Source of IL 2 was IL 2–containing supernatant absorbed neat with BALB/c Con A–activated T cells. IL 2 was added at a final concentration of 10% at the beginning of culture.
‡ Absorption by the indicated number of Con A–activated spleen cells purified to blast cells by equilibrium density gradient centrifugation was done for three hours on ice. The supernatant was then cleared and sterilized and added to culture as indicated. 3C7 is an anti–IL 2 receptor MAb obtained from Ethan Shevach.

Additional Effects of a-Ly-6.1 MAb on T Cell–Mediated Immune Responses

The results given above demonstrate that the a-Ly-6.1 antibody profoundly affects T cell proliferation in vitro. Therefore, we tested the immunoregulatory effects of the a-Ly-6.1 MAb on a number of other T cell–mediated activities in vitro. In a large number of preliminary experiments, we found first that the addition of a-Ly-6.1 MAb to cultures of BALB/c or CB6F₁ mice significantly suppressed the plaque-forming cell (PFC) response of normal spleen cells to sheep red blood cells (SRBC) up to day 3 of a five-day response (Flood et al. 1985b). Addition of the a-Ly-6.1 MAb on days 4 and 5, as well as at the time of assaying the PFC response, did not affect the magnitude of the response. Second, we found that a-Ly-6.1 MAb had significant effects on in vitro generation of various T cell subsets. While pretreatment of naive T cells with a-Ly-6.1 MAb plus C′ had no effect on the generation of mature helper (T_H), suppressor (T_S), and contrasuppressor (T_{CS}) T cells, addition of a-Ly-6.1 MAb during the generation culture or posttreatment period of mature T_H, T_S, or T_{CS} cells with a-Ly-6.1 plus C′ completely abrogated their functional activity. Therefore, while an a-Ly-6.1 MAb does not react with the precursor cells of either T_H, T_S, or T_{CS} cells, it identifies an antigen that appears during the activation of these cell populations and can interfere with the functional maturation of the cells. Finally, we found that the addition of the a-Ly-6.1 MAb to allogeneic mixed lymphocyte cultures blocks the mixed lymphocyte reaction (MLR) between BALB/c responder cells and allogeneic stimulators. a-Ly-6.1 MAb also blocks the generation of BALB/c CTL but has no effect when it is added during the cell-mediated lympholysis (CML) assay. Therefore, it appears that a-Ly-6.1 MAb could block alloantigen-induced proliferation (MLR) and CTL generation but has no effect on the functional activity of mature CTL.

We have also used the a-Ly-6.1 MAb to investigate the role of T cell activation in vivo. We have found that (1) administration of a-Ly-6.1 MAb to BALB/c animals immunized with SRBC resulted in significantly fewer PFCs when compared to immunized BALB/c animals not receiving a-Ly-6.1 MAb or B6 animals comparably immunized with SRBC with and without a-Ly-6.1 MAb, (2) administration of the a-Ly-6.1 MAb significantly inhibits the generation of tumor-specific and alloantigen-specific CTL, after appropriate immunization, (3) administration of the a-Ly-6.1 MAb significantly increases the natural killer (NK) cell activity of BALB/c but not B6 mice (Palladino M unpublished data), and (4) preliminary studies on the growth of the Meth A tumor in BALB/c mice treated with the a-Ly-6.1 MAb indicates that the antibody had a significant effect on reducing tumor growth. More interesting, however, is the observation that successful treatment of BALB/c leukemia cells, which do not bear this a-Ly-6.1 antigen, was also carried out by in vivo administration of a-Ly-6.1 MAb. This suggests that the a-Ly-6.1 MAb may be a very powerful tool in studying the contribution of T lymphocytes in systemic immunity to malignant cells and raises the possibility that successful immunotherapeutic regimens may be more dependent on the lymphocyte populations targeted by the treatment than the tumor cells themselves. We are continuing the investigations on the immunologic effects of the a-Ly-6.1 MAb in vivo to determine which subsets of cells are responsible for the increased tumor immunity in treated animals.

CONCLUSION

Our results demonstrated that the BALB/c MCA-induced fibrosarcoma Meth A expresses a seemingly tumor-specific cell surface antigen that is serologically related to a determinant found on a subset of lymphocytes. This antigen is identified by its reactivity to MAb HD-42. This antibody reacts with populations of activated T and B cells but not with populations of naive T cells, B cells, or antigen-presenting cells. We also found that the expression of the antigen is determined by genes that map in or are closely linked to the a-Ly-6.1 gene complex.

The Immunologic Role of the Ly-6 Antigen

The Ly-6 locus was first discovered, and later found to be allelic, by McKenzie et al. (1977). This anti–Ly-6 antisera killed 60–70% of lymph node lymphocytes, few if any thymocytes, and a high percentage of mitogen-activated blasts, both T and B. This sera also eliminated CTL effector cells but not their precursors. Recently, a number of other antigenic determinants have been described that appear to be present on different types of cells but also map to the Ly-6 locus. Three independent investigators reported the existence of three antigens, Ly-8, Ala-1, and DAG (Frelinger and Murphy 1976, Feeney and Hammerling 1976, Sachs et al. 1973), and their results initially suggested that strain and tissue distribution of these four antigens were different, but later more rigorous comparisons of serologic reactivity led to the conclusions that all four antigens were probably identical (Horton and Sachs 1979). The consensus that emerged suggested that Ly-6 represented a differentiation antigen encoded by a single or by closely linked genes that were present on activated T cells, B cells, neutrophils, and many nonlymphoid cells (McKenzie et al. 1977, McKenzie and Potter 1979, Frelinger and Murphy 1976, Feeney 1978, Feeney and Hammerling 1976, Sachs et al. 1973, Takei et al. 1980a,b, Auchincloss et al. 1981, Potter et al. 1979, 1980, Woody 1977, Woody et al. 1977, Horton and Sachs 1979, Horton et al. 1978, 1979, Halloran et al. 1978, Kimura et al. 1980, 1984, Seto et al. 1982, Eckhardt and Herzenberg 1980, Hogarth et al. 1984). The generation of MAbs to antigens that map to the Ly-6 locus has altered the view that Ly-6 represents the product of a single gene. While Kimura et al. (1980) and Seto et al. (1982) have reported MAbs that identify antigens whose tissue distribution closely resembles the classical Ly-6.2 antigens, other investigators report antigens whose tissue distributions are different from those previously reported for Ly-6.2. Takei et al. (1980a,b) report that a MAb to the H9/25 alloantigen is present on a high percentage of bone marrow cells, precursors of cytotoxic T cells, and activated CTL. The ThB antigen was also reportedly linked to Ly-6 (Eckhardt and Herzenberg 1980), although its tissue distribution was different from both Ly-6.2 and H9/25. Auchincloss et al. (1981) reported two MAbs that identify antigens linked to Ly-6, one of which is present in moderate amounts on spleen and lymph node cells and on virtually every Con A T cell blast and LPS B blast. The other MAb was found on less than 10% of spleen and lymph node cells, greater than 90% of bone marrow cells, and 10–20% of T and B cell blasts. Recently, Meruelo et al. (1980) described an antigen, Ly-11.2, that maps very close to, but not in, the Ly-6 gene locus. This antigen is found on 10–20% of bone marrow, lymph node, spleen, and thymus cells as well as prothymocytes and NK cells. These antigens appear to represent a large set of cell surface alloantigens, whose function and structure have yet to be elucidated.

The antigen recognized by the HD-42 MAb does not appear to be related to any of the antigens thus far mentioned. It is not found in any appreciable quantity on spleen or thymus cells from normal animals and on only a small percentage (10–30%) of normal lymph node cells. While the HD-42–identified Ly-6.1 antigen is present on virtually all Con A–activated T cell blasts (90%), it is also found on LPS-activated B cell blasts. No other antibody mentioned so far shows this differential expression pattern on activated lymphocyte cell sets. Recently, Kimura et al. (1984) have reported on the results of an extensive serologic analysis of Ly-6–related antigens with a panel of MAbs that indicate there are at least five distinct antigens encoded by the Ly-6 locus, including an antigen linked to the Ly-6.1 locus defined by the MAb SK70.94. What is immediately clear from all of these studies is that the segment of murine DNA to which this HD-42 identified antigen represents an area that regulates the expression of a large number of cell surface alloantigens. Other Ly-6 antigens, the Ly-11, Ly-27.1, and the Ly-28.2 antigens and a minor histocompatibility antigen have been mapped.

It is still not clear how the antigen on Meth A cells relates to the Ly-6.1 antigen we describe on T and B cells, as well as other Ly-6–linked antigens, including Ly-m-6.1E. Kimura et al. (1984) reported the expression of Ly-m-6.1E on all five chemically induced BALB/c sarcomas tested, Meth A, CMS 4, CMS 17, CI4, and DMS 4. The Ly-6.1 antigen we describe has a more restricted pattern of expression among sarcomas; it was found only on the Meth A sarcoma among over 20 tumors tested. Firm molecular genetic and biochemical information on Ly-6.1 antigens has not yet been obtained, but preliminary evidence suggests that the antigens precipitated from T cells and Meth A cells with a-Ly-6.1 MAb are similar to each other but different from the antigen precipitated by Ly-m-6.1E antibody. However, the exact nature of these differences remains to be elucidated.

Our studies are the first to demonstrate a possible functional role for Ly-6–linked antigens. Our results with T cell lines suggest that the Ly-6.1 antigen may be a receptor for extracellular negative signals, which signal the cell to reverse or terminate functional programming. What is most intriguing about this possibility appears to be its specificity for a particular portion of the activation process for T cells. While having little or no effect on mitogen-activated T and B cells, the a-Ly-6.1 MAb significantly inhibits the sensitivity of activated T cells to the lymphokine IL 2 with di-butyl cGMP. Therefore, it appears that Ly-6–linked antigens play a critical role in a very restricted part of the T cell activation process, the activation signal given to the T cell by IL 2. The relevance of this biologic process to fibrosarcoma cells and the function of the Ly-6.1–linked antigen on Meth A to the T cell–defined antigen remains unclear.

Relevance to Cancer

The nature of antigens expressed on tumor cells after malignant transformation has long been an area of intense interest for tumor biologists. Chemically transformed cells and cells that become malignantly transformed because of repeated exposure to ultraviolet (UV) light express unique antigens that do not appear to be expressed by other transformed or nontransformed cells of the same tissue type. The nature of these tumor-specific surface antigens has, for the most part, remained a mystery. My coworkers and I have recently been involved in studies aimed at determining the nature of tumor-specific antigens on chemically and UV-induced tumors and their relationship to normal cellular interaction molecules used by cells of the immune system to communicate. Our results have found a very strong relationship between these transformation-related antigens and lymphocyte-interaction molecules. We have found that a unique transplantation antigen on the Meth A sarcoma is serologically cross-reactive with a cell interaction molecule linked to the Igh variable region used by regulatory T cells to passage biologically active informational signals (Flood et al. 1983a,b,c, Flood 1985); that the tumor-specific rejection antigen on the regressor UV-induced sarcoma 1591 from C3H mice is a class I MHC-linked molecule (Philipps C, McMillan M, Flood PM unpublished data); and that the Ly-6.1–linked antigen on the Meth A sarcoma is a T cell activation antigen. All three cases, which represent the best-defined tumor-associated antigens currently being studied, represent antigens important in lymphocyte communication.

Clearly, more evidence is needed, including biochemical and molecular genetic data, to determine the precise relationship between antigens expressed on tumor cells to the ones expressed on the regulatory T cells. However, the evidence at hand suggests that the aforementioned tumor antigens and the polymorphic cell interaction molecules (CIM) found on lymphocyte subsets are the same or are variants of the same structural gene. The parasitic use of CIM, which may or may not be modified by the carcinogenic process, appears to be an optimal way of generating the incredible diversity reported for tumor-associated antigens, since both germ line and somatic mechanisms exist for generating such diversity. While it remains to be seen just how much diversity exists in the Ly-6.1 gene locus, the fact that at least three independently derived tumor-associated antigens are products of polymorphic lymphocyte CIM suggests that the use of these polymorphic antigens by tumor cells may be an important part of the transformation process.

The question then is why are these types of antigens expressed on tumor cells, especially on nonlymphoid tumor cells? To answer this question, we need a better understanding of the role of these antigens in cellular communication. These highly polymorphic antigens represent important self-recognition molecules that play a critical role in driving immune responses. The expression of these antigens by tumor cells may play a similar role, i.e., drive an immune response that may be beneficial for tumor development, perhaps by interfering with normal immune responses or by preferentially activating suppressor T cells. Suppressor T cell responses have been found in the response to both the Meth A tumor (North and Bursuker 1984) and the 1591 tumor (Schreiber H, Flood PM unpublished data). In addition, the Meth A transplantation antigen is involved in suppressor cell interactions (Flood 1985, Flood et al. 1983a,c), and immune responses generated to this antigen can also block immunity (Flood et al. 1983b). Further analysis of the immunoregulatory activity of these antigens may help explain why these antigens are found on malignant cells.

An equally interesting finding described above is the observation that administration of large doses of a-Ly-6.1 MAb to tumor-bearing animals increases the tumor resistance of these animals. Although the mechanisms responsible for this increased tumor resistance are unknown, the results suggest that the lymphoid population rather than the tumor cell itself was the target of the immunotherapy. The immunologic mechanisms responsible for this increased tumor immunity appear to be the elimination of regulatory T lymphocytes based on the following observations: (1) in vivo administration of a-Ly-6.1 eliminates the generation of helper, suppressor, cytolytic, and delayed-type hypersensitivity (DTH)–mediating T cells, while B cell responses to LPS in vivo appear normal, (2) a-Ly-6.1 MAb administration increases NK cell activity, (3) a-Ly-6.1 MAb does not decrease antigen-presenting cell (APC) function in treated mice, and (4) a-Ly-6.1 administration does not increase the endogenous expression of interferon or IL 2 in the serum of treated animals. Therefore, we suggest that a-Ly-6.1 MAb increases tumor immunity by eliminating host regulatory mechanisms responsible for suppressing natural immunity. Previous results in which suppressive mechanisms have been circumvented (Hamaoka and Fujuwara 1984) or eliminated with antibody (Greene et al. 1977) have shown that removal of suppression leads to increased tumor resistance. In addition to removal of suppression, the activation of contrasuppression has been suggested as a possible mechanism for increased tumor immunity (Flood et al. 1985a, Flood PM, Ron Y, Freidman A unpublished data). These results suggest, therefore, that immunotherapeutic regimens aimed at regulatory lymphocytes, rather than or in addition to malignant cells, may ultimately be more successful in treating malignant disorders. The use of reagents like a-Ly-6.1 MAb to manipulate and dissect T cell immune responses may be a valuable asset not only to immunologists

studying T cell activation but also to clinicians trying to develop immunotherapeutic techniques to treat a wide variety of malignant disorders.

REFERENCES

Auchincloss H Jr, Ozato K, Sachs DH. 1981. Two distinct murine differentiation antigens determined by genes linked to the Ly-6 locus. J Immunol 127:
1839–1843.
DeLeo AB, Shiku H, Takahashi T, John M, Old LJ. 1977. Cell surface antigens on
chemically induced sarcomas of the mouse: I. Murine leukemia virus-induced
antigens and alloantigens on cultures, fibroblasts and sarcoma cells: Description of a unique antigen on BALBc Meth A sarcoma. J Exp Med 146:720–734.
Eckhardt LA, Herzenberg LA. 1980. Monoclonal antibodies to ThB detect close
linkage of Ly-6 and a gene regulating ThB expression. Immunogenetics 11:
275–291.
Feeney AJ, Hammerling U. 1976. Ala-1, a murine alloantigen of activated lymphocytes. Immunogenetics 3:369–379.
Feeney AJ. 1978. Expression of Ly-6 activated T and B cells: Possible identity
with Ala-1. Immunogenetics 7:537–543.
Festenstein H, Schmidt W. 1981. Variation in MHC antigenic profiles of tumor
cells and its biological effects. Immunol Rev 60:85–101.
Flood PM. 1985. Investigations into the nature of Igh-V region restricted T cell
interactions using antibodies to antigens on methylcholanthrene-induced sarcomas: I. Analysis of an Ly1 I-J$^+$ suppressor-inducer factor. J Immunol 134:
1665–1672.
Flood PM, DeLeo AB, Old LJ, Gershon RK. 1983a. The relation of surface antigens on methylcholanthrene-induced fibrosarcomas to immunoglobulin heavy
chain variable region-linked T cell interaction molecules. Proc Natl Acad Sci
USA 80:1683–1687.
Flood PM, DeLeo AB, Old LJ, Gershon RK. 1983b. Inhibition of the induction
of contrasuppression by antisera against tumor-associated surface antigens on
methylcholanthrene-induced sarcomas. *In* Neth R, Gallo RC, Greaves MF,
Moore MAS, Winkler K, eds., Modern Trends in Human Leukemia V. Springer-
Verlag, Berlin, West Germany, pp. 486–489.
Flood PM, DeLeo AB, Old LJ, Gershon RK. 1983c. Similarities between trans-
plantation antigens on methylcholanthrene-induced sarcomas and T cell regulatory molecules. Ann NY Acad Sci 418:206–219.
Flood PM, Chue B, Green DR. 1985a. Control of immune responsiveness by regulatory T lymphocytes. *In* Cruse JM, Lewis RE, eds., Concepts in Immuno-
pathology. Karger, New York.
Flood PM, Murphy DB, Horowitz M, et al. 1985b. A monoclonal antibody which
recognizes an Ly-6 linked antigen inhibits the generation of functionally active
T cell subsets. J Immunol 135:63–72.
Frelinger JA, Murphy DB. 1976. A new alloantigen, Ly-8, recognized by C3H
anti-AKR serum. Immunogenetics 3:481–487.
Gorden P, Carpenter J-L, Orci L. 1981. Morphological and biochemical events in
the interaction of polypeptide hormones with target cells. *In* Middlebrook JL,
Kohn LD, eds., Receptor mediated binding and internalizations of toxins and
hormones. Academic Press, New York, pp. 251–278.

Greene MI, Dorf ME, Pierres M, Benaceraff B. 1977. Reduction of syngeneic tumor growth by an anti I-J alloantiserum. Proc Natl Acad Sci USA 74: 5118–5122.

Halloran PF, Dutton D, Chance H, Cohen Z. 1978. An Ly-like specificity with extensive nonlymphoid expression. Immunogenetics 7:185–200.

Hamaoka T, Fujuwara H. 1984. Augmented induction of tumor-specific immunity and its application to the active immunotherapy. Prog Immunol 5:1253–1260.

Henderson LA, Cianarra R, Riblet R, Forman J. 1984. H-40, an antigen controlled by an Igh-linked gene and recognized by cytotoxic T lymphocytes: II. Recognition of H-40 as a tumor antigen in leukemic animals. J Immunol 133:2778–2785.

Hogarth PM, Houlden BA, Latham SE, Suton VR, McKenzie IFC. 1984. Definition of new alloantigens encoded by genes in the Ly-6 complex. Immunogenetics 20:57–68.

Horton MA, Sachs JA. 1979. Identity of murine lymphocyte alloantigens DAG, Ala-1, Ly-8 and Ly-6. Immunogenetics 9:273–280.

Horton MA, Beverly PCL, Simpson E. 1978. Serological properties of anti-Ly 6.2 serum produced by a new immunization schedule. Immunogenetics 7: 173–178.

Horton MA, Beverly PCL, Simpson E. 1979. Expression of Ly-6 alloantigen during differentiation of cytotoxic T cells. Eur J Immunol 9:345–352.

Invernizzi G, Parmiani G. 1975. Tumor-associated transplantation antigens of chemically-induced sarcomas cross reacting with allogenic histocompatibility antigens. Nature 254:713–715.

Kimura S, Tada N, Nakayama E, Hammerling U. 1980. Studies on the mouse Ly-6 alloantigen system: Serological characterization of mouse Ly-6 alloantigen by monoclonal antibodies. Immunogenetics 11:373–381.

Kimura S, Tada N, Liu-Lam Y, Hammerling U. 1984. Studies of the mouse Ly-6 alloantigen system. Immunogenetics 20:47–56.

Malek T, Robb R, Shevach E. 1983. Identification and initial characterization of a rat monoclonal antibody reactive with the murine interleukin 2 receptor-ligand complex. Proc Natl Acad Sci USA 80:5694–5699.

McKenzie IFC, Potter T. 1979. Murine cell surface antigens. Adv Immunol 27: 229–254.

McKenzie IFC, Cherry M, Snell GD. 1977. Ly-6.2: A new lymphocyte specificity on peripheral T cells. Immunogenetics 5:25–32.

Meruelo D, Paolini A, Dlieger N, Offer M. 1980. Definition of a new T lymphocyte cell surface antigen, Ly 11.2. J Immunol 125:2713–2718.

Miyawaki T, Yachie A, Uwadana N, Ohzeki S, Nagaoki T, Taniguchi N. 1982. Functional significance of Tac antigen expressed on activated human T lymphocytes: Tac antigen interacts with T cell growth factor in cellular proliferation. J Immunol 129:2474–2478.

North RJ, Bursuker I. 1984. Generation and decay of the immune response to a progressive fibrosarcoma: I. Ly1$^+$,2$^-$ suppressor T cells down regulate the generation of Ly1$^-$, 2$^-$ effector T cells. J Exp Med 159:1295–1311.

Potter TA, Watt SM, Burgess AW, McKenzie IFC. 1979. Characterization of surface alloantigens on murine neutrophils. Immunogenetics 8:461–473.

Potter TA, McKenzie IFC, Morgan GM, Cherry M. 1980. Murine lymphocyte alloantigens: I. The Ly-6 locus. J Immunol 125:541–545.

Sachs JA, Huber B, Pena-Martinez J, Festenstein H. 1973. Genetic studies and effect on skin allograft survival of DBA/2 DAG, Ly, and M locus antigens. Transplant Proc 5:1385–1391.

Seto M, Takahashi T, Tanimoto M, Nishizuka Y. 1982. Production of monoclonal antibodies against the MM antigen: The serological identification of MM antigen with Ly-6.2 alloantigen. J Immunol 138:201–205.

Takei F, Galfre G, Alderson T, Lennox ES, Milstein C. 1980a. H9/25 monoclonal antibody recognizes a new allospecificity of mouse lymphocyte subpopulations: strain and tissue distribution. Eur J Immunol 10:241–246.

Takei F, Waldmann H, Lennox ES, Milstein C. 1980b. Monoclonal antibody H9/25 reacts with functional subsets of T and B cells: Killer, killer precursor, and plaque forming cells. Eur J Immunol 10:503–509.

Woody JN. 1977. Ly-6 is a T cell differentiation antigen. Nature 269:61–63.

Woody JN, Feldmann M, Beverly PCL, McKenzie IFC. 1977. Expression of alloantigens Ly-5 and Ly-6 on cytotoxic effector cells. J Immunol 118:1739–1743.

Symposium on Fundamental Cancer Research, Vol. 38.

10. Mutagen-induced Antigenic Variants of Tumor Cells

Thierry Boon, Aline Van Pel, Etienne De Plaen, and
Françoise Vessière

Ludwig Institute for Cancer Research and the Cellular Genetics Unit, Catholic University of Louvain, Brussels, Belgium

Tumor-associated transplantation antigens (TATA) are commonly found on rodent tumors induced by oncogenic viruses, chemical carcinogens, and ultraviolet (UV) irradiation (Gross 1943, Prehn and Main 1957, Klein et al. 1960, Kripke 1974). In contrast, spontaneous rodent tumors appear to be incapable of eliciting any rejection response in the syngeneic host (Hewitt et al. 1976, Middle and Embleton 1981). In man, there is good evidence that some tumors carry tumor-associated antigens that elicit an autologous antibody response (Pfreundschuh et al. 1978). However, it is difficult to evaluate to what extent human tumors carry surface antigens that can be the targets for an autologous rejection response.

The results to be reviewed here are based on the observation that when clonal mouse tumor cell lines are exposed in vitro to the potent mutagen N-methyl-N'-nitro-N-nitrosoguanidine (MNNG), the surviving cell population contains variants that are unable to form progressive tumors in normal adult syngeneic animals (Boon 1983) (Figure 10.1). These variants have, therefore, been named tum$^-$ to distinguish them from the tumorigenic (tum$^+$) cells from which they are derived. Tum$^-$ variants have been obtained from many different mouse tumor cell lines, including teratocarcinoma (Boon and Kellermann 1977), Lewis lung carcinoma (Van Pel et al. 1979), mastocytoma P815 (Uyttenhove et al. 1980), several spontaneous leukemias (Van Pel et al. 1983), and an adenoacanthoma (Frost et al. 1983). With a dose of MNNG allowing for approximately 0.1% survival of the initial cells, the frequency of tum$^-$ variants among the survivors usually ranges from 1–20%. Most of these variants retain the tum$^-$ phenotype in long-term culture.

TUM$^-$ ANTIGENS

The failure of tum$^-$ variants to form progressive tumors is the consequence of an immune rejection response. Tum$^-$ variants do form progressive tumors

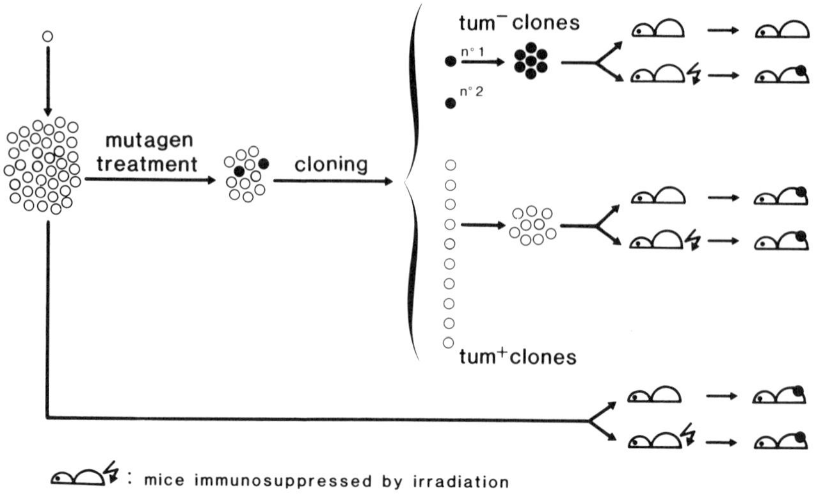

: mice immunosuppressed by irradiation

FIGURE 10.1. Production of tum⁻ clones.

in nude mice and in mice that have been immunodepressed by a sublethal dose of gamma radiation (Boon and Kellermann 1977, Van Pel et al. 1979, Uyttenhove et al. 1980, Frost et al. 1983). For mastocytoma P815, which produces ascites, it is possible to follow the fate of tum⁺ or tum⁻ cells injected in the peritoneal cavity with an agar colony test. The results indicate that the tum⁻ cells multiply exponentially during the first 10 days (Figure 10.2). Around day 12 to 15, the tumor cells are eliminated completely in a few days and a large influx of lymphocytes and macrophages into the peritoneal cavity is observed (Uyttenhove et al. 1980). Mice that have rejected a tum⁻ variant are endowed with a radioresistant immune memory that enables them to reject a challenge of the same variant even when they receive concurrent immunosuppressive irradiation (Boon and Kellermann 1977, Van Pel et al. 1979, Uyttenhove et al. 1980). This immune memory can be transferred adoptively with immune spleen T cells (Boon and Kellermann 1977).

When mice are immunized against a tum⁻ variant, they usually present a higher degree of resistance against a challenge with the same variant than against any other tum⁻ variant derived from the same tumor cell line (Boon and Van Pel 1978, Van Pel et al. 1979). This can be explained by assuming that most tum⁻ variants have acquired a new transplantation antigen that is specific for each variant. As shown below, the existence of these "tum⁻ antigens" has been confirmed in vitro.

We have been unable to obtain antibodies directed against tum⁻ antigens. This is not surprising, considering the scarcity of specific antibodies obtained against TATA of methylcholanthrene-induced tumors and against minor histocompatibility antigens. However, with some tum⁻ systems, it has been possible to observe a strong cytolytic T lymphocyte (CTL) response directed against tum⁻ antigens (Boon et al. 1980, Vessière et al. 1982). We summarize here the results obtained with P815 tum⁻ variants, since they have been the subject of the most extensive study with CTL.

When spleen cells from syngeneic mice that have rejected a tum⁻ variant are stimulated in vitro with the same variant, very active CTL are generated. In most instances, these CTL show a definite specificity for the immunizing variant, even though a significant lytic activity is observed against the tum⁺ cells and other tum⁻ variants (Boon et al. 1980). A systematic analysis of the CTL activities generated in response to more than 20 variants has led to the conclusion that most tum⁻ variants generate a variant-specific CTL activity, confirming the evidence obtained in vivo for new tum⁻ antigens. This CTL

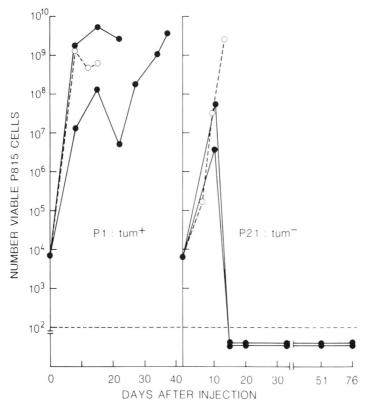

FIGURE 10.2. Mice were injected intraperitoneally with 10^4 tum⁺ or tum⁻ cells. On various days thereafter, a sample of the peritoneal fluid was collected and the number of viable tumor cells was estimated by an agar colony test.
●: normal mice
○: irradiated mice

activity is H-2 restricted (Van Snick et al. 1982). No tum⁻ antigen has been found twice among more than 15 variants expressing these antigens. Moreover, no cross-reactive lysis involving any pair of tum⁻ variants has been observed, above what can be accounted for by the TATA already present on the original tum⁺ cells. Thus, the repertoire of the tum⁻ antigens is very likely to exceed 50 and may prove to be considerably larger. In this respect, the tum⁻ antigens are similar to the methylcholanthrene-induced TATA.

It should be noted that for some tumors, strong CTL activities are observed with most tum⁻ variants, whereas for other tumors, no CTL activity is observed against any tum⁻ variants, even though the variants of both tumors are vigorously rejected. Such a lack of correlation between CTL activity and rejection response has been reported for other systems, such as the male-specific antigen H-Y (Hurme et al. 1978a,b).

The results obtained in vitro with immune spleen cells have been confirmed and extended by the clonal analysis of CTL. When stimulated in limiting dilution conditions in the presence of interleukin 2, spleen cells from mice immunized with P815 tum⁻ variants yield CTL clones at a frequency of 10^{-4} to 10^{-3} (Maryanski et al. 1982). With spleen cells that have already been stimulated in mass culture, this frequency rises to 10^{-1}. CTL clones are obtained that show a strict specificity for the immunizing tum⁻ variant (Figure 10.3).

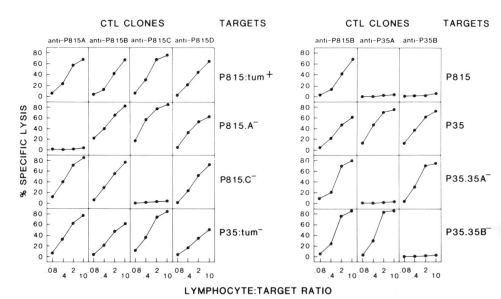

FIGURE 10.3. Lytic activity of cytolytic T lymphocyte clones directed against components of the P815 tum⁺ antigen (anti-P815A, -B, -C, -D) or tum⁻ antigen (anti-P35A, -P35B). Target cells are tum⁺ (P815), tum⁻ (P35), and antigen-loss secondary variants.

Others are directed against a TATA of P815 (tum$^+$ antigen). Many CTL clones can be expanded and maintained in culture for several months without losing their activity and specificity.

By using CTL clones directed against tum$^-$ antigens of P815, it has been possible to dissect these antigens into several components that may be lost independently of each other (Maryanski and Boon 1982). Upon incubation of some tum$^-$ variants in the presence of the appropriate anti-tum$^-$ CTL clone, stable secondary variants can be obtained that have lost the tum$^-$ antigen recognized by this CTL. In some instances, these antigen-loss variants have retained another antigenic determinant that is specific for the original tum$^-$ variant. Other CTL clones can then be obtained that are directed against this second tum$^-$ antigenic determinant (Figure 10.3). Thus, two components of the tum$^-$ antigen can be identified. Each can be selected independently of the other. When both are removed, the cells regain their ability to form tumors in normal mice (Maryanski and Boon 1982). When an occasional injection of tum$^-$ cells produces a progressive tumor, these tumor cells have also usually lost the tum$^-$ antigen or at least one of its components (Maryanski et al. 1983a).

CTL clones have also allowed the distinction of four different antigenic components in the TATA present on the tum$^+$ P815 cells (Figure 10.3). Here also, antigen-loss variants are relevant to an interesting phenomenon encountered in vivo. Sometimes an intraperitoneal inoculum of P815 is almost completely eliminated by a rejection response, but a small number of residual tumor cells persist and remain stationary in the peritoneal cavity for a period that can exceed several weeks. This phenomenon has also been observed with mouse lymphoma L5178Y and has been referred to as the tumor dormant state (Weinhold et al. 1979). Eventually the P815 tumor cells that have escaped rejection proliferate to form a progressive lethal tumor. These escaping cells have always lost one or two components of the TATA of P815 (Uyttenhove et al. 1983).

Even though it has been possible to characterize the tum$^-$ antigens with great precision using CTL clones, we have not gained much insight into the nature of these antigens. Are they related to the TATA obtained after chemical carcinogens or UV induction of tumors? By what mechanism do they arise at such extraordinarily high frequencies? Major progress in our understanding would be achieved by knowing whether the large number of different tum$^-$ antigens constitutes a family of related molecules coded by a family of genes like the immunoglobulins or the major histocompatibility class I and class II molecules. Or, are the tum$^-$ antigens carried by an array of completely unrelated molecules? Owing to the lack of antibodies, the biochemical isolation and characterization of tum$^-$ antigens has remained elusive. The cloning of the relevant genes may be easier to achieve. This could be attempted by gene transfection, since the expression of tum$^-$ antigens is dominant; somatic hybrids obtained by fusing one tum⁺ and one tum⁻ cell express the parental tum⁻ antigen (Maryanski et al. 1983b). However, it will be necessary to devise methods whereby antigen-positive transfectants can be detected with cytolytic T cells. This requires that the DNA recipient be a good target for CTL and be of the same H-2 haplotype as the tum⁻ system providing the DNA. Considering this and the possibility that the tum⁻ antigen might show tissue-specific expression, we thought that it would be best to transfect DNA from the tum⁻ variant in the original tum⁺ cell. The P815 system has the advantage of having many well-characterized tum⁻ variants and high susceptibility to CTL lysis. Unfortunately, the P815 tum⁺ cell is a very poor DNA recipient; the transfection frequency is approximately 1,000-fold lower than that of L cells.

We have, therefore, attempted to isolate a high efficiency DNA recipient from a tumor cell line derived from mouse mastocytoma P815. We reasoned that if a population of cells that are transfectable at low efficiency contains some variants transfectable at an efficiency that is much higher, then a commensurate enrichment for these variants should be found in populations of cells expressing a transfected selectable gene. Hopefully, it might then be possible to identify the high efficiency variants by a screening procedure. We therefore submitted a thymidine kinase (tk)–deficient mutant of P815 to repeated cycles of transfections with a tk gene and tk⁺ selection followed by reverse selection with bromodeoxyuridine. We were able to isolate a cell line that is transfectable at a 100-fold higher frequency than the original P815 cell line (Van Pel A, De Plaen E, Boon T unpublished data). We hope that this cell will prove useful in the isolation of tum⁻ genes.

PROTECTION CONFERRED BY TUM⁻ VARIANTS AGAINST THE ORIGINAL TUMOR CELLS

By rejecting a living inoculum of tum⁻ variant cells, mice acquire a certain degree of resistance against a challenge with the original tum⁻ clone. This protection is weak; it is usually not effective against challenges that exceed a few times the minimum tumorigenic dose. However, it has long-term effects and is specific for the original tumor (Boon and Van Pel 1978, Van Pel et al. 1983).

This protective effect was to be expected for tum⁻ variants obtained from slightly immunogenic tumors, like Lewis lung carcinoma. For P815, it is more interesting because no protection can be obtained with irradiated tum⁺ cells, even though this tumor carries TATA. But for the teratocarcinoma cell line PCC4, the protection observed is truly remarkable because this tumor does not show any immunogenicity. Not only do irradiated PCC4 cells fail to immunize, but even when living cells are injected to produce a subcutaneous tumor, which is surgically removed after three weeks, no subsequent protection is observed. Nevertheless, PCC4-derived tum⁻ variants confer a significant protection (Boon and Van Pel 1978). Thus, by immunizing with tum⁻ variants, one can obtain a rejection response directed against TATA that do not elicit a rejection response on their own.

For most weakly or nonimmunogenic tumors, a protective immunization can be obtained with living tum⁻ cells, but not with irradiated tum⁻ or tum⁺ cells. This is probably largely due to the fact that tum⁻ variants provide a way to maintain a high dose of immunogen for 10 or more days, during which time the tum⁻ cells proliferate before they are rejected. However, the results mentioned above regarding teratocarcinoma suggest that this is not the whole story, since in teratocarcinoma, a large dose of living tum⁺ cells fails to immunize. Also, we have obtained one P815 tum⁻ variant that confers protective immunity even when irradiated cells are used for immunization. The presence of a new tum⁻ antigen may therefore play a direct role in facilitating an immune response to a TATA of the tum⁺ cell. Such an associative recognition was suggested by Mitchison several years ago (Mitchison 1970, Lake and Mitchison 1976).

Since tum⁻ variants appeared to provide an efficient way to elicit an immune response against very weak TATA, it was tempting to examine whether their use could result in detection of TATA on mouse spontaneous tumors, which appear to be devoid of any immunogenicity. Tum⁻ variants have been derived from two spontaneous leukemias obtained by Hewitt in CBA/Ht mice. Some of these variants provide a significant protection against the parental tumor cell lines and also against the parental tumors that have never been adapted to culture (Van Pel et al. 1983). The protection is specific in that it applies exclusively to the parental tumor (Figure 10.4). Also, mice immunized with tum⁻ variants produce CTL directed specifically against the parental tumor. These results, which were obtained under conditions aimed at minimizing artifactual antigenicity, suggest that spontaneous tumors also carry weak TATA. The only reservation is that the spontaneous tumors used for this work had been transplanted many times. Acquisition of TATA during these transplantations cannot be excluded.

In view of the results obtained with the spontaneous tumors, it appears worthwhile to find out whether antigenic variants of human tumors could be obtained by mutagenesis and whether these variants could be used to elicit a response directed against a putative TATA on the original tumor. The possibility of obtaining tum⁻ variants in other species than the mouse has now been demonstrated by Zbar and his associates (1984), who obtained such variants by treating a guinea pig fibrosarcoma with MNNG. For human tumors, a possible scheme would be to adapt to culture tumor cells removed by surgery, clone these cells, treat them with a mutagen in vitro, clone the survivor cells, and inject a few of these clones back into the patient. Before injection, the cells would be killed by irradiation. After one or more injections, the peri-

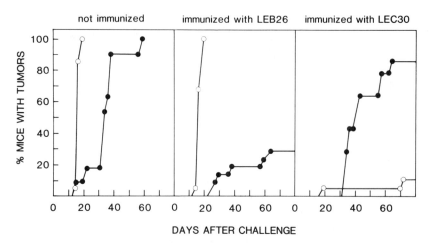

FIGURE 10.4. Challenge with spontaneous leukemias LEB(●) and LEC (○) of control mice and mice that had rejected either tum⁻ variant LEB26 derived from LEB or variant LEC30 derived from LEC.

toneal blood cells of the patients could be restimulated in mixed lymphocyte tumor cell culture conditions with the clones of mutagen-treated cells and their cytolytic activity assayed on several targets. If a group of peripheral blood lymphocytes (PBL) restimulated with one of the mutagen-treated clones showed a preferential lytic activity on that clone, this would constitute evidence for the presence of a new antigen.

We are currently studying whether this scheme can be applied to human melanoma. Initially, it appeared that the cloning of normal cells or mutagen-treated melanoma cells occurred with a very low efficiency. Also, the clones multiplied extremely slowly. However, we found that the addition of irradiated 3T3 cells markedly improved the cloning efficiency and the growth rate of the clones (Vessière et al. 1985). Because of this improvement, it is now possible to complete the cloning and mutagenesis step in less than six months. A few patients have been injected with autologous mutagen-treated melanoma cells. Hopefully, it will be possible to examine the PBL of a sufficient number of patients to find out whether tum⁻-like antigens are present on mutagen-treated human tumor cells.

REFERENCES

Boon T. 1983. Antigenic tumor cell variants obtained with mutagens. Adv Cancer Res 39:121–151.

Boon T, Kellermann O. 1977. Rejection by syngeneic mice of cell variants obtained by mutagenesis of a malignant teratocarcinoma cell line. Proc Natl Acad Sci USA 74:272–275.

Boon T, Van Pel A. 1978. Teratocarcinoma cell variants rejected by syngeneic mice: Protection of mice immunized with these variants against other variants and against the original malignant cell line. Proc Natl Acad Sci USA 75: 1519–1523

Boon T, Van Snick J, Van Pel A, Uyttenhove C, Marchand M. 1980. Immunogenic variants obtained by mutagenesis of mouse mastocytoma P815: II. T lymphocyte mediated cytolysis. J Exp Med 152:1184–1193.

Frost P, Kerbel R, Bauer E, Tartamella-Blondo R, Cefalu W. 1983. Mutagen treatment as a means for selecting immunogenic variants from otherwise poorly immunogenic malignant murine tumors. Cancer Res 43:125–132.

Gross L. 1943. Intradermal immunization of C3H mice against a sarcoma that originated in an animal of the same line. Cancer Res 3:326–333.

Hewitt HB, Blake ER, Walder A. 1976. A critique of the evidence for active host defence against cancer, based on personal studies of 27 murine tumours of spontaneous origin. Br J Cancer 33:241–259.

Hurme M, Chandler PR, Hetherington CM, Simpson E. 1978a. Cytotoxic T cell response to H-Y: Correlation with the rejection of syngeneic male skin grafts. J Exp Med 147:768–775.

Hurme M, Hetherington CM, Chandler PR, Simpson E. 1978b. Cytotoxic T cell response to H-Y mapping of the Ir genes. J Exp Med 147:758–767.

Klein G, Sjorgen H, Klein E, Hellstrom KE. 1960. Demonstration of resistance against methylcholanthrene-induced sarcomas in the primary autochthonous host. Cancer Res 20:1561–1562.

Kripke M. 1974. Antigenicity of murine skin tumors induced by ultraviolet light. JNCI 53:1333–1336.

Lake P, Mitchison NA. 1976. Regulatory mechanisms in the immune response to cell-surface antigen. Cold Spring Harbor Symp Quant Biol 41:589–595.

Maryanski J, Boon T. 1982. Immunogenic variants obtained by mutagenesis of mastocytoma P815: IV. Analysis of variant-specific antigens by selection of antigen-loss with cytolytic T cell clones. Eur J Immunol 12:406–412.

Maryanski J, Marchand M, Uyttenhove C, Boon T. 1983a. Immunogenic variants obtained by mutagenesis of mouse mastocytoma P815: VI. Occasional escape from host rejection due to antigen-loss secondary variants. Int J Cancer 31: 119–123.

Maryanski JL, Szpirer J, Szpirer C, Boon T. 1983b. Immunogenic variants obtained by mutagenesis of mouse mastocytoma P815: VII. Dominant expression of variant antigens in somatic cell hybrids. Somatic Cell Genet 9:345–357.

Maryanski J, Van Snick J, Cerottini J-C, Boon T. 1982. Immunogenic variants obtained by mutagenesis of mouse mastocytoma P815: III. Clonal analysis of the syngeneic cytolytic T lymphocyte response. Eur J Immunol 12:401–406.

Middle JG, Embleton MJ. 1981. Naturally arising tumors of the inbred WAB/Not rat strain: II. Immunogenicity of transplanted tumors. JNCI 67:637–643.

Mitchison NA. 1970. Immunologic approach to cancer. Transplant Proc 2: 92–96.

Pfreundschuh M, Shiku H, Takahashi T, et al. 1978. Serological analysis of cell surface antigens of malignant human brain tumors. Proc Natl Acad Sci USA 75:5122–5126.

Prehn R, Main J. 1957. Immunity to methylcholanthrene-induced sarcomas. JNCI 18:769–778.

Uyttenhove C, Maryanski J, Boon T. 1983. The escape of mouse mastocytoma P815 after nearly complete rejection is due to antigen-loss variants rather than immunosuppression. J Exp Med 157:1040–1052.

Uyttenhove C, Van Snick J, Boon T. 1980. Immunogenic variants obtained by mutagenesis of mouse mastocytoma P815: I. Rejection by syngeneic mice. J Exp Med 152:1175–1183.

Van Pel A, Georlette M, Boon T. 1979. Tumor cell variants obtained by mutagenesis of a Lewis lung carcinoma cell line: Immune rejection by syngeneic mice. Proc Natl Acad Sci USA 76:5282–5285.

Van Pel A, Vessière F, Boon T. 1983. Protection against two spontaneous mouse leukemias conferred by immunogenic variants obtained by mutagenesis. J Exp Med 157:1992–2001.

Van Snick J, Maryanski J, Van Pel A, Parmiani G, Boon T. 1982. Immunogenic variants obtained by mutagenesis of mouse mastocytoma P815: V. H-2 associativity of variant-specific antigens. Eur J Immunol 12:905–908.

Vessière F, Darville M, Knuth A, Boon T. 1985. Use of irradiated mouse fibroblasts to improve the cloning and adaptation to culture of human melanoma cells. Int J Cancer 35:231–235.

Vessière F, Georlette M, Warnier G, Leclerc J-C, Van Pel A, Boon T. 1982. Immunogenic variants obtained by mutagenesis of mouse Lewis lung carcinoma: Recognition of variant-specific antigens by cytolytic T lymphocytes. Eur J Cancer Clin Oncol 18:867–874.

Weinhold K, Miller D, Wheelock E. 1979. The tumor dormant state: Comparison of L5178Y cells used to establish dormancy with those that emerge after its termination. J Exp Med 149:745–757.

Zbar B, Sukumar S, Tanio Y, Terata N, Hovis J. 1984. Antigenic variants isolated from a mutagen-treated guinea pig fibrosarcoma. Cancer Res 44:5079–5085.

Symposium on Fundamental Cancer Research, Vol. 38.

11. Is the Immunotherapy of Metastasis Feasible?

Philip Frost and Robert S. Kerbel *

*Department of Cell Biology and Medicine, The University of Texas M. D. Anderson Hospital and Tumor Institute at Houston, Houston, Texas 77030, and *Department of Pathology, Queen's University, Kingston, Ontario, Canada K7L 3NJ*

Tumor immunology as an area of scientific endeavor has been associated with periods of great euphoria that have dwindled to moderate enthusiasm, only to be replaced by widespread criticism. The criticism has been based on the lack of proven effectiveness of immunotherapy and on a more serious question regarding a basic premise of tumor immunobiology, namely, whether strictly tumor-specific antigens can be definitely identified on human tumors. Without unequivocal evidence for human tumor-specific antigens, the basic tenets of tumor immunology, namely the specificity and systemic nature of immune responses, have come under serious scrutiny. The current state of pervasive cynicism regarding tumor immunology is, in our view, unwarranted and likely reflects considerable anxiety that stems from the urgent need to develop newer approaches for the therapy of neoplasia. The initial failure of broadly based immunologic approaches to tumor therapy should not deter the rational pursuit of the use of immunotherapy in the treatment of neoplasia.

Criticism of experimental tumor immunology evolved from evidence that spontaneous murine tumors elicited a weak or no immune response. This is in contrast to virally or chemically induced tumors. This observation was actually made 20 years ago (Baldwin 1966, 1973, Prehn 1963, 1976, Klein and Klein 1977) and reconfirmed more recently (Embleton and Middle 1981, Middle and Embleton 1981), but the weak response was regarded as an anomaly and not addressed. The issue of the lack of antigenicity of spontaneous tumors was, however, resurrected as a result of the publications of Hewitt et al. (1976, Hewitt 1979). After years of trying to detect tumor-specific antigens in 27 spontaneously arising murine tumors of various histologic origins, Hewitt and his coworkers could not find a single clear case of an immune response induced by any of the tumors examined. Based on these and earlier findings, they argued that the observation that virus- or carcinogen-induced tumors could induce a rejection response in the host was irrelevant to human oncology. This view undermined the basic principles that served as the foundation for specific immunotherapy.

GENERATION OF IMMUNOGENIC VARIANTS USING MUTAGENS

In 1977, Boon and Kellermann reported that the treatment of a nonimmunogenic murine teratocarcinoma with the mutagen N-methyl-N'-nitro-N-nitrosoguanidine resulted in the production of immunogenic clones at high frequency. These clones were designated as tum⁻ (subsequently designated Imm⁺ in this chapter because they are immunogenic) because of their failure to grow in normal syngeneic animals. Such clones, however, grew in immunosuppressed or nude mice (Uyttenhove et al. 1980, Maryanski et al. 1982). We subsequently confirmed these findings using a second mutagen, ethylmethane sulfonate, and eight unrelated murine tumor lines (Frost et al. 1983).

The results obtained from our studies have been consistent with those of Boon and his colleagues (1977). Imm⁺ clones were obtained from all the tumors tested, whether they were chemically induced, spontaneous, or of viral origin (Frost et al. 1983). All Imm⁺ clones were incapable of growth in syngeneic hosts but grew in immunosuppressed or nude mice. The Imm⁺ clones expressed both a unique antigen and one shared with the parent tumor and other clones from the same tumor. Van Pel and Boon (1982) clearly demonstrated this and were able to produce long-term T cell lines that were either specific for an individual Imm⁺ clone or for the shared antigen. Those cytotoxic T lymphocyte (CTL) lines specific for an individual clone were not cross-reactive with any other clone. CTL lines directed toward the common antigen were able to destroy numerous clones and the parent population. The coexistence on the same cell of the public (common antigen) and the new, mutagen-induced private antigen conferred upon the Imm⁺ clone an unusual ability to generate potent CTL responses that resulted in tumor regression. This phenomenon represents an extraordinary manifestation of tumor cell xenogenesis, for these clones behave as major histocompatibility complex (MHC)–incompatible allografted tumors, despite their rejection by strictly syngeneic hosts.

We found, as did Boon and his colleagues (1977), that preinjection of syngeneic hosts with Imm⁺ clones protected the animals against normally lethal doses of the parent tumor. They were also able to protect the mice against a lethal challenge from a spontaneous murine tumor they obtained from H. B. Hewitt. The immune protection provided by the Imm⁺ clones was specific for the tumor of origin. Imm⁺ MDAY-D2 clones (of DBA/2 mice) did not protect against a challenge with an unrelated DBA/2 tumor, such as the P815 mastocytoma, and Imm⁺ clones of P815 did not protect against a challenge with MDAY-D2 clones (Frost et al. 1983). The CTL responses generated by Imm⁺

clones were also not cross-reactive. Our results also indicated that most Imm $^+$ clones were not stable and reverted to the Imm $^-$ phenotype. This was likely a result of the loss or suppression of the expression of both copies of the genes coding for either the common or the specific antigen. Maryanski and Boon (1982) demonstrated that Imm $^-$ revertants were antigen-loss variants.

Multiple mutagen treatments appeared to enhance both the selection and stability of Imm $^+$ clones. Multiple mutagen treatments in association with selection for drug resistance also enhanced the selection of Imm $^+$ variants (Frost et al. 1983).

By generating Imm $^+$ variants from poorly or nonmetastatic tumors we were able to expand on experiments we had attempted several years earlier. At that time we had addressed the question of whether a near optimal immune response could affect the growth of established metastases. We designed a non-H2 allogeneic model to test whether a near optimal immune response could be used to eradicate metastases (Wiltrout et al. 1980, Wiltrout and Frost 1980). BALB/c mice were injected with 5×10^5 DBA/2 MDAY-D2 tumor cells. The animals were killed 14 days later; their spleens contained CTL moderately reactive with MDAY-D2 cells (functional (F) CTL). F-CTL and normal BALB/c spleen cells were then used to adoptively immunize nude mice that had been injected subcutaneously (s.c.) with 10^4 MDAY-D2 cells 12–15 days earlier. The nude mice underwent laparotomy on day 11 to document the existence of metastasis prior to cell transfer on day 12. All animals were then observed for six months, and some were sacrificed during that time to obtain histologic specimens from the liver. All control nude mice died by day 25. The nude mice whose immune systems were reconstituted with normal or immune spleen cells survived with no evidence of tumor at six months. Histologic examination confirmed a progressive infiltrate of lymphocytes around the tumor metastases and the subsequent rejection of the tumor. These experiments proved that an adequate immune response could in fact successfully remove a large and disseminated tumor load.

THE ROLE OF SUPPRESSOR CELLS

In our initial studies with the MDAY-D2 tumor, we noted that syngeneic DBA/2 mice challenged s.c. with MDAY-D2 cells produced no detectable CTL response, unless the draining peripheral lymph node cells were restimulated in vitro with mitomycin C–treated tumor cells (Frost et al. 1982). In contrast, tumor-bearing spleen cells were only marginally responsive on day 8 after tumor challenge. We, therefore, designed a series of experiments to determine whether the evanescent spleen cell response was due to the presence of suppressor T cells in the spleens of tumor-bearing animals (Frost et al. 1982). We found from these studies that spleen cells from tumor-bearing animals abrogate the in vitro generation of CTL from primed peripheral lymph

TABLE 11.1. Adoptive Immunotherapy of MDAY-D2 Metastases

Group	Number of Animals	Type of Treatment	Survival Time in Days				Survival at	
			25	35	45	60	45 Days (%)	60 Days (%)
1	40	NONE (CONTROLS)	3	1	0	0	0	0
2	24	SURG	2	1	0	0	0	0
3	24	CY	21	5	0	0	0	0
4	25	F-CTL ALONE	2	0	0	0	0	0
5	24	SURG + F-CTL	3	2	0	0	0	0
6	54	SURG + CY	38	22	14	0	26	0
7	35	SURG + CY + IL 2	34	25	18	2	51	6
8	50	SURG, CY, NSC	48	31	21	9	42	18
9	42	SURG, CY, M-CTL	41	30	26	22	62	52
10	22	SURG, CY, F-CTL	22	19	13	9	59	41
11	20	SURG, CY, NSC + M-CTL	20	15	12	8	60	40
12	27	SURG, CY, NSC + M-CTL + IL 2	27	22	15	14	56	52
13	24	SURG, CY, F-CTL + M-CTL	24	9	4	0	17	0
14	10	SURG, CY, F-CTL + M-CTL + IL 2	5	4	2	0	20	0
15	27	SURG, CY, M-CTL + IL 2	27	22	12	8	44	30
16	15	SURG, CY + ACTIVE IMM	15	13	11	9	73	60
17	15	SURG, CY + ACTIVE IMM + IL 2	15	6	4	0	27	0

DBA/2 mice were injected s.c. with 2×10^3 MDAY-D2 cells on day 0. Ten days later, the primary tumor was resected (except in Groups 1, 3, and 4) and each animal was given a single dose of 100 mg/kg cyclophosphamide on day 11 (except in Groups 1, 4, and 5). One day later, the groups received either adoptive or active immunization as described.

SURG = surgical removal of the primary tumor; CY = cyclophosphamide; F-CTL = In vitro–activated CTL; IL 2 = interleukin 2 (given intraperitoneally in gelatin); NSC = normal spleen cells; M-CTL = spleen cells from an animal that had rejected an Imm+ tumor clone.

node cells from the same animal and that this suppression is mediated by splenic T cells with the LY23$^+$ phenotype. The suppressor T cell effect was only observed if tumor-bearing splenic T cells were added before beginning 48 hours of in vitro culture of responding peripheral lymph node cells. We also found that tumor-bearing spleen cells did not suppress the mitogen responsiveness of normal cells. Animals bearing unrelated syngeneic tumors did not generate suppressor T cells capable of suppressing peripheral lymph node cells of MDAY-D2 tumor–bearing mice nor did MDAY-D2 suppressor T cells affect the in vitro response to the P815 mastocytoma. These data provided a basis for our use of cyclophosphamide as a means of inhibiting the suppressor T cell response to the MDAY-D2 tumor in the immunotherapy protocols described below.

SYNGENEIC MODEL

With the knowledge that the immune response can cope with disseminated tumor and our awareness of the role of suppressor T cells in the response to the MDAY-D2 tumor, we designed experiments that would make use of this information in conjunction with the availability of Imm$^+$ clones. Our protocols were directed toward the treatment of established metastases rather than the primary tumor so as to mimic clinical neoplasia more closely. Our protocol, therefore, included s.c. injections of tumor cells followed by resection of the primary tumor 10 days later. Animals were then treated with cyclophosphamide to inhibit suppressor T cell activity and were either adoptively or passively immunized.

Treatments for the control animals are shown in Table 11.1 (groups 1–7). The experimental groups included animals adoptively immunized with three different sources of lymphoid cells. The first source was F-CTL. These cells were actively cytotoxic at the time of adoptive transfer, that is, they had been activated in vitro with mitomycin C–treated tumor cells. The second source of lymphoid cells was memory CTL (M-CTL), which were derived from the spleens of animals immunized with an Imm$^+$ clone four to six weeks earlier. No active CTL could be detected in this population de novo, but F-CTL could be derived if the cells were restimulated in vitro (Frost P unpublished data). The final source was normal spleen cells removed from normal DBA/2 mice that had no exposure to tumor.

The results of these studies are shown in Table 11.1. There is little doubt that every single modality used alone failed to prolong survival significantly. The use of surgery in conjunction with cyclophosphamide was partially effective, but ultimately failed. We believe this happened because of the sensitivity of MDAY-D2 to the direct chemotherapeutic effect of cyclophosphamide. With this in mind, we performed several experiments (not shown in Table 11.1) in which we repeatedly treated animals bearing MDAY-

D2 with 100 mg/kg of cyclophosphamide, beginning one week after tumor challenge and then every three to five days. While life was prolonged somewhat, all animals died by day 35. Animals in whom the primary tumors were surgically resected and who received multiple cyclophosphamide injections had a mean survival comparable to those receiving a single cyclophosphamide injection. Whether this was due to the rapid development of drug resistance is not known.

What is clear from these preliminary studies is that adoptive immunotherapy can produce a reasonable percentage of "cures" in animals appropriately treated. We use the term "cure" only to mean that the animals surviving at day 60 appeared healthy, and when they were killed, they had no evidence of tumor. This was not always the case, for at day 60, all animals in group 7 and 8 had liver metastases, but these were larger and less dispersed than generally seen. Groups 9–12 had 20, 7, 13, and 12 animals free of tumor at day 60. Animals in group 15 were inadvertently destroyed without assessing the extent of their tumors.

It appears, from these preliminary studies, that M-CTL in conjunction with surgery and cyclophosphamide is, so far, the most successful regimen. However, we would stress several key points about these studies. The tumor used, MDAY-D2, is likely one of the most virulent murine tumors known. As few as 10 cells will kill an animal in 35 days after s.c. injection. The surgical resection of the primary injection site in as few as three days after challenge with 2×10^3 cells is insufficient to prevent metastases, and death occurs in 25 days. The fact that we achieved any success in treating this tumor is remarkable and, in our view, speaks well for the use of such protocols in the treatment of less aggressive tumors. We stress, also, that while we report survival data, our interest is in developing a means for curing the animals. Future experiments will, therefore, be observed for longer periods. These data are insufficient, however, for assessing the effectiveness of interleukin 2 as an adjunct to immunotherapy. The use of this lymphokine must be further analyzed. Finally, we point out that the rationale for using combinations of M-CTL and F-CTL with or without normal spleen cells remains logical. Our view is that F-CTL may have an acute effect (suppressor T cells do not affect F-CTL), while M-CTL and normal spleen cells are activated in vivo. We plan, therefore, to continue such therapy in conjunction with active immunization.

T CELL RESISTANCE AND ANTIGEN-LOSS VARIANTS

Because of evidence that tumor cells can become resistant to CTL (Fidler and Bucana 1977, Fidler 1978), we designed a series of experiments to determine if we could select a population of MDAY-D2 cells resistant to CTL generated by the MDW1 Imm$^+$ variants (Table 11.2). MDAY-D2 parent cells were exposed to CTL generated from in vivo MDW1-primed DBA/2 spleen cells,

TABLE 11.2. *Cytotoxic T Lymphocyte Resistance of MDAY-D2 Cells*

Treatment Number	Cytotoxicity (%)
1	98
2	94
3	96
4	78
5	42
6	86
7	94
8	64
9	96
10	28
11	53
12	58
13	69
14	30
15	62
16	48
17	54

MDAY-D2 cells were treated with CTL generated by the MDW1 Imm$^+$ variants. Cells surviving each treatment were retreated and assessed for their CTL sensitivity.

which were restimulated in vitro with mitomycin C–treated MDW1 cells. The MDAY-D2 cells were plated in duplicate sets; one set had radiolabeled MDAY-D2 cells and the other did not. The percentage of cytotoxicity was assessed using the radiolabeled cells. The unlabeled cells were then allowed to regrow and were subsequently used as the source of target cells in repeat CTL experiments. In all repeat experiments, previously untreated MDAY-D2 cells were used as controls. These results indicate that while there is a general trend for decreased sensitivity to CTL, most cells remain sensitive. However, we recognize the likelihood of developing antigen-loss variants and all new protocols currently include, first, the use of M-CTL sensitized to at least five individual Imm$^+$ clones. Second, they include the use of macrophage activation as an adjunct to therapy. These latter studies are based on the reports of Fidler et al. (1982), who demonstrated that the activation of macrophages by liposome-encapsulated MDP is an effective means for treating metastases. Our goal, therefore, is to use CTL as a debulking procedure followed by macrophage activation aimed at destroying putative antigen-loss variants. Finally, similar combinations of immunotherapy with chemotherapy will also be attempted.

In summary, evidence from a syngeneic murine model indicates that mutagen-induced Imm⁺ variants can be effective in generating an immune response capable of destroying metastases. In recognizing the limitations of a single-modality therapy for heterogeneous metastases, we have incorporated other means of treatment, such as surgical removal of the primary tumor, in our protocols. Future protocols will utilize additional combinations of treatments in our efforts to eradicate metastases.

ACKNOWLEDGMENT

The authors wish to thank Ms. Elaine Bauer and Ms. Rosalie Tartamella-Blondo for their excellent technical assistance.

This investigation was supported by grant number CA 28060 awarded by the National Cancer Institute, United States Department of Health and Human Services. Robert S. Kerbel is a Research Scholar of the National Cancer Institute of Canada.

REFERENCES

Baldwin RW. 1966. Tumour-specific immunity against spontaneous rat tumours. Int J Cancer 1:257–264.

Baldwin RW. 1973. Immunological aspects of chemical carcinogenesis. Adv Cancer Res 18:1–75.

Boon T, Kellermann O. 1977. Rejection by syngeneic mice of all variants obtained by mutagenesis of a malignant teratocarcinoma line. Proc Natl Acad Sci USA 74:272–275.

Embleton MJ, Middle JG. 1981. Immune responses to naturally occurring rat sarcomas. Br J Cancer 43:44–52.

Fidler IJ. 1978. Recognition and destruction of target cells by tumoricidal macrophages. Isr J Med Sci 14:177–191.

Fidler IJ, Bucana C. 1977. Mechanism of tumor cell resistance to lysis by syngeneic lymphocytes. Cancer Res 37:3945–3956.

Fidler IJ, Barnes Z, Fogler WE, Kirsh R, Bugelski P, Poste G. 1982. Involvement of macrophages in the eradication of established metastases following intravenous injection of liposomes containing macrophage activators. Cancer Res 42:496–502.

Frost P, Prete P, Kerbel RS. 1982. Eradication of the in vitro generation of the cytotoxic T cell response to a metastatic murine tumor: The role of suppressor T cells. Int J Cancer 30:211–218.

Frost P, Kerbel RS, Bauer E, Tartamella-Blondo R, Cefalu W. 1983. Mutagen treatment as a means for selecting immunogenic variants from otherwise poorly immunogenic malignant tumors. Cancer Res 43:125–132.

Hewitt HB. 1979. A critical examination of the foundations of immunotherapy of cancer. Clin Radiol 30:361–369.

Hewitt HB, Blade ER, Walder AS. 1976. A critique of the evidence for active host defense against cancer based on personal studies of 27 murine tumors of spontaneous origin. Br J Cancer 33:241–259.

Klein G, Klein E. 1977. Rejectability of virus-induced tumors and non-rejectability of spontaneous tumors: A lesson in contrasts. Transplant Proc 9:1095–1104.

Maryanski JL, Boon T. 1982. Immunogenic variants obtained by mutagenesis of mouse mastocytoma P815: IV. Analysis of variant-specific antigens by selection of antigen-loss variants with cytolytic T cell clones. Eur J Immunol 12: 406–412.

Maryanski JL, Van Snick J, Gerottini JC, Boon T. 1982. Immunogenic variants obtained by mutagenesis of mouse mastocytoma P815: III. Clonal analysis of the syngeneic cytolytic T lymphocyte response. Eur J Immunol 12:401–406.

Middle JG, Embleton MJ. 1981. Naturally arising tumors of the inbred WAB/Not rat strain: II. Immunity of transplanted tumors. JNCI 67:637–643.

Prehn RT. 1963. The role of immune mechanisms in the biology of physically induced tumors. Symp Fundam Cancer Res 16:475–485.

Prehn RT. 1976. Tumor progression and homeostasis. Adv Cancer Res 23: 203–236.

Uyttenhove C, Van Snick J, Boon T. 1980. Immunogenic variants obtained by mutagenesis of mouse mastocytoma P815: I. Rejection by syngeneic mice. J Exp Med 152:1175–1183.

Van Pel A, Boon T. 1982. Protection against a non-immunogenic mouse leukemia by an immunogenic variant obtained by mutagenesis. Proc Natl Acad Sci USA 79:4718–4722.

Wiltrout RH, Frost P. 1980. Cell-mediated cytotoxic responses induced in vivo and in vitro by a metastatic murine tumor. J Immunol 124:2254–2263.

Wiltrout RH, Frost P, Morrison MK. 1980. Immune regression of visceral metastases in athymic mice: Correlation of "low level" in vitro cell-mediated cytotoxic reactions with allograft rejection in vivo. Transplantation 29:283–286.

IMMUNOLOGIC EFFECTOR
MECHANISMS

Symposium on Fundamental Cancer Research, Vol. 38.
© 1986 by The University of Texas System Cancer Center.

12. The Complexity of Unique Tumor-Specific Antigens

Richard D. Wortzel, Hans J. Stauss, Carter Van Waes, and Hans Schreiber*

Department of Pathology, The University of Chicago, La Rabida-University of Chicago Institute, Chicago, Illinois 60649

Investigating the identity and character of tumor antigens has been a great challenge in research. Knowledge of such structures would appear to be fundamental to gaining an understanding of tumor biology and immunology. Historically, the search for tumor antigens focused on identifying antigens common to all cancers, but absent from normal cells. Although such "common" tumor antigens have not yet been detected, these earlier studies led to the most important discoveries of transplantation and differentiation molecules that are present on normal cells (for review, see Old 1982). It also became evident from this work that many tumors, particularly those induced by physical or chemical carcinogens, express antigens uniquely specific for an individual tumor, even when the tumors are of the same histologic type and genetic origin and are induced by the same carcinogen. In fact, a seemingly endless diversity of such tumor-specific antigens has been detected, the extent of which has been compared to that of immune receptors (Burnet 1970). Tumor-specific antigens were classically defined by transplant rejection experiments (Gross 1943, Foley 1953, Baldwin 1955, Prehn and Main 1957, Klein et al. 1960). It is apparent that further characterization of such structures was to a large extent limited by the lack of reliable and permanent tumor-specific probes (Klein 1978). As a result, very little is presently known about the nature and complexity of tumor-specific antigens on any single tumor. Not only are we unaware of the molecular composition and genetic origin of these structures, but even the structural complexity of the tumor antigen is poorly understood, i.e., if one or more antigens are expressed on a single tumor cell. With the recent discovery of monoclonal antibodies (Kohler and Milstein 1975) and cloned T cell lines (Gillis and Smith 1977), a careful dissection of unique tumor-specific antigens should be possible.

The murine ultraviolet (UV) light-induced tumor model (Kripke 1981) ap-

---

*Address all correspondence and reprint requests to Dr. Schreiber.

pears to be a particularly well-suited system for the study of tumor-specific antigens. UV radiation is a major etiologic factor in the pathogenesis of skin cancer (Emmett 1973), and excellent examples of immunosurveillance mechanisms have been observed with UV-induced tumors in mice (Kripke 1981) and also in man (Hardie et al. 1980, Penn 1980). The antigenicity of such tumors is advantageous to study for a number of reasons. First, strong tumor-specific transplantation antigens are expressed on murine UV-induced fibrosarcomas (Kripke 1977). Many of these highly immunogenic tumors cannot be transplanted into normal syngeneic immunocompetent hosts yet grow regularly in immunodeficient or immunosuppressed mice (Kripke 1977, Daynes and Spellman 1977, Flood et al. 1980). In contrast, many other experimental tumors, such as those often studied by early investigators, can be transplanted repeatedly into normal syngeneic hosts. It is quite possible that these earlier studies in tumor immunology were limited by this successive transplantation, since recent studies indicate that cancers can rapidly lose antigenic surface markers as a result of immunoselection of variants by the host immune response (Weinhold et al. 1979, Bosslet and Schirrmacher 1981, Urban et al. 1982a, Urban and Schreiber 1983, Uyttenhove et al. 1983). Because of the high immunogenicity of UV-induced tumors, acquisition of such tumors in their original state is almost a necessity in order to preserve the antigenicity that is to be characterized. It is therefore very important that the UV-induced tumors we studied were never passaged through immunocompetent hosts, and many have been preserved as original tumors without passage in vitro or in vivo. The reason why UV-induced tumors are so highly immunogenic is not completely understood. Studies suggest that it may result from UV-induced systemic immunosuppression (Fisher and Kripke 1977, Daynes and Spellman 1977, Roberts and Daynes 1980, Kripke 1981), as well as the immunoincompetence present in the aging UV-irradiated mice that develop the tumors (Spellman and Daynes 1978a, Flood et al. 1981).

Another advantage of the UV-induced tumor system is that many tumors are available that have been induced in pathogen-free mice of defined genetic background. With the aid of such controls, a tumor's unique specificity can be established, and any genetic drift of the responding inbred animal population (Bailey 1982) could be detected were it to occur. Antigens common to all tumors induced by UV radiation have also been suggested, and such antigens are believed to be involved with UV-induced specific immunosuppression (Spellman and Daynes 1978b, Kripke et al. 1979). However, because monoclonal probes, particularly T cell lines (Wortzel et al. 1983a,b), are available only to the unique tumor-specific antigens of UV-induced tumors, more information is currently known about the characterization of these specific structures. Therefore, the focus of this chapter will be a discussion of unique tumor-specific antigens. Specifically, we will describe the unique antigenicity of the UV-induced 1591-RE tumor. The 1591-RE is a highly immunogenic tumor that routinely regresses in normal syngeneic mice. By selectively suppressing the immune response to this tumor, it was demonstrated that host resistance depends on the generation of idiotypically restricted T cells specifically reactive to 1591-RE (Flood et al. 1980, Flood et al. 1981). Other experiments found that 1591-RE–specific T cells do not recognize variants of 1591-RE that grow progressively in normal mice (Urban et al. 1982a), and recently, it was shown that antigen-loss variants of 1591-RE that were selected in vitro with 1591-RE–specific cytolytic T cells grow progressively in the normal host (Wortzel et al. 1984). These studies indicate the importance of a tumor-specific antigen and tumor-specific T cells in the host rejection of the 1591-RE tumor.

MULTIPLICITY OF TUMOR-SPECIFIC ANTIGENS ON A SINGLE TUMOR CELL

The UV-induced 1591-RE tumor elicits a tumor-specific cytolytic T cell response in syngeneic mice (Flood et al. 1980). As mentioned above, these 1591-RE–specific T cells do not recognize host-selected progressor variants of 1591-RE (1591-PRO) (Urban et al. 1982a). An initial indication of the potential complexity of the 1591-RE tumor antigen came from the finding that cytolytic T cells generated against 1591-PRO recognized not only 1591-PRO but also the parental regressor tumor (Urban et al. 1984). One explanation for this finding was that the "antigen" expressed on the regressor parental 1591-RE tumor consisted of two antigens, one of which was retained on the host-selected progressor variants. We recently characterized the complexity of the 1591-RE antigen with the aid of tumor-specific cytolytic T cell lines and antigen-loss tumor variants (Wortzel et al. 1983a,b). The following general approach was used (Figure 12.1). First, tumor-specific cytolytic T cell lines were generated by immunizing syngeneic mice with the parental tumor. A 1591-RE–specific T cell clone (anti-A) was then isolated and used to select in vitro for antigen-loss variants of the 1591-RE tumor that did not express the A antigen (A^- variants). To determine if additional 1591-RE–specific antigens were retained by the A^- variants, these variants were used as immunogens in syngeneic mice. Upon finding a retained antigen (B) on the A^- variants, a second T cell line was generated and used to select in vitro for loss of the B antigen. By continuing this cycle of immunization, T cell line generation and variant selection, a C antigen and a D antigen were identified. Thus, the antigenicity of the 1591-RE tumor appeared to be a complex structure composed of multiple antigens. By comparing the phenotypes of five antigen-loss variants of 1591-RE (1591-V1 to 1591-V5) that express different combinations of these antigens, it is apparent that each of the multiple antigens is expressed

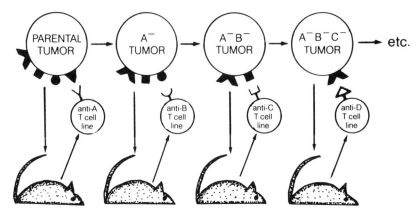

FIGURE 12.1. General approach to dissect a complex tumor-specific antigen. The antigenicity of the parental tumor is characterized by the sequential selection of antigen-loss tumor variants with tumor-specific cytolytic T lymphocyte (CTL) lines. First, a CTL line (anti-A) is generated against a parental tumor and used to select in vitro for an A⁻ tumor variant. A second mouse is immunized with the A⁻ variant to generate a second CTL line (anti-B), which is used to select in vitro for an A⁻B⁻ variant. Continuing cycles of immunization, CTL-line generation, and antigen-loss variant selection lead to the identification of additional antigens (C and D, etc.).

independently of each other (Figure 12.2). Because the 1591-RE subline 1591-RE1 was completely eliminated by each cytolytic T cell line, we showed that all four antigens could be simultaneously expressed on the same tumor cell. In addition, all of the antigens appeared to be uniquely specific for the 1591-RE lineage, since the antigen-specific cytolytic T cell lines failed to lyse a panel of unrelated syngeneic UV-induced tumors, as well as several methylcholanthrene-induced tumors and a normal syngeneic fibroblast line (Figure 12.3).

We are currently determining if additional antigens exist on the 1591-RE tumor that are recognized by cytolytic T cells, as well as identifying antigens recognized by helper T cells or possibly suppressor T cells. We have recently detected a fifth unique antigen on 1591-RE (E) that is recognized by cytolytic T cells (Wortzel RD unpublished data), indicating that other unique antigens may still be expressed on the 1591-RE tumor. Also, the A antigen has been further dissected and appears to be composed of three independent tumor-specific components (see section "Molecular Characterization of Tumor-Specific Antigens on UV-Induced Tumors"). Using a limiting dilution assay for interleukin (IL) 2 releasing helper T cells, a unique tumor-specific antigen that is distinct from the antigens recognized by the cytolytic T cells has been identified on all cells of the 1591-RE lineage (Van Waes C unpublished data). A similar antigen has also been observed in vivo using a protocol to detect

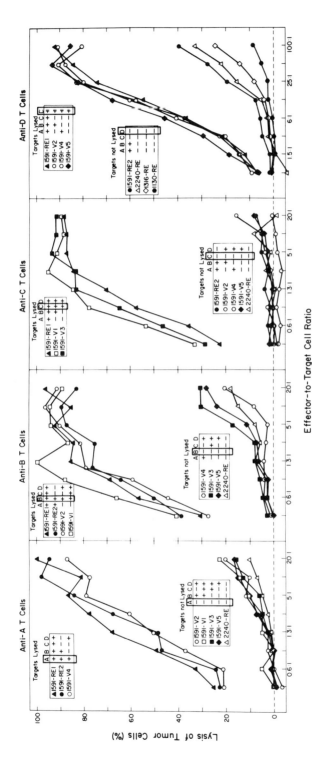

FIGURE 12.2. Multiplicity and independence of the 1591-RE–specific antigens as demonstrated by immunoselected antigen-loss variants and cytolytic T cells. Anti-A, anti-B, anti-C, and anti-D T cells were used as effectors against the indicated tumor target cells in a chromium 51 (^{51}Cr) release assay. 1591-V1 to 1591-V5 are antigen-loss tumor variants of 1591-RE selected in vitro with the tumor-specific cytolytic T cell lines (for details see Wortzel et al. 1983a). 2240-RE, 1316-RE and 1130-RE are unrelated syngeneic UV-induced fibrosarcomas. (Reproduced from Wortzel et al. 1983a with permission from MacMillan Journals Limited).

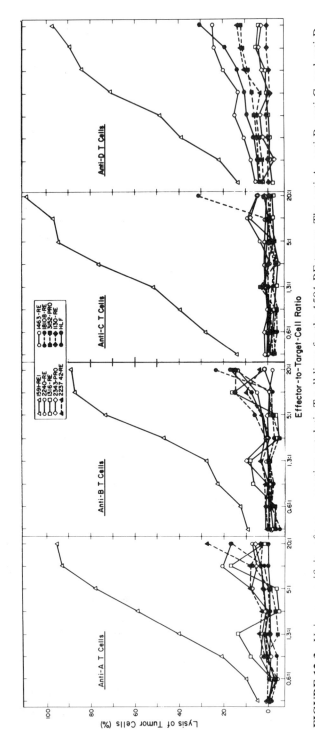

FIGURE 12.3. Unique specificity of tumor-reactive cytolytic T cell lines for the 1591-RE tumor. The anti-A, anti-B, anti-C, and anti-D T cells were used as effectors against the indicated sygeneic tumor targets in a ^{51}Cr release assay. All tumor targets were induced by UV irradiation except for 1130-RE and 3152-PRO, which were induced by 3-methylcholanthrene. HLF is an normal syngeneic fibroblast line. (Reproduced from Wortzel et al. 1983a with permission from MacMillan Journals Limited).

delayed-type hypersensitivity (DTH) responses (Van Waes C unpublished data). Efforts are currently being made to generate monoclonal probes to this "helper" antigen. In addition to antigens uniquely expressed on the 1591-RE tumor, we have identified two other antigens that are recognized by either macrophages or natural killer cells; these latter antigens are independently expressed on the tumor surface yet are not specific for the 1591-RE tumor (Urban et al. 1982a, Urban and Schreiber 1983). Thus, the antigenicity of the 1591-RE tumor is far more complex than previously anticipated, and our current understanding of this antigenicity is diagramed in Figure 12.4.

The expression of multiple tumor-specific antigens on a single tumor raises the possibility of an endless variety of unique antigens on a single cell. In this light, African trypanosomes express an enormous variety of surface antigens, although these antigens are not expressed simultaneously. It is interesting that the antigenic expression of the trypanosome appears to be affected by the environment, since upon each reinfection a particular antigen is always initially reexpressed followed by a somewhat predictable sequence of antigenic variation (Borst and Cross 1982). Thus, although the antigenicity of the 1591-RE tumor appears very stable (Wortzel et al. 1983a,b), we cannot exclude the possibility that certain environmental influences may cause the reappearance of previous "lost" antigens or the expression of new antigens. A similar multiplicity of unique tumor-specific antigens has not yet been described for other tumors, although Maryanski and Boon (1982) have shown that multiple independent tumor-associated antigens can be artificially introduced in vitro into a poorly immunogenic tumor by chemical mutagenesis of the malignant cells.

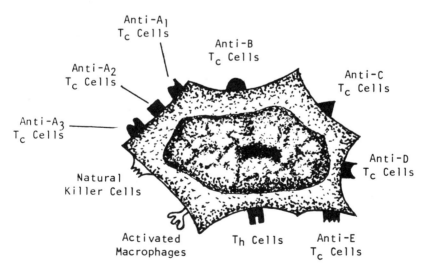

FIGURE 12.4. Multiple independent target sites on the 1591-RE tumor (for details see text).

The unique specificity of the multiple antigens for this P815 tumor, however, is somewhat difficult to assess owing to the unavailability of critical control tumor cells, i.e., control cells of similar tissue origin derived at the same time and in the same mouse strain as the tumor under investigation. Clearly, dissecting the antigenicity of a number of other tumors, both animal and human, is needed to determine how frequently multiple antigens are expressed on a single tumor.

RELEVANCE OF EACH OF THE MULTIPLE ANTIGENS IN TUMOR REJECTION

Although multiple tumor-specific antigens can be expressed on a tumor, these antigens may or may not be relevant for tumor rejection. It is conceivable, for example, that such antigens may not be targets of host rejection because they are poorly immunogenic, hidden on the cell surface, or induce some suppressor regulatory mechanism; in the last case, the resulting response may actually adversely affect rejection. One approach to determine the relevant transplantation antigens of a tumor cell is to evaluate antigenic expression before and after the tumor is passed through an immunocompetent host. Using this approach, it has been shown in a number of tumor systems, including UV-induced tumors, that cells that escape the immune defenses of the normal immunocompetent host (Bosslet and Schirrmacher 1981, Urban et al. 1982a, Urban and Schreiber 1983, Uyttenhove et al. 1983) or tumor-immune host (Weinhold et al. 1979) regularly consist of phenotypically altered variants. Such host-selected antigenic changes should represent "fingerprints" of immunologic selection pressure, and the study of these fingerprints may, therefore, give insight into the relative importance of different immune defense mechanisms operating in the host. A major shortcoming of this approach, however, is that one can only observe those changes for which probes are available. For example, with the recent application of a macrophage sensitivity assay, it was realized that progressor variants of the 1591-RE tumor not only lost a tumor-specific antigen, but also regularly became more resistant to activated macrophages (Urban and Schreiber 1983). Other unexpected changes may have also occurred, but at present remain undetected because of the unavailability of particular analytic probes. In addition, it is conceivable that several observed changes may merely be coincidental and not essential for allowing tumor escape.

We have, therefore, recently taken a different approach to study the phenotypic changes involved in allowing potentially malignant cells to grow progressively in the normal host (Wortzel et al. 1984). This approach entailed selection in vitro with cytolytic T cell lines for antigen-loss tumor variants of the regressor 1591-RE tumor and then testing the growth behavior of these variants in vivo. The intent of this protocol was to acquire tumor variants with well-defined antigenic changes such that a switch from the regressor to a progressor phenotype upon loss of a certain antigen would suggest the relevance of that antigen in tumor rejection. Two cloned tissue culture cell lines of the 1591-RE tumor, 1591-RE1 and 1591-RE2, were used for variant selection; these two lines had been independently adapted from solid tumor fragments of the fifth or first transplant generations of 1591-RE, respectively. Both 1591-RE1 and 1591-RE2 regress when transplanted into syngeneic mice; however, 1591-RE1 expresses all of the four currently defined 1591-RE–specific antigens (A, B, C, and D), while 1591-RE2 expresses only the A and B antigens (Wortzel et al. 1983a). Therefore, 1591-RE2 seemed most suitable to evaluate the individual contribution of the A and B antigens in tumor rejection, since it did not express the C and D antigens. Variants of 1591-RE2 were first selected in vitro for loss of the A or B antigens with the anti-A or anti-B cytolytic T cell lines (called AS and BS variants, respectively). The selection process was apparently specific, since all of the six variants that were selected for loss of the A antigen specifically did not express the A antigen, and all of the six variants selected for loss of the B antigen did not express the B antigen (Table 12.1). Interestingly, reactivity with the anti-C and anti-D T cell lines was observed with several of these variants, although these antigens were not detected in the parental 1591-RE2 tumor population. This unexpected reactivity will be discussed below.

The 1591-RE variants that specifically lost either the A or B antigens were then tested for their growth behavior in vivo. This was done by first growing the tissue culture cells to a solid tumor in congenic nude mice, and then challenging 5- to 10-week-old syngeneic mice subcutaneously in each inguinal area with two 2-mm^3 fragments of the solid tumor. This approach ensured that the tumor variants that were selected in vitro had not lost the capability of growing progressively in the immunodeficient host. Table 12.1 shows that four out of the six AS variants grew progressively. This growth behavior was in contrast to that of the regressor parental tumor. Selection for loss of the B antigen, however, did not affect growth in vivo, since all of the six BS variants regressed when transplanted into normal mice. Similarly, all 10 of the random clones of the parental 1591-RE2 tumor (SUB1 to SUB10) were rejected by the normal hosts. Therefore, expression of the A antigen was always associated with regression while its absence allowed the tumor to grow progressively in four out of six cases. In contrast, expression of the B and D antigens did not prevent malignant growth, since these antigens were present on the four AS variants that grew progressively in normal mice. Additional experiments using this same approach demonstrated the importance of the C antigen in the rejection of 1591-RE (Wortzel et al. 1984) and therefore may explain why one of the two AS variants, AS2 ($A^-B^+C^+D^+$), was still regressive after loss of the A antigen.

Thus, the selective loss of certain of the multiple antigens expressed on the

TABLE 12.1. *1591-Variants Selected In Vitro for Loss of the A Antigen*

Derivation	Designation	A	B	C	D	Tumor Incidence (%)[†]
Parental	1591-RE2	+	+	−	−	1/300 (0)
Anti-A selected	AS1	−	+	−	+	7/7 (100)
	2	−	+	+	+	0/7 (0)
	3	−	+	−	+	5/7 (71)
	4	−	+	−	+	7/7 (100)
	5	−	+	−	+	7/7 (100)
	6	−	+	−	−	0/7 (0)
Anti-B selected	BS1	+	−	−	−	0/5 (0)
	2	+	−	−	ND	0/5 (0)
	3	+	−	−	ND	0/7 (0)
	4	+	−	−	ND	0/5 (0)
	5	+	−	−	ND	0/5 (0)
	6	+	−	−	ND	0/5 (0)
Randomly selected	SUB1	+	+	−	ND	0/7 (0)
	2	+	+	−	ND	0/7 (0)
	3	+	+	−	ND	0/6 (0)
	4	+	+	−	ND	0/6 (0)
	5	+	ND	−	ND	0/7 (0)
	6	+	ND	−	ND	0/7 (0)
	7	+	ND	−	ND	0/7 (0)
	8	+	ND	−	ND	0/7 (0)
	9	+	ND	−	ND	0/7 (0)
	10	+	ND	−	ND	0/7 (0)

Reproduced from Wortzel et al. 1984 with permission from the National Academy of Sciences of the United States of America.
*Expression of the A, B, C and D antigens as determined by cytolysis of the designated tumor cells with the anti-A, anti-B, anti-C, and anti-D T cell lines.
[†]Number of mice with progressively growing tumors six weeks after tumor challenge/number of mice challenged. Parentheses indicate the percentage of mice with progressively growing tumors. All animals that had tumors at six weeks eventually died because of progressive tumor growth.
ND = not done.

1591-RE tumor was sufficient to allow this potentially malignant tumor to grow progressively in normal syngeneic mice. To critically evaluate the relevance of each of the 1591-RE antigens, it was necessary that the antigen-loss variants expressed well-defined antigenic changes. Several findings indicated this. First, we have shown that each T cell line selected only for loss of the appropriate antigen and never for loss of the other T cell–recognized antigens (Wortzel et al. 1984) or for loss of other cell surface structures such as H-2 K or D (Wortzel et al. 1983a). In addition, the tumor's sensitivity to other purported defense cells against cancer, such as activated macrophages or natural killer cells, was not affected by the selection process (Wortzel et al. 1984); this is in contrast to the progressor variants, selected in vivo by the host, that display a decreased sensitivity to activated macrophages (Urban and Schreiber 1983). Although we describe antigenic changes that appear to be well defined, we cannot exclude the possibility that during selection in vitro, other antigens not yet identified were concomitantly lost along with the T cell–recognized antigens.

In contrast to antigenic changes that were appropriate and anticipated, several variants unexpectedly expressed antigens that were not detected on the population from which the variants were selected. For example, AS2 (C$^+$) was selected from 1591-RE2 (C$^-$), and the D antigen was present on variants (AS1, AS2, AS3, AS4, and AS5) selected from 1591-RE2 (D$^-$). This finding was particularly surprising, since the expression of the 1591-RE antigens was stable by continuous passage in culture and in congenic nude mice for over four months (Wortzel et al. 1983a,b). It is conceivable that these newly expressed antigens were present on an undetectably small percentage of the parental population or were possibly induced during the selection process. Because the antigens were identified solely by monoclonal T cell probes, it is not even clear if the newly expressed antigens are molecularly identical to the original antigen molecules. The mechanism of this antigenic "reexpression" currently remains unresolved because first, 1591-RE cells are not available immediately after the original cloning, and second, the antigens have not yet been molecularly characterized.

The above studies indicate that the expression of multiple tumor-specific antigens that are recognized by cytolytic T cells can be critical in the rejection of the 1591-RE tumor. It is still unclear, however, why one of the 1591-RE variants, AS6 (A$^-$B$^+$C$^-$D$^-$), has a regressor phenotype, since this variant does not express either of the two 1591-RE antigens (A and C) associated with regressive behavior. One possibility for this anomaly is that other rejection antigens that are as yet unidentified are expressed on this tumor variant. Such antigens may be recognized by immune cells other than cytolytic T cells (DTH or help-inducing T cells) and have therefore not been detected by our cytolytic tumor-specific probes. In this light, the role of T cell subsets other than cytolytic T cells have been implied to be of primary importance in allograft and tumor rejection (Loveland et al. 1981, Bhan et al. 1981), although the relative importance of these subsets is still uncertain (Mills and North 1983). It is possible that this hypothetical antigen is usually lost from the parental tumor along with the A and C antigens, but in the case of AS6, it remained behind. Other immunologic host defense cells may also be involved in the rejection of this tumor by the normal host, although we find that two likely candidates, activated macrophages and natural killer cells, do not seem to play a critical role. It is clear that further evaluation of the host response to such variants as AS6 will aid in elucidating the mechanisms responsible for the rejection of 1591-RE.

PECKING ORDER AMONG MULTIPLE TUMOR-SPECIFIC ANTIGENS

It would appear that the expression of multiple transplantation antigens on a single tumor would be advantageous to the host for effective tumor rejection. This is because if the host simultaneously recognizes multiple antigens, immune escape should be less likely, since the tumor would have to simultaneously lose multiple antigens in order to evade the host response. For example, we have shown that loss of a single antigen occurs at a frequency of less than 10^{-4} tumor cells (Wortzel et al. 1983a,b). Therefore, a tumor variant that has simultaneously lost four independent antigens would be extremely rare, having a frequency of approximately 10^{-16}. However, in contrast to such a potentially effective host defense, we have demonstrated that the host does not recognize all of the multiple independent antigens on 1591-RE simultaneously (Wortzel et al. 1983b, Urban et al. 1984). For example, as shown in Figure 12.5 (lower panel), immunization with the 1591-RE2 tumor $(A^+B^+C^-D^-)$, which expresses both the A and B antigens, elicited a cytolytic immune response that did not lyse 1591-PRO $(A^-B^+C^-D^-)$, indicating that the host did not generate an anti-B response. However, an immune response could be generated against the B antigen when the immunizing tumor was A^-B^+, as in the 1591-PRO variant (Figure 12.5, upper panel), since the response generated lysed both 1591-PRO and 1591-RE. Thus a hierarchy or "pecking order" appears to exist in the host response to these two antigens, the A antigen being "immunodominant" and the B antigen "immunorecessive." With respect to the two other tumor-specific antigens that are currently identified by T cells on the 1591-RE tumor (C and D), preliminary studies suggest that the C antigen is immunodominant like the A antigen, and the D antigen is immunorecessive like the B antigen (Wortzel RD unpublished data).

A hierarchy in the immune response to multiple antigens has been described in a number of systems, including minor histocompatibility antigens (Wettstein and Bailey 1982) and viral antigens (Zinkernagel et al. 1978, Pfizenmaier et al. 1980). The mechanism for the immunologic preference that we and others observe is unclear. In the 1591-RE model, it is possible that the B antigen is immunorecessive simply because the precursor frequency or affinity of the T cells reactive with the B antigen may be lower than that for the immunodominant A antigen. However, this explanation alone seems unlikely,

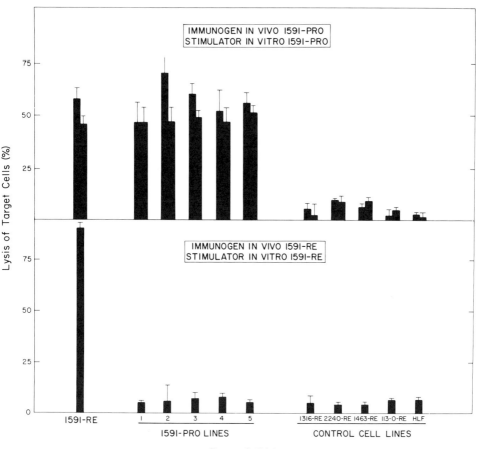

FIGURE 12.5. Hierarchy in the host response to the A and B antigens as demonstrated by differences in the reactivity pattern of cytolytic T cells derived from mice immunized with either 1591-RE $(A^+B^+C^-D^-)$ or 1591-PRO $(A^-B^+C^-D^-)$. Spleen cells from mice immunized with 1591-RE (lower panel) or 1591-PRO (upper panel; double bars represent two independently derived 1591-PRO tumors) were restimulated in vitro with the same tumor cells and were used as cytolytic effectors in a ^{51}Cr release assay against the indicated tumor target cells. 1591-PRO1 to 1591-PRO5 (all A^-B^+) are five independently derived host-selected progressor variants of 1591-RE2. 1591-RE2 is referred to here as 1591-RE. A description of the control cell lines is provided in Figure 3. (Reproduced from Urban et al. 1984 with permission from Verlag Chemie GmbH).

since the immunorecessive B antigen remains unrecognized by the host cytolytic response even after repeated immunizations with a tumor that expresses both the A and B antigens (Urban et al. 1984). It is also unlikely that the B antigen is simply hidden on the cell surface, since the B antigen as well as the A antigen are accessible on the parental tumor as targets and stimulators for cytolytic T cells in vitro (Wortzel et al. 1983b). As a third explanation, it is conceivable that the A and B antigens may compete for antigen presentation and thus bias immune recognition. This has been postulated for the hierarchy detected for viral antigens (Zinkernagel et al. 1978, Doherty et al. 1978, Kurrle et al. 1978) and minor histocompatibility antigens (Wettstein and Bailey 1982, Gordon et al. 1977). Finally, it is also possible that immunoregulatory cells are induced by the immunodominant antigen. The immunoregulatory cells favor this antigen and possibly also suppress the immune response to the immunorecessive antigen.

A pecking order in the host response to multiple independent tumor-specific antigens should have several important consequences. As alluded to above, it would appear that tumor escape would be facilitated by sequential rather than simultaneous selection. Consistent with this, recent experiments have shown that when the 1591-RE tumor grows progressively, antigenic changes occur in sequence (Urban JL unpublished data). The antigens evaluated in such studies were the A and B antigens, as well as the antigens recognized by activated macrophages; the latter were lost independently of the A antigen (Urban and Schreiber 1983). The protocol entailed challenging UV-irradiated mice with the 1591-RE regressor tumor and at various times excising the developing tumors, adapting the tumors to culture, and then reanalyzing their sensitivity to activated macrophages or to the cytolytic anti-A and anti-B T cells. UV-irradiated mice were chosen as the ideal hosts for this study, since antigenic variants are isolated from such mice at a particularly high frequency, possibly because these animals are partially immunosuppressed, but they retain enough immunity to exert an immunoselective pressure without eliminating the tumor (Urban et al. 1982b). The results clearly showed that the independent markers were lost in sequence and not simultaneously: first the macrophage-recognized target, then the A antigen, and last the B antigen (Urban JL unpublished data). It is possible that this sequential selection, as compared to simultaneous selection, allows for tumor escape by selecting for the more frequent "single-loss" variants rather than the far less frequent "multiloss" variants.

While a hierarchy in the immune response to multiple antigens may apparently favor tumor escape, such immunologic preference would also lead to the retention of tumor-specific antigens on the progressor variants. These retained antigens, being tumor specific, may be useful therapeutically by providing targets for passive or active immunotherapy. In addition, because more than one tumor-specific antigen may be retained on the progressor variants, as found in the 1591-RE system, escape from such immunotherapy may be less likely with the use of immunologic probes simultaneously directed against several of these independent target structures. In addition, by gaining a better understanding of the regulatory events involved in this hierarchy, we may also discover new approaches for manipulating the immune system to improve tumor rejection.

MOLECULAR CHARACTERIZATION OF TUMOR-SPECIFIC ANTIGENS ON UV-INDUCED TUMORS

Although unique tumor-specific antigens have been demonstrated on many tumors induced by physical and chemical carcinogens, nothing is currently known about the molecular nature or genetic origin of any of these antigens. A characterization of such surface structures will obviously aid in understanding the mechanism of tumor escape and the host antitumor response. Monoclonal antibodies are apparently the most suitable immunologic probes for purifying and characterizing these antigens. Recently, two 1591-RE–specific monoclonal antibodies (called CP28 and CP3F4) have been isolated (Philipps et al. 1985a). These antibodies did not bind 37 syngeneic unrelated UV-induced tumors or normal syngeneic adult or embryonic cells, as determined by quantitative cytofluorometry. In addition, the antibodies displayed a reactivity pattern identical to the anti-A cytolytic T cell line (Wortzel et al. 1984), as determined by recognition of 1591-RE antigen-loss variants that were selected with either the antibodies or anti-A T cell line, as well as recognition of host-selected progressor variants of 1591-RE. Thus it appears likely that the antibodies recognize the A antigen or at least a tumor-specific antigen closely linked to the A antigen.

Using immune precipitation of radiolabeled antigen followed by two-dimensional gel electrophoresis, Philipps et al. (1985a) showed that the 1591-RE–specific monoclonal antibodies recognized a 45-kDa molecule, which had the typical appearance of a class I molecule, and that this 45-kDa molecule was associated with a 12-kDa molecule that had a pI consistent with that of β_2 microglobulin. This finding is interesting in light of earlier studies that showed that many tumors react with alloantigen-specific immunologic probes, suggesting the existence of alien major histocompatibility complex (MHC) class I molecules on malignant cells. These previous studies were inconclusive, however, because the antigens studied were not molecularly characterized (Invernizzi and Parmiani 1975, Bortin and Truitt 1980, 1981, Bach and Bortin 1981, Festenstein and Schmidt 1981, Callahan et al. 1983). Also, it was unclear if such antigens were related to unique tumor antigens because of the absence of syngeneic monoclonal tumor-specific antibody probes. Using the 1591-RE–specific monoclonal antibodies, we have shown that when they were tested for reactivity with lymphocytes from other strains of mice, these antibodies reacted with public specificities controlled by class I genes of the MHC locus. The specificity of this cross-reactivity was confirmed with alloantigen class I gene–transfected cells (Stauss et al. 1985). We also tested to see if, conversely, alloantigen-specific probes would react with unique tumor-specific antigens. Such studies showed that, indeed, some alloantigen-specific monoclonal antibodies, e.g., those reactive with "L-like" molecules (Sharrow et al. 1984), cross-reacted with a unique 1591-RE–specific antigen. However, the antigenic similarity of any allogeneic class I gene product and the tumor-specific antigen was always partial, i.e., some, but never all epitopes were shared, indicating that the antigens had different molecular structures. Further analysis of the 1591-RE–specific class I antigens revealed that the "A antigen" is actually composed of at least three unique independent components that each appear to be novel class I molecules (Stauss HJ unpublished data). Thus, we demonstrate that unique tumor-specific antigens recognized by the syngeneic host can be novel class I molecules. We expect that unique tumor-specific class I antigens will be found on other tumors and that the earlier widespread observation of "alien" class I MHC tumor antigens is related to our findings.

At present, it is not clear if the other T cell–recognized antigens on the 1591-RE tumor (B, C, and D) belong to a similar family of novel class I molecules, since these antigens have not been characterized with antibody probes. However, because at least three of the 1591-RE–specific antigens are novel class I molecules, it appears appropriate to discuss possible mechanisms for the origin of such surface structures. One explanation for the abnormal expression of alien class I genes on the 1591-RE tumor is that 1591-RE may not have originated in an inbred mouse strain (Bailey 1982). This is highly unlikely, however, because 1591-RE still expresses the normal class I H-2 K and D specificities and isoenzymes of the C3H/HeN mouse strain from which this tumor originated (Philipps et al. 1985b). In addition, a characteristic C3H/HeN pattern was revealed by a Southern blot analysis of *Bam*H1-digested 1591-RE tumor DNA, using cDNA probes specific for class I genes (Stauss HJ unpublished data). A second explanation that appears more likely is that the novel class I antigens on the 1591-RE tumor result from subtle somatic changes that occurred during or after exposure to UV radiation. For example, gene derepression or recombinational events among the numerous homologous class I genes might account for the expression of novel class I antigens. Simple activation of preexisting genes, however, would probably not generate sufficient variability to account for the enormous pleomorphism of tumor antigens, since the genome contains only about 30 class I genes (Steinmetz et al. 1982, Weiss et al. 1984). On the other hand, recombinational events in the MHC region should have the potential to provide sufficient antigenic diversity by activating previously silent class I DNA sequences, as well as by generating novel class I genes that bear new unique antigenic sites on the expressed molecules. In this light, it is interesting that one of the 1591-RE–specific antigens is an L-like class I molecule, since L molecules are normally never expressed in the C3H/HeN mouse strain from which the 1591-RE tumor originated (Steinmetz et al. 1982). The inability to express the L antigen may be due to a lack of the functional flanking sequence necessary for antigen expression. It is therefore conceivable that a recombinational event may have allowed the expression of the L molecule on 1591-RE.

Upon characterizing the other unique tumor-specific antigens on the 1591-RE tumor, we hope to determine whether or not the multiple antigens belong to a family of related gene products. The only other unique tumor-specific antigen comparatively well described appears to be the methylcholanthrene-induced fibrosarcoma Meth A. The expression of the Meth A antigen is closely linked to the Ig gene cluster (Pravtcheva et al. 1981, Flood et al. 1983). Since the Ig and MHC genes belong to the same supergene family of cell-cell recognition sites (Steinmetz and Hood 1983), it is attractive to speculate that many tumor-specific antigens may be related to an alteration in cell-cell recognition molecules that regulate normal growth and differentiation (Moscona 1962, Boyse 1970, Hood et al. 1977). In this way, changes in such cell surface molecules may be involved with malignant behavior (Boyse 1970, Sondel and Bach 1980). Gene cloning and gene transfection experiments are clearly invaluable tools for the further characterization of tumor-specific antigens, and this approach may also be useful in determining the possible relationship of these antigens to malignant potential.

CONCLUDING REMARKS

Dissection of the complex antigen on a UV-induced tumor, as an experimental model, suggests that the antigenicity of malignant cells can be composed of multiple components that are all independently expressed and tumor specific. This unexpected antigenic complexity should not only influence future studies that investigate the nature of the tumor antigen but may also be consequential in the effectiveness of potential immunotherapy. For example, the expression of multiple independent tumor antigens would appear to favor effective rejection by making tumor escape less likely, provided that the host recognizes the multiple independent target structures simultaneously. However, we find that the host response focuses on a limited number of tumor antigens and that this antigenic hierarchy actually favors tumor progression. It would therefore be advantageous for the therapist to attempt to overcome this hierarchy in the host response by manipulating the immune system to recognize the multiple antigens simultaneously. Such therapy might be approached by idiotype-specific manipulations (Schreiber 1984). In contrast to this apparent disadvantage, the antigenic hierarchy may be therapeutically useful by allowing the retention (at least temporarily) of tumor-specific antigens on progressor variants that could be the target sites of effective passive immunotherapy.

The mechanism responsible for generating the extensive antigenic diversity among different tumors is at present unclear, but any model must now account for the antigenic diversity that can be expressed on an individual tumor cell. The tumor-specific antigens currently best characterized (1591-RE and Meth A) appear to be related to two gene families known to have extensive pleomorphism (MHC and Ig, respectively), and the abnormal expression of these genes may suggest a possible mechanism for the antigenic variation among tumor antigens. It is also interesting that the MHC and Ig gene families code for cell surface molecules involved in cell-cell interactions, for this suggests a possible relationship between the tumor antigen and malignant behavior.

ACKNOWLEDGMENT

This work was supported by grants RO1-CA-22677 and PO1-CA-19266, awarded by the National Cancer Institute, United States Department of Health and Human Services. H.S. was supported by the Research Career Development Award CA-00432, R.D.W. and C.V.W. by the National Institute of General Medical Sciences grant PHS-T32-GM-07281, and H.J.S. by the National Cancer Cytology Center.

REFERENCES

Bach FH, Bortin MM. 1981. Alien histocompatibility antigens and alloimmunization: Conceptual and practical considerations. Transplant Proc 13:1975–1978.

Baldwin RW. 1955. Immunity to methylcholanthrene-induced tumors in inbred rats following implantation and regression of implanted tumors. Br J Cancer 9:652–657.

Bhan AK, Perry LL, Cantor H, McCluskey RT, Benacerraf B, Greene MI. 1981. The role of T cell sets in the rejection of a methylcholanthrene-induced sarcoma (S1509a) in syngeneic mice. Am J Pathol 102:20–27.

Bailey DW. 1982. How pure are inbred strains of mice? Immunology Today 3:210–214.

Borst P, Cross GAM. 1982. Molecular basis for trypanosome antigenic variation. Cell 29:291–303.

Bortin MM, Truitt RL. 1980. First international symposium on alien histocompatibility antigens on cancer cells: Introduction. Transplant Proc 12:1.

Bortin MM, Truitt RL. 1981. Second international symposium on alien histocompatibility antigens on cancer cells: Introduction. Transplant Proc 13:1751–1752.

Bosslet K, Schirrmacher V. 1981. Escape of metastasizing clonal tumor cell variants from tumor-specific cytolytic T lymphocytes. J Exp Med 154:557–562.

Boyse EA. 1970. Organization and modulation of cell membrane receptors. *In*

Smith RT, Landy M, eds., Immune Surveillance. Academic Press, New York, London, pp. 5–48.

Burnet FM. 1970. A certain symmetry: Histocompatibility antigens compared with immunocyte receptors. Nature 226:123 126.

Callahan GN, Pardi D, Giedlin MA, Allison JP, Morizot DM, Martin WJ. 1983. Biochemical evidence for expression of a semi-allogeneic, H-2 antigen by a murine adenocarcinoma. J Immunol 130:471–479.

Daynes RA, Spellman CW. 1977. Evidence for the generation of suppressor cells by ultraviolet radiation. Cell Immunol 31:182–187.

Doherty PC, Biddison WE, Bennink JR, Knowles BB. 1978. Cytotoxic T cell responses in mice infected with influenza and vaccinia viruses vary in magnitude with H-2 genotype. J Exp Med 148:534–543.

Emmett EA. 1973. Ultraviolet radiation as a cause of skin tumors. CRC Crit Rev Toxicol 2:211-255.

Festenstein H, Schmidt W. 1981. Variation in MHC antigenic profiles of tumor cells and its biological effects. Immunol Rev 60:85–127.

Fisher MS, Kripke ML. 1977. Systemic alteration induced in mice by ultraviolet light irradiation and its relationship to ultraviolet carcinogenesis. Proc Natl Acad Sci USA 74:1688–1692.

Flood PM, DeLeo AB, Old LJ, Gershon RK. 1983. Relation of cell surface antigens on methylcholanthrene-induced fibrosarcomas to immunoglobulin heavy chain complex variable region-linked T cell interaction molecules. Proc Natl Acad Sci USA 80:1683–1687.

Flood PM, Kripke ML, Rowley DA, Schreiber H. 1980. Suppression of tumor rejection by autologous anti-idiotypic immunity. Proc Natl Acad Sci USA 77:2209–2213.

Flood PM, Urban JL, Kripke ML, Schreiber H. 1981. Loss of tumor-specific and idiotype-specific immunity with age. J Exp Med 154:275–290.

Foley EJ. 1953. Antigenic properties of methylcholanthrene-induced tumors in mice of the strain of origin. Cancer Res 13:835–843.

Gillis S, Smith KA. 1977. Long term culture of tumor-specific cytotoxic T cells. Nature 268:154–156.

Gordon RD, Samelson LE, Simpson E. 1977. Selective response to H-Y antigen by F1 female mice sensitized to F1 male cells. J Exp Med 146:606–610.

Gross L. 1943. Intradermal immunization of C3H mice against a sarcoma that originated in an animal of the same line. Cancer Res 3:326–333.

Hardie IR, Strong RW, Hartley LCJ, Woodruff PWH, Clunie GJA. 1980. Skin cancer in Caucasian renal allograft recipients living in a subtropical climate. Surgery 87:177–183.

Hood L, Huang HV, Dreyer WJ. 1977. The area-code hypothesis: The immune system provides clues to understanding the genetic and molecular basis of cell recognition during development. Journal of Supramolecular Structure 7:531–559.

Invernizzi G, Parmiani G. 1975. Tumor-associated transplantation antigens of chemically induced sarcomata cross reacting with allogeneic histocompatibility antigens. Nature 254:713–714.

Klein G. 1978. Commentary and overview. *In* Mitchison NA, Landy M, eds. Manipulation of the Immune Response in Cancer. Academic Press Inc., London, pp. 339–353.

Klein G, Sjogren HO, Klein E, Hellstrom KE. 1960. Demonstration of resistance against methylcholanthrene-induced sarcomas in the primary autochthonous host. Cancer Res 20:1561–1572.

Kohler G, Milstein C. 1975. Continuous cultures of fused cells secreting antibody of predefined specificity. Nature 256:495–497.

Kripke ML. 1977. Latency, histology, and antigenicity of tumors induced by ultraviolet light in three inbred mouse strains. Cancer Res 37:1395–1399.

Kripke ML. 1981. Immunologic mechanisms in UV radiation carcinogenesis. Adv Cancer Res 34:69–106.

Kripke ML, Thorn RM, Lill PH, Civin CI, Pazmino NH, Fisher MS. 1979. Further characterization of immunologic unresponsiveness induced in mice by ultraviolet radiation. Transplantation 28:212–217.

Kurrle R, Rollinghoff M, Wagner H. 1978. H-2-linked murine cytotoxic T cell responses specific for sendai virus-infected cells. Eur J Immunol 8:910–912.

Loveland BE, Hogarth PM, Ceredig RH, McKenzie IFC. 1981. Cells mediating graft rejection in the mouse: I. Lyt-1 cells mediate skin graft rejection. J Exp Med 153:1044–1057.

Maryanski JL, Boon T. 1982. Immunogenic variants obtained by mutagenesis of mouse mastocytoma 815: IV. Analysis of variant-specific antigens by selection of antigen-loss variants with cytolytic T cell clones. Eur J Immunol 12:406–412.

Mills CD, North RJ. 1983. Expression of passively transferred immunity against an established tumor depends on generation of cytolytic T cells in recipient: Inhibition of suppressor T cells. J Exp Med 157:1448–1460.

Moscona AA. 1962. Cellular interactions in experimental histogenesis. Int Rev Exp Pathol 1:371–428.

Old LJ. 1982. Cancer immunology: The search for specificity. Natl Cancer Inst Monogr 60:193–209.

Penn I. 1980. Immunosuppression and skin cancer. Clin Plast Surg 7:361–368.

Pfizenmaier K, Pan S, Knowles BB. 1980. Preferential H-2 association in cytotoxic T cell responses to SV40 tumor-associated specific antigens. J Immunol 124:1888–1891.

Philipps C, McMillan M, Flood PM, et al. 1985a. A tumor-unique class I major histocompatibility complex (MHC)-like molecule as a unique tumor-specific antigen (Abstract). Fed Proc 44:550.

Philipps C, McMillan M, Flood PM, et al. 1985b. Identification of a unique tumor-specific antigen as a novel class I major histocompatibility molecule. Proc Natl Acad Sci USA 82:5140–5144.

Pravtcheva DD, DeLeo AB, Ruddle FH, Old LJ. 1981. Chromosome assignment of the tumor-specific antigen of a 3-methylcholanthrene-induced mouse sarcoma. J Exp Med 154:964–977.

Prehn RT, Main JM. 1957. Immunity to methylcholanthrene-induced sarcomas. JNCI 18:769–778.

Roberts LK, Daynes RA. 1980. Modification of the immunogenic properties of chemically-induced tumors arising in hosts treated concomitantly with ultraviolet light. J Immunol 125:438–447.

Schreiber H. 1984. Idiotype network interactions in tumor immunity. Adv Cancer Res 41:291–321.

Sharrow SO, Flaherty L, Sachs DH. 1984. Serologic cross-reactivity between class I MHC molecules and an H-2-linked differentiation antigen as detected by monoclonal antibodies. J Exp Med 159:21–40.

Sondel PM, Bach FH. 1980. The alienation of tumor immunity· Alien-driven diversity and alien-selected escape. Transplant Proc 12:211–215.

Spellman CW, Daynes RA. 1978a. Immunoregulation by ultraviolet light: III. Enhancement of suppressor cell activity in older animals. Exp Gerontol 13: 141–146.

Spellman CW, Daynes RA. 1978b. Ultraviolet light induced suppressor lymphocytes dictate specificity of anti-ultraviolet tumor immune responses. Cell Immunol 38:25–34.

Stauss HJ, Goodenow RS, McMillan M, et al. 1985. Differences between alien and tumor-specific class I major histocompatibility complex (MHC) molecules defined by the analysis of gene transfectants (Abstract). Proceedings of the American Association for Cancer Research 26:312.

Steinmetz M, Hood L. 1983. Genes of the major histocompatibility complex in mouse and man. Science 222:727–733.

Steinmetz M, Winoto A, Minard K, Hood L. 1982. Clusters of genes encoding mouse transplantation antigens. Cell 28:489–498.

Urban JL, Burton BC, Holland JM, Kripke ML, Schreiber H. 1982a. Mechanisms of syngeneic tumor rejection: Susceptibility of host-selected progressor variants to various immunologic effector cells. J Exp Med 155:557–573.

Urban JL, Holland M, Kripke ML, Schreiber H. 1982b. Immunoselection of tumor cell variants by mice suppressed with ultraviolet light. J Exp Med 156:1025–1041.

Urban JL, Schreiber H. 1983. Selection of macrophage-resistant progressor tumor variants by the normal host: Requirement for concomitant T cell–mediated immunity. J Exp Med 157:642–656.

Urban JL, Van Waes C, Schreiber H. 1984. Pecking order among tumor-specific antigens. Eur J Immunol 14:181–187.

Uyttenhove C, Maryanski J, Boon T. 1983. Escape of mouse mastocytoma P815 after nearly complete rejection is due to antigen-loss variants rather than immunosuppression. J Exp Med 157:1040–1052.

Weinhold KJ, Miller DA, Wheelock EF. 1979. The tumor dormant state: Comparison of L5178Y cells used to establish dormancy with those that emerge after its termination. J Exp Med 149:745–757.

Weiss EH, Golden L, Fahrner K, et al. 1984. Organization and evolution of the class I gene family in the major histocompatibility complex of the C57BL/10 mouse. Nature 310:650–655.

Wettstein PJ, Bailey DW. 1982. Immunodominance in the immune response to "multiple" histocompatibility antigens. Immunogenetics 16:47–58.

Wortzel RD, Philipps C, Schreiber H. 1983a. Multiple tumor-specific antigens expressed on a single tumor cell. Nature 304:165–167.

Wortzel RD, Urban JL, Philipps C, Fitch FW, Schreiber H. 1983b. Independent immunodominant and immunorecessive tumor-specific antigens on a malignant tumor: Antigenic dissection with cytolytic T cell clones. J Immunol 130: 2461–2466.

Wortzel RD, Urban JL, Schreiber H. 1984. Malignant growth in the normal host after variant selection in vitro with cytolytic T cell lines. Proc Natl Acad Sci USA 81:2186–2190.

Zinkernagel RM, Althage A, Cooper S, et al. 1978. Ir-genes in H-2 regulate generation of anti-viral cytotoxic T cells: Mapping to K or D and dominance of unresponsiveness. J Exp Med 148:592–606.

Symposium on Fundamental Cancer Research, Vol. 38.

13. Macrophage Recognition of Self from Nonself: Implications for the Interaction of Macrophages with Neoplastic Cells

Isaiah J. Fidler and Alan J. Schroit

Department of Cell Biology, The University of Texas M. D. Anderson Hospital and Tumor Institute at Houston, Houston, Texas 77030

Since the discovery of the lymphocyte and its pivotal role in host immunity and chronic inflammatory responses, the macrophage has received far less attention than biologic relevance would dictate. For well over a century, detailed microscopic studies have allowed investigators to conclude that fixed or free phagocytic mononuclear cells or both are associated with processes of tissue turnover. These processes include tissue remodeling during embryogenesis and metamorphosis, tissue destruction and repair subsequent to injury or infection, and tissue renewal following the removal of damaged or senescent cells. Since most of this earlier work was based upon morphologic observations, it was generally accepted that the primary mechanism by which macrophages accomplished their tasks involved a nonsophisticated process of phagocytosis and intracellular disposal. There is now, however, an overwhelming body of data to suggest that this is an oversimplified interpretation of the true nature and role of the macrophage. In fact, the macrophage, a remarkably well-conserved cell in evolution that is responsible for maintaining homeostasis in multicellular organisms, is probably one of the most versatile cells in the body.

The macrophage is unique because of its multiple roles in diverse physiologic processes (Van Furth 1975). Although certain animals can survive without the benefit of an intact lymphocyte system, e.g., invertebrates, athymic mice, athymic and asplenic mice, and bursectomized birds, it is doubtful that animals could survive without an intact macrophage system. Indeed, cells of the macrophage-histiocyte series are an essential component of homeostasis. In both vertebrates and invertebrates, the primary function of macrophages could well be to discriminate between "self" and "nonself." For example, macrophages recognize, phagocytose, and ultimately dispose of effete cells, cellular debris, and foreign invaders. Moreover, the removal of effete red blood cells (RBC) from the circulation is a continuous process that requires that macrophages distinguish young from old cells, as well as healthy from damaged cells. Macrophages are continuously involved in the controlled metabolism of lipids and iron and in host response to injury, i.e., inflammation. Frequently, macrophages that line body cavities provide the first line of defense against microbial infections and parasitic infestations and participate in the second line of defense against foreign invaders. Macrophages frequently regulate both the afferent and efferent arms of the immune system, which probably primarily evolved to aid macrophages in host defense. For this reason, reference to macrophages as accessory cells for lymphocytes is biologically inaccurate. T cells and B cells evolved far later than the macrophage. More appropriately then, T and B cells are accessory to macrophages.

During the past decade, we and others have been interested in elucidating the role that macrophages play in host defense against cancer in general and cancer metastasis in particular. In order to understand the mechanism by which macrophages discriminate between normal cells and tumor cells (see below), it is imperative to determine the requirements for macrophage recognition of "nonself." It is therefore necessary to define those surface moieties responsible for the binding to macrophages, and the conditions that might influence macrophage attachment to its target. In this chapter, we describe both our published work and some unpublished observations on the interaction of macrophages with synthetic phospholipid membranes, normal cells, modified RBC, sickled RBC, virus-infected cells (herpes simplex virus type 2, HSV-2), and neoplastic cells. In several of these systems the data suggest that membrane phospholipids could serve as a moiety that provides the signal for recognition of "altered self" by macrophages.

THE ACTIVATION OF CYTOTOXIC PROPERTIES IN MACROPHAGES

Macrophage function can be divided into two categories. The first consists of functions that are carried out continuously, e.g., removal of effete RBC from the circulation, and the second category involves macrophage function that is far less frequent, e.g., participation in host defense against infections, parasites, and cancer (for review, see Fidler and Poste 1982, Fidler 1984). These latter functions require the recruitment and "activation" of macrophages to perform a specific task. Once this task is completed, the cells can revert to the "nonactivated" state and can be reactivated if necessary. It should be noted that the use of "activated" to describe macrophages is a working definition, and its use in the literature is extended to describe a large number of macrophage phenotypes that may or may not be related to the increased capacity of macrophages to recognize and destroy microorganisms, parasites, or cancer cells.

There are two major physiologic pathways by which macrophages can be activated to become cytotoxic against infectious agents (bacteria, parasites) or cancer. Macrophages are readily activated to become bactericidal upon *immediate* interaction with certain microorganisms or their products, e.g., endotoxins, certain bacteria cell wall skeletons, and muramyl dipeptide. The quick reactivity of macrophages to microorganisms appears to be extremely well conserved in evolution. In fact, one method for detection of endotoxins in biologic materials relies on the *Limulus* amebocyte lysate assay. Thus, the phagocytes of both a "living fossil" like the horseshoe crab and of man react alike when confronted with endotoxins.

The chemical composition of those cell wall components of microorganisms responsible for activation of macrophages is poorly understood, and their use in vivo is often accompanied by significant toxicity. The notable exceptions in this category are the synthetic moieties N-acetyl-L-alanyl-D-isoglutamine (MDP) (Chedid et al. 1979) and N-acetyl-muramyl-L-ananyl-D-isoglutamyl-L-alanyl-phosphatidyl-ethanolamine (MTP-PE) (Gisler et al. 1979, Fidler et al. 1982a,b), which have potent effects on a variety of host defense cells, including the capacity to activate macrophages (Parant 1979, Lederer 1980, Sone and Fidler 1981). Although MDP and MTP-PE influence several macrophage functions in vitro (Sone and Fidler, 1981, Fidler et al. 1982b) comparable effects have not been observed in vivo because these drugs are rapidly excreted after parenteral administration (Parant et al. 1979, Fogler et al. 1985). Even when injected at very high doses, MDP does not significantly induce macrophage-mediated antitumor activity in situ (Fidler et al. 1981).

The other category of macrophage-activating agents with the potential for in vivo therapeutic use is the lymphokines. Antigen- and mitogen-stimulated T lymphocytes release lymphokines that interact in a highly specific fashion with target cells bearing appropriate receptors. In the case of macrophages, activation is produced by a family of lymphokines generally referred to as macrophage activation factors (MAF) (Fidler and Raz 1981), which include, among others, gamma interferon (IFN-γ) (Kleinerman et al. 1984). The therapeutic use of lymphokines (MAF, IFN-γ) has been hindered by either the lack of purified preparations or by the extremely short half-life of intravenously administered materials. Moreover, only a small fraction of the mononuclear phagocyte system can respond to free lymphokines (Poste 1979, Poste and Kirsh 1979), and even the few responding macrophages can be activated by lymphokines only within a short period of time after the extravasation of the macrophages from the circulation (Poste and Kirsh 1979). Finally, the tumoricidal properties of MAF-activated macrophages are short-lived (two to three days), and these cells become refractory to reactivation by free lymphokines (Poste 1979, Poste and Kirsh 1979, Poste et al. 1979a,b).

Efforts to activate macrophages by treatment with agents that stimulate T lymphocytes to produce MAF may also be unproductive. Recent data have shown that the lymphocytes of animals bearing large progressive tumors are deficient in their ability to release lymphokines that recruit and activate macrophages (Fidler and Raz 1981). If such a defect is a common occurrence in the tumor-bearing host, administration of agents that seek to augment host antitumor responses by stimulating lymphokine production in situ may be of little value because of a preexisting functional lesion in "target" lymphocytes. In addition, this approach does not overcome the problem described above, in which a substantial fraction of the available macrophage population at any one time may be refractory to activation by lymphokines (Poste 1979).

Fortunately, many of the problems with activating macrophage tumoricidal properties in vivo with compounds such as MDP, MTP-PE, MAF, and IFN-γ can be overcome with the use of liposome-based drug delivery systems. Studies in many laboratories have demonstrated the utility of liposomes as carrier vehicles for drug delivery in vivo (Gregoriadis et al. 1977, Gregoriadis and Allison 1980, Nicolau and Paraf 1981). Moreover, liposomes provide a particularly convenient nontoxic carrier (Hart et al. 1981) for the delivery of biologically active materials to mononuclear phagocytes in vivo. Following intravenous administration, the majority (80–90%) of liposomes are taken up by reticuloendothelial (RE) cells in the liver and spleen and by circulating monocytes (Poste et al. 1982, Fidler et al. 1980, Schroit and Fidler 1982, Schroit et al. 1983a). By exploiting this localization pattern, we can target liposome-encapsulated materials to macrophages in vivo (Schroit et al. 1983b).

Indeed, it has been shown that lymphokines (MAF, IFN-γ) and muramyl peptides (MDP, MTP-PE) encapsulated within liposomes are highly effective in activating mouse and human macrophages in vitro and mouse and rat macrophages in vivo (Fidler 1980, 1984, Sone and Fidler 1980, Fidler et al. 1982a,b, Fidler and Fogler 1982, Fidler and Schroit 1984,). Development of the tumoricidal state requires phagocytic uptake of the liposomes, which is followed by a lag period of four to eight hours before tumoricidal activity is expressed (Fidler and Raz 1981, Fidler et al. 1981, Raz et al. 1981). Studies on the mechanism of activation by liposome-encapsulated compounds indicated that participation of cell surface receptors is not required, suggesting that activation results from the interaction of MAF or MDP with an intracellular site or sites (Poste and Kirsh 1979, Poste et al. 1979a,b, Fidler and Raz 1981, Fidler et al. 1981, Raz et al. 1981). Although it has been shown that MAF-induced activation (in free form) requires binding to a fucoglycolipid receptor on the macrophage surface (Poste et al. 1979b), liposome-encapsulated lymphokines can activate macrophages lacking these receptors (Poste et al. 1979a,b, Poste and Kirsh 1979). Moreover, lymphokines encapsulated within liposomes can induce activation of subpopulations of tissue and intratumoral macrophages that are completely refractory to activation by free (unencapsulated) lymphokines (Poste et al. 1979b). In addition to the highly efficient, targeted delivery of activation agents to macrophages in vivo, encapsulation of labile, immunogenic molecules within liposomes not only prevents their premature inactivation or degradation of these molecules but also reduces the likelihood of undesirable immune sensitization.

RECOGNITION PATTERNS

Recognition of Phospholipids by Macrophages

In order for liposomes to serve as vehicles for the delivery of compounds to cells of the RE system, they must avidly bind to and be phagocytosed by the cells. Extensive experimentation has revealed that macrophages might be able to recognize certain classes of phospholipids. This conclusion is based upon the many observations that the inclusion of negatively charged phospholipids in liposomes greatly enhances their binding to and subsequent phagocytosis by mouse peritoneal macrophages (Poste et al. 1979b, Raz et al. 1981), mouse Kupffer cells (Scherphof et al. 1983, Xu et al. 1984, Xu and Fidler 1984), mouse or rat alveolar macrophages (Fidler et al. 1980, Schroit and Fidler 1982), human alveolar macrophages (Sone and Tsubura 1982), and human peripheral blood monocytes (Mehta et al. 1982, Kleinerman et al. 1983a,b). Specifically, negatively charged liposomes containing phosphatidylserine (PS) are phagocytosed 5 to 10 times faster than are liposomes of the same size and configuration consisting only of phosphatidylcholine (PC) (Figure 13.1). The addition of another negatively charged phospholipid similar to PS, phosphatidylglycerol, to liposomes also produces significant enhancement in liposome binding to and phagocytosis by macrophages (Mehta et al. 1982).

The in vivo interaction of liposomes with circulating monocytes or with fixed macrophages is also influenced by the size of the liposome and by its lipid composition. Thus, large multilamellar vesicles or liposomes constructed by reverse evaporation are arrested in lung vasculature more frequently than small unilamellar liposomes of identical lipid composition (Table 13.1). After intravenous injection, liposomes of the same structural class are more efficiently arrested in the lung when they contain negatively charged phospholipids (PS) than when they contain only neutral phospholipids (PC) (Fidler et al. 1980, Schroit and Fidler 1982).

Recognition of RBC

The average life span of RBC in mammals is 120 days, and effete RBC are removed from the circulation by cells of the RE system. It is reasonable to assume that effete cells must acquire a specific determinant that triggers their

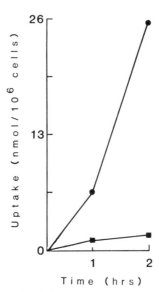

FIGURE 13.1. Phagocytosis of phosphatidylcholine (PC) and PC/phosphatidyl-serine (PS) (7:3 mol ratio) multilamellar vesicles. Macrophage monolayers were incubated with multilamellar vesicles and washed, and the amount of cell-associated liposomes was determined. Circles, PC/PS; squares, PC.

TABLE 13.1. *Lung Retention of Liposomes of Differing Size and Phospholipid Composition after Intravenous Administration into Mice*

Liposome Structure	Lipid Composition (mol ratio)	Intravenously Injected Dose Retained in Lungs (%)
MLV	PC	2.2
SUV	PC	0.5
REV	PC/PS (7/3)	7.2
SUV	PC/PS (7/3)	0.9
MLV	PC/PS (9/1)	2.2
MLV	PC/PS (8/2)	2.3
MLV	PC/PS (7/3)	6.6

Mice were injected intravenously with liposome preparations containing iodinated lipids (2 μmol in 0.2 ml saline), the lung radioactivity was monitored four hours later.
MLV = multilamellar vesicles; SUV = small unilamellar vesicles; REV = reverse evaporation phase vesicles; PC = phosphatidylcholine; PS = phosphatidylserine.

recognition and in situ removal by mononuclear phagocytes. Several very attractive mechanisms have been proposed over the years that either directly (Danon and Marikovsky 1964, Danon et al. 1971, Bocci 1976) or indirectly (Kay 1975, 1980, Alderman et al. 1981) involve modification of endogenous RBC carbohydrates by removal of sialic acid. These mechanisms may operate directly, by macrophage recognition of the altered surface charge (loss of sialic acid) or indirectly, by binding of autologous antibodies to previously masked RBC antigens such as asialoglycophorin (Alderman et al. 1981) or band 3 (Low et al. 1985) followed by Fc receptor-mediated binding (Alderman et al. 1981, Kay 1980). Collectively, these data suggest that the recognition of effete RBC by macrophages involves carbohydrates and proteins.

Little attention, however, has been given to the possibility that RBC membrane phospholipids might also play a role in this process. Because of our interest in the interaction of macrophages with phospholipid liposomes (see preceding section), we were intrigued by the observation that RBC membrane phospholipids are distributed asymmetrically. Of the four major phospholipids—PC, PS, phosphatidylethanolamine (PE) and sphingomyelin—that constitute the RBC membrane, only PS is found exclusively in the inner bilayer leaflet (Gordesky and Marinetti 1973, Verkleij et al. 1973, Rothman and Lenard 1977), possibly suggesting an important physiologic role in the preservation of this asymmetry. There is a precedent for this possibility. The asymmetric distribution of phospholipids in biologic membranes has been implicated in a variety of biologic phenomena, such as sickle cell anemia (Chiu et al. 1979, Lubin et al. 1981), platelet aggregation, and cell transformation (Rothman and Lenard 1977, Op den Kamp 1979, Fontaine and Schroeder 1979). These data and our particular interest in PS that contains liposomes raised the obvious question as to whether the presence or absence of PS from the outer leaflet of the cell membrane participates in the recognition process of RBC by macrophages.

In an attempt to answer this question, we have investigated the capability of macrophages cultivated in vitro to recognize RBC containing exogenously supplied phospholipid analogs (Tanaka and Schroit 1983), sickled RBC (Schwartz et al. 1985), and inside-out RBC ghosts displaying endogenous PS in their outer leaflet (Schroit et al. 1984). More recently, we have completed studies on the in vivo clearance of RBC displaying outer leaflet PS (Schroit et al. 1985).

In the first set of experiments, we investigated whether macrophages could recognize PS that was localized in the outer leaflet bilayer of RBC. Experimental procedures were developed to define those conditions under which exogenously supplied self-quenching fluorescent PS and PC analogs (Struck and Pagano 1980, Pagano et al. 1981, Schroit and Pagano 1981) would transfer to and become incorporated into the plasma membrane of RBC, as opposed to their mechanisms of vesicle-cell interactions (Pagano et al. 1981, Raz et al.

TABLE 13.2. *Binding and Phagocytosis of RBC Treated with Fluorescent Lipids by Macrophages and Inhibition of the Process by PC/PS Liposomes*

	RBC Uptake (%)		
Type of RBC	Without SUV	With SUV	Inhibition (%)
Control (untreated)	1.9	2.2	—
NBD-PC–treated	2.3	2.0	13
NBD-PS–treated	10.2	4.1	60

Macrophage monolayers ($\sim 10^5$ cells) were incubated with a 60-fold excess of ^{51}Cr-labeled RBC for 1 hour at 37°C. Inhibition was carried out by pretreatment of the macrophages with PC/PS SUV (7:3 mol ratio; 10 nmoles lipid) for 30 minutes at 37°C. The cultures were then washed and incubated with the various RBC preparations for an additional 1 hour at 37°C.
RBC = red blood cells; PC = phosphatidylcholine; PS = phosphatidylserine; SUV = small unilamellar vesicles; NBD = 1-acyl-2[(N-Y-nitro-benzo-2-oxa-1, 3 diazole) aminocaproyl].

1981). Under appropriate conditions, it was determined that approximately 90% of the total cell-associated lipid was diluted in the RBC membrane (Tanaka and Schroit 1983). Fluorescence microscopy of RBC treated in this manner revealed the presence of bright, uniform peripheral ring fluorescence, corroborating lipid dequenching of the initial nonfluorescent donor vesicles. The uptake of RBC treated with 1-acyl-2[(N-4-nitro-benzo-2-oxa-1,3 diazole) aminocaproyl]-phosphatidylserine (NBD-PS) (at NBD-PS concentrations where essentially all of the cell-associated lipid analog was confirmed to be properly inserted in the outer leaflet) by in vitro cultivated mouse peritoneal macrophages at 37°C was four to five times greater than that of either NBD-PC–treated or –untreated control RBC (Table 13.2). This observation was also confirmed by fluorescence microscopy, which revealed typical fluorescent RBC-macrophage rosettes in NBD-PS–treated RBC (Figure 13.2) (Tanaka and Schroit 1983).

In order to directly compare the ultrastructural characteristics and possible differences of PS-mediated macrophage binding and the well-known high-affinity binding of opsonized RBC to macrophages, scanning and transmission electron photomicrographs of both preparations were carried out (Schroit et al. 1984). Both NBD-PS and opsonized RBC formed typical rosettes, although the degree of RBC clustering was clearly more pronounced in the opsonized RBC. In addition, the opsonized RBC had a distorted and crowded appearance, suggesting very strong adhesion to the macrophage surface, whereas the binding of NBD-PS–treated RBC appeared to be more delicate, with little or no morphologic aberrations in the attached RBC (Figure 13.3).

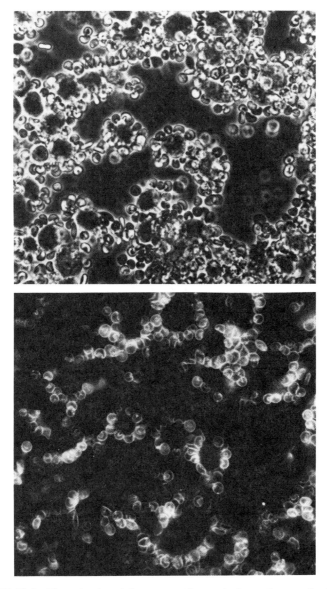

FIGURE 13.2. Phase (top) and fluorescent (bottom) photomicrograph of NBD-phosphatidylserine–treated RBC-macrophage rosettes.

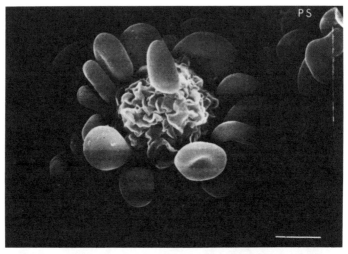

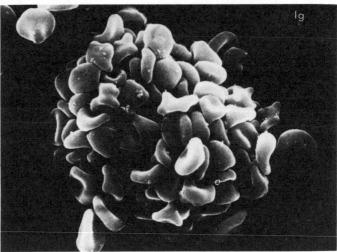

FIGURE 13.3. Scanning electron micrograph of mouse macrophages incubated with NBC-phosphatidylserine (PS)–treated RBC (PS, top) or opsonized RBC (Ig, bottom). Bar = 5 μ.

Evidence indicating the possibility of PS involvement in the physiologic recognition and clearance of RBC with outer leaflet PS has recently been published (Schroit et al. 1984, 1985). In these experiments, syngeneic mice were injected intravenously with ^{51}Cr-labeled RBC containing outer leaflet NBD-PS and the clearance of the cells from the peripheral blood was examined.

TABLE 13.3. *Clearance of Control, NBD-PC– and NBD-PS–Treated RBC from the Circulation*

Type of RBC	RBC Injected (cpm × 10^{-3})	RBC Remaining in Peripheral Blood (cpm × 10^{-3})	Clearance (%)
Control (untreated)	557	524	0
NBD-PC–treated	605	493	14
NBD-PS–treated	574	255	53

Control or vesicle-treated ^{51}Cr-labeled mouse RBC (0.2 ml = 4 × 10^9, RBC = 10^5 cpm) were injected intravenously. One hour later, aliquots of blood (0.2 ml) were counted. Total blood volume was determined by the following relationship by using control untreated RBC. Total blood volume = [(cpm injected × 0.2) – cpm in 0.2 ml]. The percent clearance was calculated by using control RBC as a 0% clearance reference.
RBC = red blood cells; PC = phosphatidylcholine; PS = phosphatidylserine; NBD = 1-acyl-2[(N-Y-nitro-benzo-2-oxa-1, 3 diazole) aminocaproyl].

Within one hour after injection, more than 50% of the injected NBD-PS–treated RBC were cleared and found to localize in the liver and spleen (Table 13.3). In contrast, NBD-PC–treated RBC and untreated control RBC were not cleared from the circulation to any significant extent.

Collectively, these data suggest that a normal lipid constituent of biologic membranes, PS, can play a role in the process of in vitro and in vivo recognition of RBC by macrophages.

The Recognition of Sickled Human RBC by Peripheral Blood Monocytes

The average life span of circulating sickled RBC is considerably shorter than that of normal RBC (McCurdy 1969). Recent observations that sickled RBC are unusually adherent to artificial lipid vesicles (Schwartz et al. 1983), cultured endothelial cells (Hoover et al. 1979, Hebbel et al. 1980), and macrophages (Hebbel and Miller 1984) have suggested that sickled RBC may display a membrane abnormality that could increase their propensity for cell-to-cell interaction. Interestingly, in normal RBC, PS is found exclusively in the inner leaflet of the plasma membrane (see above), whereas in irreversibly sickled RBC or reversibly sickled RBC, PS is localized in both the inner and outer membrane leaflets (Chiu et al. 1979, 1981, Lubin et al. 1981).

We have, therefore, recently determined whether the abnormal exposure of outer leaflet PS in sickled RBC could also explain the increased interaction of sickled RBC with macrophages (Schroit et al. 1984, Schwartz et al. 1985). In these experiments, normal RBC, irreversibly sickled RBC, and reversibly sickled cells were incubated with blood monocytes. Deoxygenation of sickled RBC resulted in increased binding to monocytes as compared to oxygenated (PS expressed only in the inner leaflet) sickled RBC, and oxygenated or deoxygenated normal RBC (PS expressed only in the inner leaflet). Morphologic examination of this interaction has revealed the presence of sickled RBC-monocyte rosettes and provided confirmation of the quantitative binding data (Schroit et al. 1984).

It seems, therefore, that PS in the outer leaflet of the sickled RBC membrane served as a recognition moiety by monocytes. Indeed, this conclusion is supported by inhibition studies wherein treatment of monocytes with PS liposomes resulted in an approximate 60% inhibition of sickled RBC adherence to the monocytes. No similar inhibition could be obtained by preincubating the monocytes with PC liposomes. These findings suggest that qualitative abnormalities in the organization of RBC membrane phospholipids may have significant pathophysiologic implications.

Recognition and Lysis of Herpesvirus-infected but Not Uninfected Cells

Although viral diseases of man and domesticated animals are a major cause of morbidity and mortality, early hopes for antiviral treatment similar to that for bacteria have not been fulfilled. The lack of success in treating viral diseases has resulted in part from the fact that viral replication is associated with normal host cells' biosynthetic pathways (Vilcek 1979). Another obstacle to effective viral therapeutics is the difficulty in delivering antiviral agents to the site of virus replication. Several groups of viruses infect cells of the RE system, and virus replication in macrophages is often an integral factor in the pathogenesis of severe systemic virus infections (Mims 1964, Morgensen 1977, Koff and Fidler 1985).

Most acute viral infections are characterized by an inflammatory response with characteristic perivascular infiltration of mononuclear phagocytes (Johnson 1982). Macrophages are important components of the host's first line of defense against virus infections, and their accumulation at sites of primary virus infection is enhanced by the release of chemotactic stimuli produced at foci of virus replication (Allison 1974, Glasgow 1979). In viral reinfections, the interaction of virus-coded proteins with sensitized lymphocytes could trigger the release of lymphokines with chemotactic activity and lymphokines that can also activate the macrophages for antiviral effects (McFarland et al. 1972). Subsequent to interaction with various factors, macrophages can become cytostatic and cytotoxic against virus infected cells (Morahan et al. 1977, 1980, Goldman and Hogg 1978, Chapes and Tompkins 1979, Koff et al. 1983).

For these reasons, we have recently proposed that targeting liposomes to mononuclear phagocytes (Schroit et al. 1983a,b, Alving 1983) could be used to deliver antiviral agents or immunomodulators to macrophages in situ for the treatment of viral disease (Koff and Fidler 1985). The suggested use of liposomes is based in part on our own data showing that liposomes containing various immunomodulators can activate human blood monocytes to distinguish between HSV-2–infected cells and uninfected normal cells (Koff et al. 1984). Highly purified human blood monocytes were incubated with liposomes containing immunomodulators such as lymphokines, IFN-γ, and MTP-PE. After 24 hours of incubation, the cultures were washed and the monocytes were tested for their ability to lyse uninfected and HSV-2–infected normal human cells or normal mouse cells. Monocytes incubated with control (unactivated) medium were not cytotoxic against any of the targets. In contrast, activated monocytes lysed HSV-2–infected cells but did not harm uninfected normal cells (Table 13.4). In addition, the systemic administration of liposomes containing MTP-PE but not control liposomes can protect a high proportion of mice from a lethal infection with HSV-2. We base this conclusion upon the data of very recent experiments in which mice infected with HSV-2 (intraperitoneally or intravenously) were given multiple intravenous injections of liposomes containing balanced salt solutions or MTP-PE. A high proportion of mice treated with liposome–MTP-PE survived the lethal HSV-2 infection (Koff et al. 1985), indicating that the delivery of macrophage activators to cells of the RE system via liposomes could bring about significant therapeutic benefits in the management of an acute viral infection (Koff et al. 1985).

The mechanisms by which macrophages discriminate virus-infected from uninfected cells is unknown, although virus-induced changes in the com-

TABLE 13.4. *Monocyte Mediated Lysis of HSV-2–Infected Cells but Not of Uninfected Cells*

	Target Cell Lysis by Activated Monocytes (%)	
Target cells	Free–MAF	Liposome–MAF
Uninfected WHE (human)	8	3
HSV-2–infected WHE (human)	28	21
Uninfected 10E2 (mouse)	1	14
HSV-2–infected 10E2 (mouse)	0	22

Human monocytes were activated by free or liposome encapsulated MAF prior to interaction with ^{51}Cr-labeled target cells. Percent cytotoxicity was derived from comparison with target cells cultured alone.
HSV-2 = type 2 herpes simplex virus; MAF = macrophage activation factors.

position of the host cell plasma membranes might play a role in this process (Shillitoe and Rapp 1979). Recent studies with recombinant reoviruses have suggested that recognition of reovirus-infected target cells by mouse peritoneal cells is via the virus hemagglutinin protein (Letvin et al. 1982). In any event, the finding that macrophages activated via liposomes containing immunomodulators recognize and destroy tumorigenic cells (see below) and HSV-2 infected cells but not normal cells (Hibbs 1974a, Fidler 1978, Fidler et al. 1978, Fidler and Kleinerman 1984), suggests the possibility that the recognition moiety might be similar.

Recognition and Destruction of Neoplastic Cells

Macrophages activated by free or liposome–containing immunomodulators such as MDP, MAF, or IFN-γ acquire the ability to recognize and lyse neoplastic cells by a mechanism that requires direct cell-to-cell contact (Figure 13.4) (Hibbs 1974b, Bucana et al. 1976, 1983, Marino and Adams 1980a,b). The ability of tumoricidal macrophages to discriminate between tumorigenic and normal cells has been studied in several systems, including syngeneic and allogeneic mouse tumors, syngeneic rat tumors, and syngeneic guinea pig tumors (Hibbs 1974b, Fidler 1978, Fidler et al. 1978, Hamilton and Fishman 1981, 1982). These data indicate that, at least in vitro, tumoricidal macrophages of rodents can discriminate between neoplastic and nonneoplastic cells by a process that is independent of transplantation antigens, species-specific antigens, tumor-specific antigens, cell cycle time, or various phenotypes associated with transformation. Moreover, data obtained in various murine systems suggest that the susceptibility of tumor cells to destruction by tumoricidal macrophages is also independent of in vivo biologic behavior of the tumor cells, such as invasiveness, metastatic potential, growth rate, and resistance to lysis by lymphocytes, natural killer cells, or cytotoxic drugs (for review, see Fidler 1984).

Most studies on the interaction of macrophages with tumor cells have been carried out in systems with isolated cultures of tumorigenic cells (Mantovani et al. 1979, Sone and Tsubura 1982, Kleinerman et al. 1983a,b, Fogler and Fidler 1985). However, since metastatic cells proliferate among normal host cells, it was essential to determine whether human blood monocytes could also discriminate between tumorigenic and nontumorigenic human target cells under cocultivation conditions because these conditions would more closely resemble in vivo conditions (Fidler and Kleinerman 1984).

Highly purified preparations of peripheral blood monocytes isolated from normal human donors were activated in vitro by incubation with human lymphokines encapsulated in multilamellar liposomes. The cytotoxic properties of these monocytes against several tumorigenic and nontumorigenic allo-

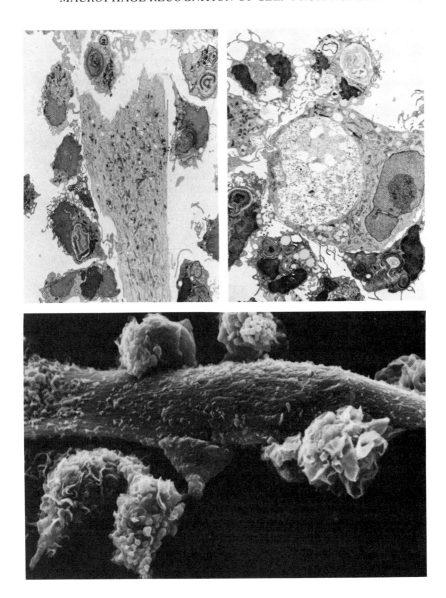

FIGURE 13.4. Transmission (top) and scanning electron micrographs (bottom) of activated macrophage-tumor cell interaction. Note endocytosed liposomes in the transmission micrographs.

TABLE 13.5. *Selective Monocyte-Mediated Cytotoxicity against Tumorigenic Cells Cocultivated with Nontumorigenic Targets*

Target Cells Labeled with [³H] thymidine		Target Cells Labeled with [¹⁴C] thymidine	
A375 melanoma	(58%)	Dermal fibroblasts	(0%)
Dermal fibroblasts	(−8%)	A375 melanoma	(53%)
HT-29 carcinoma	(44%)	Lung cells	(−2%)
Lung cells	(3%)	HT-29 carcinoma	(52%)
NAT-glioblastoma	(38%)	Lung cells	(0%)
Lung cells	(−1%)	NAT-glioblastoma	(45%)
A375 melanoma	(48%)	NAT glioblastoma	(47%)
A375 melanoma	(41%)	HT-29 carcinoma	(49%)
A375 melanoma	(51%)	A375 melanoma	(33%)
Lung cells	(0%)	Dermal fibroblasts	(1%)
Lung cells	(1%)	Kidney cells	(2%)
Kidney cells	(0%)	Dermal fibroblasts	(0%)

In these experiments, target cells were cultured alone, with monocytes incubated with liposomes containing medium, or with liposomes containing lymphokines. Control monocytes were not cytotoxic to any of the targets. The number in parentheses is the percentage of target cell lysis as compared with that of control monocytes and target cells ($P < .001$).

geneic target cell populations were assessed by an in vitro radioisotope-release assay. Various combinations of three tumorigenic (A375 melanoma, HT-29 carcinoma, and NAT glioblastoma) and three nontumorigenic target-cell populations (lung cells, skin cells, and kidney cells) labeled with either [³H]thymidine or [¹⁴C]thymidine were mixed and plated onto monolayers of blood monocytes. When possible, we attempted to pair tumor cells with physiologically acceptable normal counterparts. We therefore used both epithelial cells and fibroblasts as normal controls for tumors of endodermal, ectodermal, and mesenchymal origin. In all combinations used, activated monocytes specifically lysed only allogeneic neoplastic cells and left non-tumorigenic cells unharmed (Table 13.5).

These data demonstrate that, in common with other mammalian macrophages, human blood monocytes that are activated in vitro by interaction with liposomes containing immunomodulators can selectively lyse neoplastic cells in mixed cultures. It should be noted that the selective lysis of tumorigenic cells was not merely because of an inherent resistance of normal cells to lysis mediated by immune cells, but was associated with activated monocytes, since both tumorigenic and nontumorigenic cells were equally susceptible to in vitro lysis mediated by stimulated peripheral blood lymphocytes.

Recognition of Tumorigenic Cells with Temperature-dependent
Transformed Phenotypic Characteristics

To determine whether any of the altered cell surface properties commonly
present in virus-transformed cells provide the basis for macrophage recognition, we tested the ability of tumoricidal macrophages to recognize and destroy cell lines transformed by polyoma virus or simian virus 40 (SV-40) in
which several of the surface characteristics associated with the transformed
phenotype are only expressed at specific temperatures (Fidler et al. 1978). We
reasoned that if macrophages recognized target cells by a surface moiety that
is associated with transformation, destruction of temperature-sensitive transformed cells would occur at the permissive (33°C) but not at the nonpermissive (39°C) temperatures for transformation. To do so, macrophage mediated cytotoxicity was determined at both 33°C and 39°–40°C (Table 13.6).
Specifically, we used baby hamster kidney cells transformed by the ts-3 mutant of polyoma virus, rat embryo 3Y1 cells transformed by a temperature-
sensitive A cistron mutant of SV-40 and the ts-H6-15 line of SV-40–transformed
mouse 3T3 cells. All target cells were lysed in vitro by activated mouse or rat
macrophages at both the permissive and nonpermissive temperatures for

TABLE 13.6. *In Vitro Cytolysis Mediated by Tumoricidal Mouse*
Macrophages against Untransformed, Wild-Type Transformed and
Temperature-Sensitive Mutant Cells.

Target Cells		Macrophage Mediated Cytotoxicity (%)	
Source	*Type*	*33°C*	*39°C*
Mouse	3T3 (untransformed)	0	1
	SV-40 3T3 (wild, transformed)	63	62
	ts-H6-15 (ts mutant)	56	60
Hamster	BHK/c13 (untransformed)	1	2
	PY-BHK (wild, transformed)	50	51
	ts-3 PY-BHK (ts mutant)	53	61
Rat	3Y1-B1 (untransformed)	3	2
	SV-68/3Y1 (wild, transformed)	72	91
	ts-640/3Y1 (ts mutant)	53	87

Target cells were cultured with control and lymphokine activated macrophages
for 72 hours at either the permissive temperature (33°C) or nonpermissive temperature (39°C) for expression of the transformation phenotypes. Percent macrophage mediated cytotoxicity was derived from comparison of target cell
survival with normal noncytotoxic macrophages.

expression of the transformed phenotype. The target cells transformed by wild-type SV-40 or polyoma virus were also lysed at both temperatures, but untransformed target cells were not harmed by the macrophages. Since the macrophages killed target cells with temperature-dependent phenotypic characteristics equally well at both temperatures, we concluded that phenotypic characteristics of transformation, such as expression of cell surface high molecular weight (>200,000) glycoproteins, Forssman antigen, surface changes for lectin agglutination, expression of SV-40 T antigen, low saturation density, or density-dependent inhibition of DNA synthesis are all unlikely to contribute to the mechanism by which macrophages recognize and destroy transformed cells, at least in vitro (Fidler et al. 1978).

CONCLUDING REMARKS

The macrophage is a cell whose primary function, phagocytosis, has been well conserved throughout evolution. In multicellular organisms, it is probably one of the most versatile cells; the macrophage's function in both vertebrates and invertebrates is to discriminate between "self" and "nonself" and thus to recognize, phagocytose, and dispose of effete cells, cellular debris, and foreign invaders.

The mechanism responsible for the remarkable ability of mononuclear phagocytes to discriminate between young and old cells, healthy and damaged cells, and normal and tumorigenic cells is not known. It is tempting to speculate that cells recognized as "nonself" must exhibit a new and specific, recognizable membrane determinant that provides the signal for their removal by phagocytic cells. It is inconceivable that mononuclear phagocytes have the ability to recognize the potentially infinite diversity presented by modified polypeptide and carbohydrate sequences, which have been shown to be different between normal cells and a variety of pathologic cells, especially when one considers that macrophages can easily discriminate tumor cells (a property related solely to the tumorigenic phenotype) and virus-infected cells from "normal" cells.

Throughout phylogenetic development, macrophages have retained the primitive function of endocytosis. It is therefore conceivable that these cells must be able to recognize a moiety that has not undergone numerous evolutionary modifications. This assumption would, therefore, imply a minor role for carbohydrates and polypeptides in the early phylogenetic appearance of the endocytotic process and would suggest that phospholipids might be one of the earliest and most primitive moieties providing a signal for recognition of "altered self" by macrophages.

Certainly, there is no question that macrophages can recognize carbohydrates and proteins on their targets (Cohn 1978, Karnovsky and Lazdins

1978), and we do not imply that recognition of altered surface charge does not play a role in macrophage recognition of senescent or damaged cells. We do believe, however, that our results suggest that a normal lipid constituent of biologic membranes, PS, plays a prominent role in the process of macrophage recognition of synthetic phospholipid membranes, RBC, and perhaps neoplastic cells.

Could this observation indicate that macrophages have retained an "undifferentiated," primordial, recognition system? Indeed, recent data from our laboratory indicate that this may be the case. We have shown that the binding of liposomes containing PS by adherent insect plasmacytes isolated from the hemolymph of the lepidopteran *Heliothis virescens* is more avid than the binding of liposomes composed exclusively of PC, a finding strikingly similar to that seen in studies of mammalian macrophages (Ratner S unpublished data).

In conclusion, the data presented here do suggest that PS can serve as a signal for triggering macrophage recognition of various targets. While these findings do not imply that evolutionarily more sophisticated recognition systems, such as protein- and carbohydrate-related processes, are not as important, they do suggest that a simpler recognition mechanism may be operative, a system that has endured at least several steps of phylogenetic development.

ACKNOWLEDGMENT

The data reviewed in this manuscript are from many collaborators, whose invaluable help we wish to acknowledge. We thank Corazon Bucana, William Fogler, Eugenia Kleinerman, Wayne Koff, John Madsen, George Poste, Stuart Ratner, Avraham Raz, Saburo Sone, Robert Schwartz, and Yutaka Tanaka for their invaluable contributions.

REFERENCES

Alderman EM, Fudenberg HH, Lovins RE. 1981. Isolation and characterization of an age-related antigen present on senescent human red blood cells. Blood 50:341–349.

Allison AC. 1974. On the role of mononuclear phagocytes in immunity against viruses. Prog Med Virol 18:15–31.

Alving CR. 1983. Delivery of liposome-encapsulated drugs to macrophages. Pharmacol Ther 22:407–424.

Bocci V. 1976. The role of sialic acid in determining the life span of circulating cells and glycoproteins. Experientia 32:135–140.

Bucana C, Hoyer LC, Hobbs B, Breesman S, McDaniel M, Hanna MG Jr. 1976. Morphological evidence for the translocation of lysosomal organelles from cytotoxic macrophages into the cytoplasm of tumor target cells. Cancer Res 36:4444–4458.

Bucana CD, Hoyer LC, Schroit AJ, Kleinerman E, Fidler IJ. 1983. Ultrastructural studies of the interaction between liposome-activated human blood monocytes and allogeneic tumor cells in vitro. Am J Pathol 112:101–111.

Chapes SK, Tompkins WAF. 1979. Cytotoxic macrophages induced in hamsters by vaccinia virus: Selective cytotoxicity for virus-infected targets by macrophages collected late after immunization. J Immunol 123:303–309.

Chedid L, Carelli L, Audibert F. 1979. Recent developments concerning muramyl dipeptide, a synthetic immunoregulating molecule. J Reticuloendothel Soc 26:631–641.

Chiu D, Lubin B, Shohet SB. 1979. Erythrocyte membrane lipid reorganization during the sickling process. Br J Haematol 41:223–234.

Chiu D, Lubin B, Roelofsen B, Van Deenen LLM. 1981. Sickled erythrocytes accelerate clotting in vitro: An effect of abnormal membrane lipid asymmetry. Blood 58:398–401.

Cohn Z. 1978. The activation of mononuclear phagocytes: Fact, fancy, future. J Immunol 121:813–861.

Danon D, Marikovsky Y. 1964. Determination of density distribution of red cell populations. J Lab Clin Med 64:668–674.

Danon D, Marikovsky Y, Skutelsky E. 1971. In Ramot B, ed., Red Blood Cell Structure and Metabolism. Academic Press, New York, pp. 23–28.

Fidler IJ. 1978. Recognition and destruction of target cells by tumoricidal macrophages. Isr J Med Sci 14:177–191.

Fidler IJ. 1980. Therapy of spontaneous metastases by intravenous injection of liposomes containing lymphokines. Science 208:1469–1471.

Fidler IJ. 1981. The in situ induction of tumoricidal activity in alveolar macrophages by liposomes containing muramyl dipeptide is a thymus-independent process. J Immunol 127:1719–1720.

Fidler IJ. 1984. The MAF dilemma. Lymphokine Research 3:51–54.

Fidler IJ, Fogler WE. 1982. Activation of tumoricidal properties in macrophages by lymphokines encapsulated in liposomes. Lymphokine Research 1:73–77.

Fidler IJ, Kleinerman ES. 1984. Lymphokine-activated human blood monocytes destroy tumor cells but not normal cells under cocultivation conditions. J Clin Oncol 2:937–943.

Fidler IJ, Poste G. 1982. Macrophage-mediated destruction of malignant tumor cells and new strategies for the therapy of metastatic disease. Springer Semin Immunopathol 5:161–174.

Fidler IJ, Raz A. 1981. The induction of tumoricidal capacities in mouse and rat macrophages by lymphokines. In Pick E, ed., Lymphokines, vol. 3. Academic Press, New York, pp. 345–363.

Fidler IJ, Schroit AJ. 1984. Synergism between lymphokines and muramyl dipeptide encapsulated in liposomes: In situ activation of macrophages and therapy of spontaneous cancer metastasis. J Immunol 133:515–518.

Fidler IJ, Roblin RO, Poste G. 1978. In vitro tumoricidal activity of macrophages against virus-transformed lines with temperature-dependent transformed phenotypic characteristics. Cell Immunol 38:131–146.

Fidler IJ, Raz A, Fogler WE, Kirsh R, Bugelski P, Poste G. 1980. The design of liposomes to improve delivery of macrophage-augmenting agents to alveolar macrophages. Cancer Res 40:4460–4466.

Fidler IJ, Sone S, Fogler WE, Barnes ZL. 1981. Eradication of spontaneous metastases and activation of alveolar macrophages by intravenous injection of liposomes containing muramyl dipeptide. Proc Natl Acad Sci USA 78: 1680–1684.

Fidler IJ, Barnes Z, Fogler WE, Kirsh R, Bugelski P, Poste G. 1982a. Involvement of macrophages in the eradication of established metastases following intravenous injection of liposomes containing macrophage activators. Cancer Res 42:496–501.

Fidler IJ, Sone S, Fogler WE, et al. 1982b. Efficacy of liposomes containing a lipophilic muramyl dipeptide derivative for activating the tumoricidal properties of alveolar macrophages in vivo. J Biol Response Mod 1:43–55.

Fogler WE, Fidler IJ. 1985. Nonselective destruction of murine neoplastic cells by syngeneic tumoricidal macrophages. Cancer Res 45:14–18.

Fogler WE, Wade R, Brundish DE, Fidler IJ. 1985. Distribution and fate of free and liposome-encapsulated [^{3}H]nor-muramyl dipeptide and [^{3}H]muramyl tripeptide phosphatidylethanolamine in mice. J Immunol 135:1372–1377.

Fontaine RN, Schroeder F. 1979. Plasma membrane aminophospholipid distribution in transformed murine fibroblasts. Biochim Biophys Acta 558:1–12.

Gisler RH, Dietrich FM, Baschang G, et al. 1979. *In* Turk JL, Danker D, eds., Immune Responsiveness. The MacMillan Press Ltd., London, pp. 133–160.

Glasgow LA. 1979. Biology and pathogenesis of viral infections. *In* Galasso GJ, Merigan TC, Buchanan RA, eds., Antiviral Agents and Viral Diseases of Man. Raven Press, New York, pp. 39–76.

Goldman R, Hogg N. 1978. Enhanced susceptibility of virus-infected fibroblasts to cytostasis mediated by peritoneal exudate cells. J Immunol 121:1657–1663.

Gordesky SE, Marinetti GV. 1973. The arrangement of phospholipids in the human erythrocyte. Biochem Biophys Res Commun 50:1027–1031.

Gregoriadis G, Allison AC, eds. 1980. Liposomes in Biological Systems. Wiley Interscience, New York.

Gregoriadis G, Nefrungen DE, Hunt R. 1977. Fate of liposome-associated agents injected into normal and tumor-bearing rodents. Life Sci 21:357–370.

Hamilton TA, Fishman M. 1981. Characterization of the recognition of target cells sensitive or resistant to cytolysis by activated rat peritoneal macrophages. J Immunol 127:1702–1707.

Hamilton TA, Fishman M. 1982. Characterization of the recognition of target cells sensitive to or resistant to cytolysis by activated macrophages. Cell Immunol 68:155–164.

Hart IR, Fogler WE, Post G, Fidler IJ. 1981. Toxicity studies of liposome-encapsulated immunomodulators administered intravenously into dogs and mice. Cancer Immunol Immunother 10:157–166.

Hebbel RP, Miller WJ. 1984. Phagocytosis of sickle erythrocytes: Immunologic and oxidative determinants of hemolytic anemia. Blood 64:733–741.

Hebbel RP, Yamuda O, Moldow CF, Jacob HS, White JG, Eaton JW. 1980. Abnormal adherence of sickle erythrocytes to cultured vascular endothelium: Possible mechanism for microvascular occlusion in sickle cell disease. J Clin Invest 65:154–160.

Hoover R, Rubin R, Wise G, Warren R. 1979. Adhesion of normal and sickle erythrocytes to endothelial monolayer cultures. Blood 54:872–876.

Hibbs JB Jr. 1974a. Discrimination between neoplastic and non-neoplastic cells in vitro by activated macrophages. JNCI 53:1487–1492.

Hibbs JB Jr. 1974b. Heterocytolysis by macrophages activated by bacillus Calmette-Guerin: Lysosome exocytosis into tumor cells. Science 184:468–471.

Johnson RT. 1982. Viral Infections of the Nervous System. Raven Press, New York.

Karnovsky ML, Lazdins JK. 1978. Biochemical criteria for activated macrophages. J Immunol 121:809–813.

Kay MMB. 1975. Mechanism and removal of senescent cells by human macrophages in situ. Proc Natl Acad Sci USA 72:3521–3525.

Kay MMB. 1980. Cells, signals and receptors: The role of physiological anti-antibodies in maintaining homeostasis. Adv Exp Med Biol 129:171–200.

Kleinerman ES, Erickson KL, Schroit AJ, Fogler WE, Fidler IJ. 1983a. Activation of tumoricidal properties in human blood monocytes by liposomes containing lipophilic muramyl tripeptide. Cancer Res 43:2010–2014.

Kleinerman ES, Schroit AJ, Fogler WE, Fidler IJ. 1983b. Tumoricidal activity of human monocytes activated in vitro by free and liposome-encapsulated human lymphokines. J Clin Invest 72:1–12.

Kleinerman ES, Zicht R, Sarin PS, Gallo RC, Fidler IJ. 1984. Constitutive production and release of a lymphokine with macrophage-activating factor activity distinct from gamma-interferon by a human T-cell leukemia virus-positive cell line. Cancer Res 44:4470–4475.

Koff WC, Fidler IJ. 1985. The potential use of liposome-mediated antiviral therapy. Antiviral Res 228:495–497.

Koff WC, Showalter SD, Seniff DA, Hampar B. 1983. Lysis of herpesvirus-infected cells by macrophages activated with free or liposome-encapsulated lymphokine produced by a murine T cell hybridoma. Infect Immun 42:1067–1072.

Koff WC, Fidler IJ, Showalter SD, et al. 1984. Human monocytes activated by immunomodulators in liposomes lyse herpes virus infected but not normal cells. Science 224:1007–1009.

Koff WC, Showalter SD, Hampar B, Fidler IJ. 1985. Protection of mice against Herpes simplex type 2 infection by liposomes containing muramyl tripeptide. Science 228:495–497.

Lederer E. 1980. Synthetic immunostimulants derived from the bacterial cell wall. J Med Chem 23:819–825.

Letvin NL, Kauffman RS, Finberg R. 1982. An adherent cell lyses virus-infected targets: Characterization, activation, and fine specificity of the cytotoxic cell. J Immunol 129:2396–2401.

Low PS, Waugh SM, Zinke K, Dremckhahn D. 1985. The role of hemoglobin denaturation and Band 3 clustering in red blood cell aging. Science 227:531–533.

Lubin B, Chiu D, Bastacky J, Roelofsen B, Van Deenen LLM. 1981. Abnormalities in membrane phospholipid organization in sickled erythrocytes. J Clin Invest 67:1643–1649.

Mantovani A, Jerrells TR, Dean JH, Herberman R. 1979. Cytolytic and cytostatic activity on tumor cells of circulating human monocytes. Int J Cancer 23:18–27.

Marino PA, Adams DO. 1980a. Interaction of Bacillus Calmette-Guerin–activated macrophages and neoplastic cells in vitro: I. Conditions of binding and its selectivity. Cell Immunol 54:11–25.

Marino PA, Adams DO. 1980b. Interaction of Bacillus Calmette-Guerin–activated macrophages and neoplastic cells in vitro: II. The relationship of selective binding to cytolysis. Cell Immunol 54:26–35.

McCurdy PR. 1969. ^{32}DFP and ^{51}Cr for measurement of red cell life span in abnormal hemoglobin syndromes. Blood 33:214–224.

McFarland HF, Griffin DE, Johnson RT. 1972. Specificity of the inflammatory response in viral encephalitis: I. Adoptive immunization of immunosuppressed mice infected with Sindbis virus. J Exp Med 136:216–226.

Mehta K, Lopez-Berestein G, Hersh EM, Juliano RL. 1982. Uptake of liposomes and liposome-encapsulated muramyl dipeptide by human peripheral blood monocytes. J Reticuloendothel Soc 32:155–164.

Mims CA. 1964. Aspects of the pathogenesis of virus diseases. Bacteriological Reviews 28:30–71.

Morahan PS, Glasgow LA, Crane JL Jr, Kern ER. 1977. Comparison of antiviral and antitumor activity of activated macrophages. Cell Immunol 28:404–415.

Morahan PS, Morse SS, McGeorge MB. 1980. Macrophage extrinsic anti-viral activity during herpes simplex virus infection. J Gen Virol 46:291–300.

Morgensen S. 1977. Role of macrophages in hepatitis induced by herpes simplex virus types 1 and 2 in mice. Infect Immun 15:686–691.

Morgensen SC. 1979. Role of macrophages in natural resistance to virus infections. Microbiol Rev 43:1–26.

Nicolau C, Paraf A, eds. 1981. Liposomes, Drugs and Immunocompetent Cell Functions. Academic Press, London.

Op den Kamp JAF. 1979. Lipid asymmetry in membranes. Ann Rev Biochem 48:47–71.

Pagano RE, Schroit AJ, Struck DK. 1981. Interactions of phospholipid vesicles with mammalian cells in vitro: Studies of mechanism. *In* Knight CG, ed., Liposomes: From Physical Structure to Therapeutic Applications. Elsevier, North Holland Biomedical Press, Amsterdam, pp. 323–348.

Parant M, Parant F, Chedid L, Yapo A, Petit JF, Lederer E. 1979. Fate of the synthetic immunoadjuvant, muramyl dipeptide (^{14}C-labelled) in the mouse. Int J Immunopharmacol 1:35–41.

Poste G. 1979. The tumoricidal properties of inflammatory tissue macrophages and multinucleate giant cells. Am J Pathol 96:595–606.

Poste G, Kirsh R. 1979. Rapid decay of tumoricidal activity and loss of responsiveness to lymphokines in inflammatory macrophages. Cancer Res 39:2582–2590.

Poste G, Kirsh R, Fidler IJ. 1979a. Cell surface receptors for lymphokines. Cell Immunol 44:71–88.

Poste G, Kirsh R, Fogler W, Fidler IJ. 1979b. Activation of tumoricidal properties in mouse macrophages by lymphokines encapsulated in liposomes. Cancer Res 39:881–892.

Poste G, Bucana C, Raz A, Bugelski P, Kirsh R, Fidler IJ. 1982. Analysis of the fate of systemically administered liposomes and implications for their use in drug delivery. Cancer Res 42:1412–1422.

Raz A, Bucana C, Fogler WE, Poste G, Fidler IJ. 1981. Biochemical, morphological and ultrastructural studies on the uptake of liposomes by murine macrophages. Cancer Res 41:487–494.

Rothman JE, Lenard J. 1977. Membrane asymmetry. Science 195:743–753.

Scherphof G, Roerdink F, Dijkstra J, Ellens H, de Zanger R, Wisse E. 1983. Uptake of liposomes by rat and mouse hepatocytes and Kupffer cells. Biology of the Cell 47:47–58.

Schroit AJ, Fidler IJ. 1982. Effects of liposome structure and lipid composition on the activation of the tumoricidal properties of macrophages by liposomes containing muramyl dipeptide. Cancer Res 42:161–167.

Schroit AJ, Pagano RE. 1981. Capping of a phospholipid analog in the plasma membrane of lymphocytes. Cell 23:105–112.

Schroit AJ, Galligioni E, Fidler IJ. 1983a. Factors influencing the *in situ* activation of macrophages by liposomes containing muramyl dipeptide. Biology of the Cell 47:87–94.

Schroit AJ, Hart IR, Madsen J, Fidler IJ. 1983b. Selective delivery of drugs encapsulated in liposomes: Natural targeting to macrophages involved in various disease states. J Biol Response Mod 2:97–100.

Schroit AJ, Tanaka Y, Madsen J, Fidler IJ. 1984. The recognition of red blood cells by macrophages: Role of phosphatidylserine and possible implications of membrane phospholipid asymmetry. Biology of the Cell 51:227–238.

Schroit AJ, Madsen JW, Tanaka Y. 1985. In vivo recognition and clearance of red blood cells containing phosphatidylserine in their plasma membranes. J Biol Chem 260:5131–5138.

Schwartz RS, Duzgunes N, Chiu DT-Y, Lubin B. 1983. Interaction of phosphatidylserine-phosphatidylcholine liposomes with sickle erythrocytes: Evidence for altered membrane surface properties. J Clin Invest 71:1570–1580.

Schwartz RS, Tanaka Y, Fidler IJ, Chiu D, Lubin B, Schroit AJ. 1985. Increased adherence of sickled and phosphatidylserine enriched human erythrocytes to cultured human peripheral blood monocytes. J Clin Invest 75:1965–1972.

Shillitoe EJ, Rapp F. 1979. Virus-induced cell surface antigens and cell-mediated immune responses. Springer Semin Immunopathol 2:237–259.

Sone S, Fidler IJ. 1980. Synergistic activation by lymphokines and muramyl dipeptide of tumoricidal properties in rat alveolar macrophages. J Immunol 125:2454–2460.

Sone S, Fidler IJ. 1981. In vitro activation of tumoricidal properties in rat alveolar macrophages by synthetic muramyl dipeptide encapsulated in liposomes. Cell Immunol 57:42–50.

Sone S, Tsubura E. 1982. Human alveolar macrophages: Potentiation of their tumoricidal activity by liposome-encapsulated muramyl dipeptide. J Immunol 129:1313–1317.

Struck DK, Pagano RE. 1980. Insertion of fluorescent phospholipids into the plasma membrane of a mammalian cell. J Biol Chem 255:5404–5410.

Tanaka Y, Schroit AJ. 1983. Insertion of fluorescent phosphatidylserine into the plasma membrane of red blood cells: Recognition by autologous macrophages. J Biol Chem 258:11335–11343.

Van Furth R. 1975. Mononuclear Phagocytes in Immunity, Infection, and Pathology. Blackwell Scientific Publications, Oxford.

Verkleij AJ, Zwaal RFA, Roelofsen B, Comfurius P, Kastelijn D, Van Deenen LLM. 1973. The asymmetric distribution of phospholipids in the human red cell membrane. Biochim Biophys Acta 323:178–193.

Vilcek J. 1979. Fundamentals of virus structure and replication. *In* Galasso GJ, Merigan TC, Buchanan RA, eds., Antiviral Agents and Viral Diseases of Man. Raven Press, New York, pp. 1–38.

Xu ZL, Fidler IJ. 1984. The in situ activation of cytotoxic properties in murine Kupffer cells by the systemic administration of whole *Mycobacterium bovis* organisms or muramyl tripeptide. Cancer Immunol Immunother 18:118–122.

Xu ZL, Bucana CD, Fidler IJ. 1984. In vitro activation of murine Kupffer cells by lymphokines or endotoxins to lyse syngeneic tumor cells. Am J Pathol 117: 372–380.

Symposium on Fundamental Cancer Research, Vol. 38.

14. Interleukin 2–Activated Cytotoxic Lymphocytes in Cancer Therapy

Elizabeth A. Grimm, Steven K. Jacobs, Louis A. Lanza,* Gilbert Melin, Jack A. Roth,* and Debra J. Wilson

*Surgical Neurology Branch, National Institutes of Neurological, Communicative Disorders and Stroke, and *Surgery Branch, National Cancer Institute, National Institutes of Health, Bethesda, Maryland 20205*

Human interleukin (IL) 2 is a 15,000 dalton glycoprotein secreted by helper T lymphocytes in response to various immunologic stimuli, including antigens and mitogens. The currently accepted role for IL 2 is as a growth factor (IL 2 was previously called T cell growth factor or TCGF), causing the proliferation and expansion of antigen-primed lymphocytes that express IL 2–specific receptors (Cantrell and Smith 1983). Recently, while employing IL 2 to provide this "second signal" in hopes of generating antitumor cytotoxic T lymphocytes (CTL) from cancer patients' peripheral blood lymphocytes (PBL), we discovered the IL 2 alone caused the activation of cytotoxicity (Grimm and Rosenberg 1984). We named this phenomenon the lymphokine-activated killer cell (LAK) system (Grimm et al. 1982).

The LAK system is characterized by the need for at least 48 hours of activation. LAK activation is sensitive to inhibitors of differentiation and proliferation, such as irradiation and mitomycin C, as well as hydrocortisone (Grimm et al. 1985a). The cytotoxic lymphocytes resulting from the IL 2–mediated activation express the unique function of being able to efficiently lyse a variety of natural killer (NK)–resistant fresh tumor target cells (sarcoma, melanoma, adenocarcinoma, glioma, lymphoma) in short-term chromium 51 release cytotoxicity assays. A number of other criteria that establish the LAK system and LAK cells as distinct from the classical CTL or the naturally occurring NK activity have been recently reviewed (Grimm et al. 1983b). These criteria include precursor phenotype, activation conditions, effector phenotype, and specificity of cytotoxicity. Since our realization of the unique nature of the LAK system in 1982, it has been rapidly accepted as one with new and significant potential for the therapeutic armamentarium against cancer.

METHODS USED TO APPROXIMATE IN VIVO CONDITIONS

Several of the methods used to generate and to test LAK activity are critical. While these methods have been described in detail elsewhere (Grimm and Rosenberg 1984), I will briefly review the salient aspects. LAK can be generated from any sample of PBL, from either healthy people or cancer patients, and neither macrophages, T cells, NK cells, nor B cells are required in the lymphocyte population. By current criteria, LAK develop from immature null cells that can be found in the bone marrow. The responding PBL are suspended in culture medium containing either human AB serum or autologous serum. Bovine sera are to be avoided. Cultures of PBL at 1×10^6 ml are incubated with the addition of IL 2 only. Purified IL 2 is preferable, and the units should be titrated. In our recent work we have used natural IL 2 (Delectinated TCGF, Cellular Products, Buffalo, NY) or recombinant IL 2 (Cetus Corp., Emeryville, CA) (Rosenberg et al., 1984).

After culturing of the PBL and IL 2 for at least 48 hours, and preferably three to five days, the culture contents are harvested, washed, and used as effectors in a four-hour chromium 51 release assay against fresh noncultured human tumor cells. LAK will lyse NK-sensitive and murine tumor cells, but these are to be avoided because they are also lysed by non-LAK cells. Fresh tumor target cells are obtained by digestion of fresh surgical specimens in a mixture of enzymes including collagenase, hyaluronidase, and DNase. The resulting viable tumor cells are then purified and cryopreserved in human serum and 10% dimethyl sulfoxide (DMSO) until needed. A four-hour assay is optimal for LAK testing (Grimm et al. 1985b).

While the methods for production and testing of LAK are relatively simple, they are critical. The use of human serum and fresh tumor cells as targets is necessary for proper interpretation of results, in view of the potential for application in vivo.

HUMAN LAK ACTIVATION BY IL 2 AND ITS INHIBITION BY ANTIBODIES TO THE IL 2 RECEPTOR

Culturing normal, nonimmunized PBL in medium supplemented only with IL 2 is sufficient for LAK activation. A minimal requirement for serum of 1% has been noted. Whether the serum contributes another growth factor or just nutrients is not yet known. The IL 2 units needed are equivalent to 5 BRMP (Biological Response Modifiers Program Interim IL 2 standard) units or 100 Cetus recombinant IL 2 (rIL 2) U/ml.

We have previously reported that the monoclonal antibody, anti-Tac, to the receptor for IL 2 blocks activation of LAK (Grimm et al. 1983c). Recently, another antibody to a separate epitope on the Tac molecule has been identified

TABLE 14.1. *Monoclonal Antibodies to the Receptor for IL 2 Block Activation of LAK*

Culture Additives*		Lysis of Fresh Sarcoma Tumor (%)		
rIL 2 Units	MAb[†], dilution	80:1[‡]	20:1	5:1
50	—	43	29	4
50	anti-Tac, 200^{-1}	46	33	4
50	anti-Tac, 1000^{-1}	44	22	5
50	anti-7G7, 200^{-1}	1	−8	−10
50	anti-7G7, 1000^{-1}	−3	−6	−9
10	—	24	10	−2
10	anti-Tac, 200^{-1}	5	−2	−2
10	anti-Tac, 1000^{-1}	11	3	−1
10	anti-7G7, 200^{-1}	1	−4	−5
10	anti-7G7, 1000^{-1}	−5	−4	−5
0	—	−9	−4	−9

*Peripheral blood lymphocytes were incubated for five days with the additives listed.
†The monoclonal antibody (MAb) anti-Tac was generously provided by Tom Waldmann and the anti-7G7 by David Nelson, Metabolism Branch, National Cancer Institute.
‡Ratios are effector to target cells.
IL 2 = interleukin 2; LAK = lymphokine-activated killer cell system; rIL 2 = recombinant IL 2.

and also blocked LAK activation. This monoclonal antibody, named 7G7, binds an epitope of the receptor distinct from that of Tac and from the IL 2 binding site (Rubin et al. 1985). Table 14.1 is a representative experiment of these findings. Blocking by both antibodies is significant only at suboptimal levels of IL 2, presumably because the IL 2 has a higher affinity for the receptor.

LAK ACTIVATION IN THE PRESENCE OF TUMOR CELLS

Tumor cells secrete a number of immunosuppressive factors, including those that inhibit IL 2 production, as well as IL 2 responses (Roth et al. 1982, 1983, Fontana et al. 1984). Therefore, we tested whether LAK could be activated in the presence of a growing glioma tumor cell line. PBL with or without the addition of exogenous IL 2 at the standard 100 U/ml were added to the adherent glioma cell culture. We could generate LAK (Figure 14.1), but the level per cell was significantly lower than that in the absence of tumor.

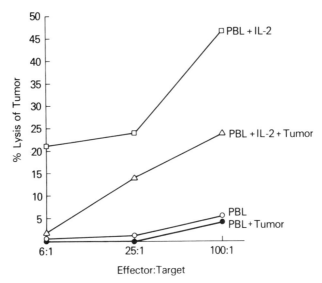

FIGURE 14.1. LAK can be generated in the presence of tumor. Results of a four-hour chromium 51 release cytotoxicity test of glioma tumor cells using LAK created under conditions of PBL + IL 2 at 100 U/ml; PBL + IL 2 at 100 U/ml + tumor at ratio of 2:1; PBL + tumor at 2:1 ratio; and PBL alone.

MAINTENANCE OF LAK LYTIC ACTIVITY IN THE CONTINUOUS PRESENCE OF SUSCEPTIBLE TUMOR CELLS

For LAK to be therapeutically useful, it is important to determine whether LAK would be able to lyse tumor cells when continuously exposed to them, as might occur in vivo. Therefore, LAK were generated under standard conditions, and on day 4, fresh LAK-sensitive tumor cells were added, along with fresh medium and IL 2. On days 7, 11, and 14, aliquots of the culture were taken and viable LAK and tumor cells were counted, tested for lysis of fresh tumor (the same as that added to the culture), and then the entire culture contents was refed with medium, IL 2, and more tumor cells (Table 14.2). Lytic activity and growth of LAK was maintained until day 14 when the experiment was terminated, owing to exhaustion of the sterile fresh tumor cell supply. It would be of interest to determine how much longer the LAK activity could be maintained under these conditions.

THE UNDEFINED LAK PRECURSOR CELL

No positive marker for the LAK precursor cell has yet been identified. Initially, LAK precursors were distinguished from monocytes, NK cells, T cells, and memory CTL because they were negative for the antigens recognized by

TABLE 14.2. *LAK Maintenance by IL 2 during Continuous Culture with Tumor in a Closed System*

Day	Recovery (%)	Lytic Units/10^6 *	Culture Contents
0	—	NT	PBL + rIL 2[†]
4	45	NT	LAK + tumor[‡] + rIL 2
7	89	20	LAK + tumor + rIL 2
11	111	NT	LAK + tumor + rIL 2
14	100	25	—

*Lytic unit is number of LAK required for 33% lysis of 5×10^3 tumor cells.
[†]rIL 2 was used at 170 Cetus units/ml.
[‡]Tumor to LAK ratio = 1:10.
Controls: Tumor + rIL 2 yielded no growth of tumor.
        Day 11 LAK + rIL 2 (no tumor) yielded 60% recovery on day 14
        and 19 lytic units.
rIL 2 = recombinant interleukin 2; LAK = lymphokine-activated killer cell system; NT = not tested; PBL = peripheral blood lymphocytes.

monoclonal antibodies to these cells (Grimm et al. 1982, 1983b). As new monoclonal antibodies have become available, they have been tested either with complement lysis or by binding with protein A Sepharose 6MB. None of three newly described monoclonal antibodies significantly or reproducibly decreased the LAK precursors NK-9 (Nieminen and Saksela 1984, the generous gift of P. Nieminen), B73.1 (Perussia et al. 1983, the generous gift of B. Perussia), and Leu-11 (Itoh et al. 1985, Becton Dickinson, Paramus, NJ).

LYSIS OF HUMAN TUMOR CELLS BY LAK EFFECTORS

Because of the broad target cell spectrum susceptible to lysis by LAK, we tested whether allogeneic fresh and cultured tumor cells would inhibit lysis of autologous tumor in unlabeled target inhibition assays. Using three patient-tumor combinations with known allogeneic mismatches, the allogeneic tumors totally inhibited the lysis of the autologous tumor (Figure 14.2). These results confirm that LAK are polyspecific in their recognition of tumor cells, i.e., they are not restricted by the human leukocyte antigen, and they cross-react at the binding stage required prior to cytolysis of tumors.

LYSIS OF LAK BY HUMAN ONCOGENE–TRANSFECTED MURINE 3T3 CELLS

Oncogenes are DNA sequences that may cause acquisition of the transformed phenotype by normal cells when integrated in the normal cell genome. Such

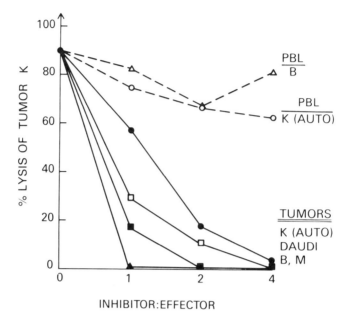

FIGURE 14.2. Inhibition of LAK lysis of autologous tumor by allogeneic fresh and cultured tumor cells. LAK prepared by PBL of patient K were tested by lysis of tumor K at a 40:1 effector: target ratio. Unlabeled tumor from patients K, B, and M, as well as the cultured lymphoma, Daudi, and PBL from patients B and K were titrated into the assay as competitors. The HLA typing of patient B is A28,-; B8,W44(W4,W6); C W4,W7. That of patient K is A2,28; BW51,W60(W4,W6); C W3,W6,DR3,W10; MB1,3; MTL,2 and for patient M is A2,3; B7,-(W6); CW7,-; DR2,5; MB1,3; MT2,3.

transfected cells have many growth and phenotypic characteristics similar to human tumor cells, but their characteristics as immunologic targets have not been defined. Therefore, to determine the pattern of cytolysis of human oncogene–transfected cells and to determine whether it resembles human tumors, we tested the lysis of these cells by LAK (Figure 14.3). Murine LAK from either the BALB/c or nu/nu mice strain lysed NIH 3T3 cells transformed by the c-Ha-*ras* or N-*ras* human oncogenes (Yuasa et al. 1983). These transfectants were grown as fresh tumor in nu/nu mice prior to use as targets. All of these transfected cells were resistant to NK lysis mediated by fresh splenocytes, even though the NK-sensitive target Yac was lysed (Lanza LA, Roth JA, Grimm EA unpublished data). Thus, *ras* oncogene–transfected murine fibroblasts exhibit the same susceptibility to murine LAK cytolysis as fresh human tumors do to human LAK.

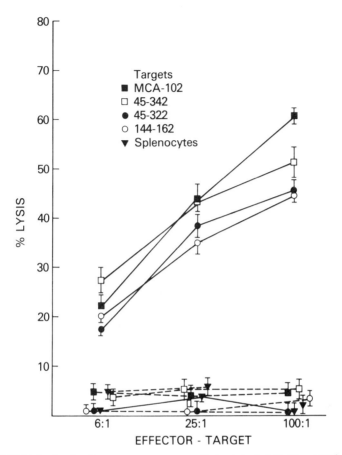

FIGURE 14.3. Lysis of human oncogene transfectants by LAK. Five ×10³ target cells were assayed for lysis by either LAK or identical splenocytes cultured in parallel with the LAK cells but without IL 2 or with fresh splenocytes in standard four-hour ⁵¹Cr-release assays at effector: target cell ratios of 100:1, 25:1, and 6.25:1. Results shown are percentage of cytolysis as determined by ⁵⁴Cr release at four hours. LAK effectors ————, splenocyte effectors — — — — — , using the H-*ras* tertiary transfectant tumor cell lines as targets. Identical results were found with N-*ras* transfectants. Significant cytolysis was demonstrated consistently against all targets except normal splenocytes by LAK cells but no lysis by the cultured splenocytes without IL 2 or by fresh splenocytes demonstrating NK lysis of Yac. Transfectant tumors were generously provided by S. A. Aaronson, National Cancer Institute.

CLINICAL EFFICACY OF LAK THERAPY

Our current understanding of the LAK system has revealed that LAK are extremely potent killers of human tumor cells in vitro, but spare normal tissue cells. Reports on murine models of LAK immunotherapy indicate that LAK (Grimm et al. 1983a, Mazumder and Rosenberg 1984) or LAK plus subsequent injections of IL 2 (Mulé et al. 1984) are effective in significantly reducing or eliminating the tumor burden of melanoma or sarcoma cells forming lung colonies after intravenous injections of the tumor cell suspension. LAK have not been successful for the treatment of tumors outside the capillary bed of the vascular system, though these same tumors could be reduced by therapy with specific CTL. The failure of LAK to have an impact on subcutaneous or intramuscular tumors is most likely due to the large size of LAK, preventing them from leaving the vasculature.

Based on the above findings, we hypothesized that LAK might be therapeutic for human tumors, if injected or placed in the tumor site. Because human malignant gliomas are resistant to all currently available chemotherapy and since surgery is, for the most part, palliative, we have proposed to treat glioma patients at the time of surgical debulking of tumor by injecting LAK with and without IL 2 into the peritumor area. Preliminary tests of intracranial injections of LAK and of IL 2 into rats have shown no deleterious effects (Jacobs SK, Grimm EA unpublished data). As part of our preclinical studies, we found that LAK are extremely efficient killers of fresh, as well as cultured

TABLE 14.3. *Lysis of Autologous Tumor Cells by Glioma Patient LAK*

	Lysis (%)		
Autologous Target Cells	Brain Tumor Cultured	Brain Tumor Fresh	Peripheral Blood Lymphocytes (PBL)
Effectors*			
1. PBL	6	6	NT
LAK	61	37	NT
2. PBL	−8	1	4
LAK	71	55	3
3. PBL	6	5	8
LAK	84	25	11
4. PBL	1	−6	−3
LAK	96	37	7

*PBL from four glioma patients were either used when fresh, untreated, or cultured with IL 2 to generate LAK.

glioma tumor cells (Jacobs SK, Grimm EA unpublished data). Table 14.3 lists the results from the testing of four glioma patients' autologous LAK for lysis of tumor.

SUMMARY AND CONCLUSIONS

LAK are cytolytic lymphocytes with the unique capacity for killing NK-resistant fresh human tumor cells in short-term assays. LAK kill autologous as well as allogeneic tumors with complete cross-reactivity. Initial studies on the classification of LAK conclude that LAK are distinct from the classical NK and T lymphocyte systems, based on a number of criteria including surface phenotype, activation conditions, and a spectrum of susceptible target cells.

LAK kill *ras* oncogene–transfected fibroblasts like they kill fresh tumors. As yet, the target cell determinant responsible for susceptibility to LAK lysis is unknown. Activation of LAK requires only IL 2 and is blocked by monoclonal antibodies to the IL 2 receptor.

Because only IL 2 alone is sufficient for LAK activation, we have done in vitro testing to determine whether fresh PBL could be activated in the presence of tumor, as might be desirable in vivo. LAK were activated sufficiently to mediate significant destruction of fresh tumor. We also tested whether LAK could be maintained in the presence of large tumors, providing IL 2 was added. Again, results were positive, suggesting that LAK either recycle or are a self-renewing population that depend on IL 2 for continued functions.

Because of these and other findings, we have initiated a clinical protocol to test whether LAK made from the PBL of patients with brain tumor could eliminate residual glioma tumor cells. Autologous LAK plus rIL 2 to maintain lytic ability are injected during surgery. Preclinical studies in a rat glioma model have shown this approach to be safe, and previous in vivo murine studies have concluded that LAK kill tumors in Winn-type lung colony formation tests (Kedar et al. 1982). Much work is needed before we can understand the LAK phenomenon and determine its usefulness in cancer therapy, as well as its inherent biologic role. We hope that this chapter will stimulate both interest and the basic research needed to realize LAK potential.

REFERENCES

Cantrell DA, Smith KA. 1983. Transient expression of interleukin-2 receptors: Consequence for T cell growth. J Exp Med 158:1895–1911.

Fontana A, Hengartner H, de Triblet N, Weber E. 1984. Glioblastoma cells release interleukin-1 and factors inhibiting interleukin-2 mediated effects. J Immunol 132:1837–1844.

Grimm EA, Rosenberg SA. 1984. The human lymphokine-activated killer cell phenomenon. *In* Pick E, ed., Lymphokines, vol. 9. Academic Press, New York, pp. 279–311.

Grimm EA, Mazumder A, Zhang HZ, Rosenberg SA. 1982. The lymphokine activated killer cell phenomenon: Lysis of NK resistant fresh solid tumor cells by IL-2 activated autologous human pheripheral blood lymphocytes. J Exp Med 155:1823–1841.

Grimm EA, Gorelik E, Rosenstein MM, Rosenberg SA. 1983a. The lymphokine-activated killer cell phenomenon: *In vitro* and *in vivo* studies. *In* Cohen S, Oppenheim J, eds., Interleukins, Lymphokines, and Cytokines. Academic Press, New York, pp. 739–746.

Grimm EA, Ramsey K, Mazumder A, Wilson DJ, Djeu J, Rosenberg SA. 1983b. Lymphokine-activated killer cell phenomenon: II. The precursor phenotype is serologically distinct from peripheral T lymphocytes, memory CTL, and NK cells. J Exp Med 157:884–897.

Grimm EA, Robb RJ, Roth JA, et al. 1983c. The lymphokine-activated killer cell phenomenon: III. Evidence that IL-2 alone is sufficient for direct activation of PBL into LAK. J Exp Med 158:1356–1361.

Grimm EA, Muul LM, Wilson DJ. 1985a. Cyclosporine and hydrocortisone exert differential inhibitory effects on the activation of human cytotoxic lymphocytes by recombinant IL-2 versus allospecific CTL. Transplantation 39:537–540.

Grimm EA, Rayner AA, Wilson DJ. 1985b. Human NK resistant tumor cell lysis is effected by IL-2 activated killer cells. Adv Exp Med Biol 184:161–175.

Itoh K, Tilden AB, Kumagai K, Balch CM. 1985. Leu-11 lymphocytes with natural killer (NK) activity are precursors of recombinant interleukin 2 (rIL-2)-induced activated killer cells. J Immunol 134:802–807.

Kedar E, Herberman RB, Gorelik E, Sredni B, Bonnard GO, Navarro N. 1982. Antitumor reactivity *in vitro* and *in vivo* of mouse and human lymphoid cells cultured with T cell growth factor. *In* Fefer A, Goldstein A, eds., The Potential Role of T Cells in Cancer Therapy. Raven Press, New York, pp. 173–189.

Mazumder A, Rosenberg SA. 1984. Successful immunotherapy of natural killer-resistant established pulmonary melanoma metastases by the intravenous adoptive transfer of syngeneic lymphocytes activated *in vitro* by interleukin-2. J Exp Med 159:495–507.

Mulé JJ, Shu S, Schwarz SL, Rosenberg SA. 1984. Successful adoptive immunotherapy of established pulmonary metastases of multiple sarcomas with lymphokine-activated killer cells and recombinant ïnterleukin-2. Science 225:1487–1489.

Nieminen P, Saksela E. 1984. A shared antigenic specificity of human large granular lymphocytes and precursors of NK-like and allospecific cytotoxic effector cells. J Immunol 133:702–708.

Perussia B, Starr S, Abraham S, Fanning V, Trinchieri G. 1983. Human natural killer cells analyzed by B73.1, a monoclonal antibody blocking Fc receptor functions: I. Characterization of the lymphocyte subset reactive with B73.1. J Immunol 130:2133–2141.

Rosenberg SA, Grimm EA, McGrogan N, Doyle M, Kawasaki E, Koths K, Mark DF. 1984. Biologic activity of recombinant human interleukin-2 produced in *E. coli*. Science 223:1412–1415.

Roth JA, Grimm EA, Gupta RK, Ames RS. 1982. Immunoregulatory factors derived from human tumors: I. Immunological and biochemical characterization of factors that suppress lymphocyte proliferation and cytotoxic responses *in vitro*. J Immunol 128:1955–1962.

Roth JA, Grimm EA, Osborne BA, Ames RS. 1983. Suppressive immuno-regulatory factors produced by tumors. Lymphokine Research 2:61–73.

Rubin LA, Kurman CC, Biddison WE, Goldmann ND, Nelson DL. 1985. Monoclonal antibody 767-B6 binds to an epitope on the human interleukin-2 receptor that is distinct from that recognized by IL-2 or anti-Tac. Hybridoma (In press).

Yuasa Y, Srivastava SK, Dunn CY, Rham JS, Reddy EP, Aaronson SA. 1983. Acquisition of transforming properties by alternate point mutations within c-*bas*/*has* human proto-oncogene. Nature 303:775–780.

Symposium on Fundamental Cancer Research, Vol. 38.
© 1986 by The University of Texas System Cancer Center.

15. Natural Killer and Other Effector Cells

Osias Stutman and Edmund C. Lattime

*Immunology Program, Memorial Sloan-Kettering Cancer Center,
New York, New York 10021*

Natural cell–mediated cytotoxicity (NCMC), of which natural killer (NK) cells are the prototypic effectors, has attracted much attention since the early 1970s. NK cells have even excited the allegorical writing gifts of many and have been called such things as an "immunologist's fancy" (Gupta 1980) and an "odyssey in biology" (Oldham 1983). Extensive activity has marked this field since the NK cell terminology was coined (Kiessling et al. 1975), which also implied that the phenomenon was being accepted as a reputable research endeavor. Once accepted, a vast amount of information was generated in a relatively short time. For example, two large volumes on NCMC have been compiled (Herberman 1980, 1982a), as well as multiple reviews and smaller volumes, with new ones in the making. To give a dimension of the outpouring of new information, the first volume on NK cells contained 84 papers and 13 summaries in 1309 pages (Herberman 1980), and the second contained 219 papers in 1546 pages (Herberman 1982a), which almost tripled the number of studies in less than two years. Whether this activity has clarified the issues or is just an example of the ease with which NK cells can be tested in vitro using NK cell–sensitive targets in humans and animals are issues beyond the scope of this review.

We could agree that in spite of the amount of published material on NCMC, most of it only descriptive, we are still faced with important unanswered questions about effector cell lineage, recognition structures, and overall function. In sum, we still do not know what NK cells are, what they see (and how), and what they do (and how). An additional emerging problem is the amount of redundant research that is being generated in the field, with repetitive papers published at an alarming rate. Although we will venture some interpretative opinions and define some problem areas in the field, this chapter will concentrate on NK and related cells, with a certain inclination for discussing animal studies that is based on our first-hand experience. This is not intended to be a comprehensive review and will be composed of brief essays dealing with various features of NCMC.

Prior to the middle 1970s, NCMC was viewed as a major, and unexpected, nuisance that complicated the attempts to detect tumor-specific cell-mediated cytotoxicity in cancer patients, since lymphoid cells from the normal control subjects proved to be efficient killers of tumor cells in vitro (Rosenberg et al. 1972, Takasugi et al. 1973, McCoy et al. 1973). The response to this situation, which certainly did not fit within the dominant conceptual framework of cancer immunology of that time, ranged from the simple elimination of the incriminating controls to the selection of "negative" normal controls that failed to lyse the particular target cells used. Since the expected result was some type of selective tumor killing by cells from the tumor-bearing patients (Hellstrom and Hellstrom 1974), the killing by normal cells was considered artifactual and due to improper preparation of the effector cells (for example, see Bean et al. 1975). When the unwanted reactivity could not be dismissed by simple technical arguments, alternative interpretations were produced. Probably the first published description of NCMC was the study by Rosenberg et al. (1972), who detected cytotoxicity against leukemic cells by lymphoid cells from the nonleukemic pair of identical twins. The interpretation of the results, however, was that the responses in the normal control subjects were due to in vivo sensitization to putative leukemia viruses, which in turn were responsible for the leukemia-associated antigens in the target cells. It goes without saying that the interpretation that cytotoxicity had to be directed against tumor-associated antigens was the prevalent one for most of the in vitro cytotoxicity data against tumors (Hellstrom et al. 1971, Hellstrom and Hellstrom 1974). As a matter of fact, the first two papers on NK cells in mice also implied that the response was directed against antigens coded by an endogenous leukemia virus (Kiessling et al. 1975, Herberman et al. 1975). Previous studies on NCMC in normal mice interpreted the presence of NCMC as related to ongoing responses to endogenous viruses (Herberman et al. 1975, Gomard et al. 1974) or to a manifestation of autoimmunity (Greenberg and Playfair 1974). However, it soon became clear that NK cell activity was not directed against murine leukemia virus determinants and that killing showed no major histocompatibility complex (MHC) restriction (Becker et al. 1976). It took a few more years to accept NCMC as immunologically interesting; its acceptance was marked by the appearance of a volume of *Immunological Reviews* dedicated to the subject (Moller 1979). The demonstration that NK cell activity could be augmented in vivo in mice (Herberman et al. 1977) and that the interferons (IFN) were the apparent mediators of such augmentation in humans (Trinchieri and Santoli 1978) and mice (Gidlund et al. 1978) were important events in the analysis of NCMC regulation and function, and they involved NCMC in the temporary "IFN-mania" of the 1980s (Bloom 1982).

It is worth noting that the antitumor effect of normal murine lymphoid cells activated by IFN was initially described in 1970, before NCMC was recognized (Chernyakhovskaya et al. 1970).

There is agreement that NK and similar NCMC effector cells do not follow some of the accepted guidelines of other cytotoxic mechanisms, such as MHC restrictions, immunologic memory, and (probably) clonality, as is the case with cytotoxic T cells (Ortaldo and Herberman 1984). However, an interesting development in NCMC has been its acceptance as a special category of immune response and not simply as an in vitro curiosity related to the killing of certain tumor cell lines.

DEFINITION OF NCMC

In a recent workshop on NK cells (Koren and Herberman 1983), a minimum terminology was agreed upon and was aimed at controlling the development of the acronyms related to NCMC effectors. Two main categories of NCMC effectors were established: natural killer (NK) and activated killer (AK) cells (note that the proposed AK terminology is not included as such in the Koren and Herberman 1983 summary and was agreed upon in another workshop in 1984). NK cells are obtained fresh and have spontaneous cytotoxicity against a variety of target cells, are lymphoid in appearance, are different from granulocytes, macrophages, and cytotoxic T cells, and show no MHC-related restriction for killing. This group includes other subclasses of effectors, such as NK subsets (Kumar et al. 1979, Minato et al. 1981, Lust et al. 1981, Biron and Welsh 1982), natural cytotoxic (NC) cells (Stutman et al. 1978, Burton 1980, Burton et al. 1981, 1982, Lust et al. 1981), and NK cells killing virus-infected targets (Harfast et al. 1977, Welsh and Hallenbeck 1980, Lopez et al. 1982), in addition to the classical NK cells. AK cells are even a more heterogeneous group that encompasses *any* type of non-MHC–restricted cell-mediated killing that is produced after in vitro culture.

These pragmatic and working definitions imply, to some extent, that NK cells are indeed a unique category of effectors. Acronyms appear as obligatory abbreviations needed for editorial purposes, but they can also create confusion. For example, MHC means for most immunologists "major histocompatibility complex," but for other scientists it also means "myosin heavy chain" (Mahdavi et al. 1982). Similarly, in the NCMC field, AK was used to describe the "anomalous killers" generated in culture (Karre and Seeley 1979) that are but a subclass of the AK cells discussed above, and NC was used to describe the "null cell" compartment in human peripheral blood that contains NK effectors and from which cloned NK cell lines can be derived (Hercend et al. 1982), in addition to being the acronym for natural cytotoxic cells (Stutman et al. 1978).

In summary, the two main features of NCMC are that they are mediated by lymphoid cells, which are not conventional T cells, macrophages, monocytes, and granulocytes and that they exhibit no MHC restriction for killing. A third feature, as it applies especially to the NK category proper, is the detection of the activity in fresh samples from normal individuals without prior sensitization. A fourth and minor feature would be the absence of immunologic memory as observed after priming in conventional immune responses. This applies both to the cells found spontaneously in normal individuals (NK) and to the variety of nonconventional in vitro–generated effectors (AK). In the terminology utilized in this review, NCMC defines the broad category of non–MHC-restricted cell-mediated cytotoxic responses detected, using either fresh or cultured cells, in normal individuals.

A Problem with NCMC

In our view, the main problem in animal and human NCMC studies is that a certain activity—the capacity to kill some selected tumor targets in vitro—is equated to the specific function of NCMC in vivo. It is commonly stated that cells that kill Yac-1 targets in mice and K-562 in humans are NK cells, by definition, and that the properties of the cells that kill such targets are those characteristic of the NK effectors. As this was, and still is, a common conceptual evil, we will not single out any specific reference to support these views. Attempts to address this problem have just begun and are symbolized by the agreement that the definition of NK cells ought to stress that the effector cells should ". . .lack the properties of classical macrophages, granulocytes or cytotoxic T lymphocytes. . ." (Koren and Herberman 1983 p. 785). Similarly, while Herberman's first book (1980) dealt with almost any cell capable of killing the prototype NK-susceptible targets, the second volume tried to concentrate on NK and related effectors (Herberman 1982a).

However, this conceptual problem has persisted despite the fact that a variety of other recognizable effector cells, especially cells of the monocyte series and T cells induced in culture and probably polyclonally activated, can also kill the same NK-susceptible targets. In summary, not everything that kills an NK-susceptible target is actually an NK effector.

The best examples of this situation follow: (1) promonocytes (Lohmann-Matthes et al. 1979), (2) fresh blood monocytes (Fischer et al. 1981), (3) activated polymorphonuclear cells (Abrams and Brahmi 1984), (4) basophil cell lines (Galli et al. 1982), (5) cloned cytotoxic T cell lines (Brooks 1983), and (6) the variety of T-like and non-T killer cells produced in culture (Cohen et al. 1971, Cohen and Wekerle 1973, Zielske and Golub 1976, Shustick et al. 1976, Burton et al. 1978, Jondal and Targan 1978, Zarling et al. 1978, Poros and Klein 1978, Seeley and Golub 1978, Karre and Seeley 1979, Paciucci et al. 1980, Klein 1982, Kedar et al. 1982, Lopez-Botet et al. 1982, Shain et al. 1982, Dorfman et al. 1982, Grimm et al. 1982, 1983, Brooks et al. 1983a,b, Macphail et al. 1984. This citation is an incomplete listing of illustrative examples in murine and human systems; some of them were described before NK cells were defined). The effectors within the last category have been called by various names, such as autosensitive, promiscuous, and anomalous killers and could certainly fall within the AK category described above.

From this conceptual problem, two unfortunate conclusions have been drawn: first, that the properties of the cells that kill Yac-1 and K-562 are the prototypic features of NK effector cells, and second, that NCMC effectors, especially of the NK type, must have some antitumor function in vivo, since they kill tumor cells in vitro. A third conclusion, derived to some extent as a reaction to the strictures of the first one, was that the NCMC effectors that did not fulfill the characteristics of the classical NK cells represented either a special subset or a distinct but related effector cell (Stutman et al. 1978, 1981, Paige et al. 1978, Kumar et al. 1979, Burton 1980, Burton et al. 1981, Lust et al. 1981, Minato et al. 1981, Patek et al. 1983, Lin et al. 1983). From these distinct but apparently NK-related effectors, the concept of heterogeneity of NCMC effectors has emerged (Stutman et al. 1978, Burton 1980, Lust et al. 1981, Minato et al. 1981, Hercend et al. 1983, Ortaldo and Herberman 1984), but still remains an unresolved issue.

Thus, two possible levels of heterogeneity can be defined. Firstly, finding several types of NCMC effectors capable of killing different targets in a non–MHC-restricted manner suggests a family of distinct but related effectors, as we originally proposed (Stutman et al. 1978), and secondly, a spurious heterogeneity is derived from killing NK-susceptible targets by a variety of other, unrelated effector cells. A good example of the latter is the situation in which the murine promonocyte and the NK cell both readily kill Yac target cells, although it is evident that they represent distinct populations. Normal promonocyte activity is observed in mice with impaired NK cell function, such as NK-low strains (Lohmann-Matthes et al. 1979) or beige mice (Roder et al. 1979). However, some properties of the promonocyte, such as the presence of the surface marker Mph 1 (Lohmann-Matthes et al. 1979), which is absent from NK and NC cells (Stutman et al. 1980b), are listed as part of the characteristics of the NK cell compartment (Minato et al. 1981). The same could be said of the killing mechanism. A report on the oxidative bursts in NK killing (Roder et al. 1982) inspired an editorial on macrophages masquerading as lymphoid NK cells (Babior and Parkinson 1982). However, it was later shown that NK killing does not involve oxidative bursts (Abrams and Brahmi 1984) and that such bursts, when detected, could be due to contaminating monocytes in the NK cell preparations.

Thus, the central problem is that all of the properties of the NCMC system have been defined by utilizing the in vitro killing of a selected target tumor cell line as the final read out. It is conceivable that such killing activity is not representative of the actual function of NCMC. For example, the function of NCMC effectors could be important indeed in homeostasis and regulation of normal cells, especially of the hematopoietic system (Hansson and Kiessling 1983), or could be involved in the control of some conventional immune functions (Nabel et al. 1982, Abruzzo and Rowley 1983) or transplantation responses (Herberman 1982b). The NCMC could also act as part of the early defense mechanisms against a variety of foreign invaders (for the possible involvement of NK cells in defense against *Trypanosoma cruzi*, *Cryptococcus*, herpesvirus 1, murine cytomegalovirus, *Babesia*, and murine hepatitis 3, see the articles by different authors on pages 1091, 1105, 1445, 1451, 1459, 1477, and 1483 in Herberman 1982a, see also Herberman 1983). In many of the early responses to a variety of infectious agents, the effector cells do not seem to be classical NK cells but are certainly different from conventional T cells, B cells, or macrophages (Bennett et al. 1976, Bennett and Baker 1977, Campbell 1976, Biron and Welsh 1982). It is also apparent that resistance to a particular agent is unlikely to be mediated exclusively by a single effector mechanism and probably involves complex interactions ranging from target cell properties to factors such as lymphokine, monokine, and cytokine production, antibody, macrophage, polymorph, eosinophil, mast cell, basophil activation, and complement components. Consequently, to ascribe a whole defense process to a single protagonist is viewed as a naive simplification. Unfortunately, such a naive simplification, which we have strongly criticized in the past (Stutman 1981a, 1983a,b), has been persistently applied in tumor immunology. The star-crossed notion that cells are "good" and antibodies are "bad" in tumor immunology (Hellstrom and Hellstrom 1974) still persists—good or bad means favoring the host or the tumor, respectively. A good example of the single-mechanism "simplification fallacy" has used the evidence that NK cells can lyse extracellular *Trypanosoma cruzi* (Hatcher and Kuhn 1982), which is evidence for the importance of the NK cells' resistance to parasites (Herberman 1983). However, *T. cruzi* are also lysed by macrophages activated via a thymus-dependent mechanism, as well as by antibodies and B cell–related effects, to cite just two other mechanisms (Nogueira and Cohn 1979, Rodriguez et al. 1981). Hatcher and Kuhn (1982) clearly indicate that NK cells are but one component of the complex responses to the parasite. Thus, the simplification fallacy is not incurred by the scientists that actually do the work but by the commentators who discuss their studies in a more general manner. As we stated in an earlier review (Stutman and Lattime 1983), these types of studies should alert us that there is probably no single mechanism that exclusively mediates any defense response, whether it is directed to parasites, bacteria, or tumors.

In summary, and returning to NCMC, the following are possible: (1) that the capacity to kill certain tumor targets may merely reflect but a single in vitro activity of a system possessing other biologic functions in vivo, (2) that such in vitro killing activity of tumor targets may represent only one compartment of NCMC rather than defining the general characteristics of NCMC as a whole, and (3) that in all probability, none of these defense responses, whether directed against tumors or not, may be actually mediated by a single protagonist mechanism.

On the other hand, the conventional murine NK cells appear to play an important role in the control of blood-borne metastatic spread, whether experimenting with artificially induced or spontaneous lung metastatic models (Gorelik et al. 1979, 1982, Hanna 1980, Hanna and Fidler 1981, Hanna and Burton 1981, Talmadge et al. 1981). However, as we pointed out (Stutman and Cuttito 1981), NK cells appear to be operative in the control of lung metastasis of lymphoid or nonlymphoid tumors, while metastases to other sites, such as lymph nodes, do not seem to be affected by NK cell deficiencies (Talmadge et al. 1981). These topics are mentioned only as examples of the difficulties with generalizations concerning the in vivo correlates of the in vitro NCMC activity. For further comments on the in vivo antitumor effects of NK and other NCMC effectors see Stutman (1981a,b, 1982, 1983a,b, 1984a,b,c, 1985).

Finally, it is worth stressing that most of the phenomenology defined as NCMC in experimental animals and in humans is derived from the analysis of the interaction of at least three variables. The first variable is the donor providing the effector cells, second is the type of target cells utilized, and third is the type and duration of the in vitro assay employed. For example, upon comparing the first reports on murine NK cells, it is apparent that the Yac targets used by Kiessling et al. (1975) were much more sensitive to NK killing in vitro than any of the lymphoma targets used in other laboratories (Herberman et al. 1975, Sendo et al. 1975, Zarling et al. 1975). A fourth, and often forgotten, variable is the type of procedure used to isolate and prepare the effector cells (see Stutman 1982 and Stutman and Lattime 1983 for further comments). The first of these variables is probably the most difficult to control, since at any given time, a variety of stimuli may augment or depress NCMC activity, especially when measured in a single tissue, such as peripheral blood lymphocytes in the human studies and spleen in the animal experiments. The studies by Pross and Baines (1982) are a good and sobering example of the margin of variation that can be observed when the same group of normal volunteers are tested periodically over several years. The latter comment is particularly appropriate in relation to the myriad papers now appearing that describe high, low, or normal levels of NK activity in the blood of patients with a variety of diseases, papers that attempt to match the superficiality and redundancy of the multiple publications on T4:T8 ratios in different diseases.

NK, NC, AND OTHER EFFECTOR CELLS

Effector cells that are capable of lysing certain tumor targets in vitro and that were obtained from normal donors can be divided into two main groups, the NK and other effectors found in freshly harvested lymphoid preparations from naive individuals and the AK effectors that are produced through a variety of in vitro culture techniques using normal lymphoid cells as the source and that have been called NK-like because of their capacity to lyse target cells that are syngeneic or autologous to the effector cells and, in most cases, include NK-susceptible target cell lines.

The NCMC effector system has certain unique properties that set it apart from the conventional T cell–, B cell–, or macrophage-mediated responses. These properties are that (1) once the system has developed, it exists at high levels in normal hosts with no need for priming, especially in such tissues as the blood and spleen, (2) it exhibits no evidence of immunologic memory; however, it may manifest a certain "selectivity" or "specificity" for a particular target, although most analyses of the repertoire suggest that it is polyclonal, (3) the effector cells show no MHC-restriction for target lysis, (4) levels and types of NCMC activity are regulated or directed by complex genetic influences that are different from those regulating conventional immune responses, (5) levels and types of NCMC activity are strongly affected by IFN and other lymphokines, and (6) NCMC activity is mediated by a heterogeneous population of effector lymphocytes of still undefined lineage that shows a certain degree of marrow dependency (Stutman et al. 1981). In addition to the books edited by Herberman (1980, 1982a), several reviews provide useful summaries of the earlier as well as the more recent studies on NK cells and other NCMC effectors, including those by Herberman and Holden (1978), Kiessling and Wigzell (1979), Clark and Harmon (1980), Roder et al. (1981), Herberman (1983), Timonen (1983), and Ortaldo and Herberman (1984), to cite but a few.

While studying the specific cell-mediated cytotoxic responses to anchorage-dependent nonlymphoid fibrosarcomas, we observed that lymphoid cells from normal mice would lyse syngeneic tumors in a similar way that NK cells would lyse lymphoid tumors in suspension cultures (Stutman et al. 1978, Paige et al. 1978). Our studies showed that the "natural" effector cell against the anchorage-dependent targets had properties different from the NK cells, although they shared the above-outlined criteria used to define NCMC. We designated such effectors as natural cytotoxic cells (Stutman et al. 1978, 1980b, 1981, Paige et al. 1978). In earlier publications, we included detailed comparative listings of the properties of NK and NC cells in mice, showing both the differences and the similarities, which will not be repeated here (see Stutman et al. 1978, 1980b, 1981, Paige et al. 1978, Stutman and

Cuttito 1981, Stutman 1982, Stutman and Lattime 1983, Lattime et al. 1981, 1982a,b,c,d, 1983a,b, Lattime and Stutman 1983).

We will concentrate these comments on characteristics that both define and contrast the NK and NC cell populations and, where appropriate, comment on the other cells with NK-like activities.

Assay Systems

NC-mediated lysis requires a long-term assay (18–24 hours) in contrast to NK cells, which lyse most of the susceptible targets in four-hour assays (Stutman et al. 1978, 1980b, Burton 1980, Patek et al. 1983). One possible explanation for this time difference is the capacity of the targets to repair the early lytic lesion (Collins et al. 1981, Patek et al. 1983). Such "counterlysis" is mediated by active metabolism of the target and may well account for the need for longer assays in a variety of in vitro cytotoxic systems, including those mediated by NK cells (Collins et al. 1981, Kunkel and Welsh 1981). The requirement for prolonged assays to identify NC activity also suggests that an activation step of the effectors could be required, in which the target itself or some of the in vitro conditions either activates the NC cells or generates activated NK cells. However, preincubation studies, as well as analysis of the surface phenotype of the effector cells at all stages of the assay, demonstrate that killing of the NC-susceptible targets is mediated exclusively by NC cells and that there is no evidence of an in vitro activation step during the assay itself (Lattime et al. 1982b). Incubation of NC cells and targets for periods of up to 18–24 hours (which produced successful killing of such targets) does not change the kinetics of lysis of new targets by those same cells. If NK activation had occurred during the first round of killing, accelerated four hours, the killing kinetics would have been expected in the second round (Lattime et al. 1982b). The killing activity is mediated by cells that were negative for the surface marker Qa-5 (Lattime et al. 1981, 1982b). Qa-5 is a monoclonal antibody reactive with NK cells in all their stages, precursor, effector, and activated effector (Chun et al. 1979, Minato et al. 1981, Lattime et al. 1981, 1983a,b) but absent from NC precursors, as well as resting and activated NC cells (Lattime et al. 1981, 1982b, 1983a,b). Such experiments also indicate that, as in the case of NK cells, NC cells are not inactivated after one cycle of killing (Lattime et al. 1982b). In addition, recent studies have shown that NC targets have the same susceptibility to lysis and require long-term assays at all stages of their cell cycle (Bykowsky et al. 1985).

Another interesting but still unresolved issue is that of anchorage-dependent versus suspension cultures. Some of the prototypic NC targets, such as Meth A and Meth 113 (Stutman et al. 1978) are readily killed when grown as adherent targets but are poorly susceptible when tested by isotope release in suspension assays (Stutman et al. 1980b). However, another prototypic NC target, WEHI-164 (Burton 1980), a sarcoma that grows in suspension cultures, can be used in cytotoxicity assays measured by ^{51}Cr release, although it also requires a long-term assay. One interesting and perhaps important finding is that NC targets, such as Meth A and Meth 113, become quite susceptible to NK-like killing in suspension cultures when infected with mycoplasmas (Herberman et al. 1984). Using Percoll fractionated spleen cells, the mycoplasma-infected cells are killed by effectors in the same large granular lymphocyte (LGL)–enriched fraction as those active with the NK-susceptible Yac-1 targets (Herberman et al. 1984). The mycoplasma-free Meth A or Meth 113 cells in suspension were not lysed by any of the Percoll effector fractions (Herberman et al. 1984), a point that supports our findings with unseparated spleen effectors (Stutman et al. 1980b). Thus, mycoplasma-free adherent cells derived from those same NC susceptible targets are readily killed by NC cells in 18–24 hours [^{3}H] proline assays (Stutman et al. 1978, 1980b) but not killed in 18–24 hour ^{51}Cr-release assays using the same NC cells in suspension (Stutman et al. 1980b, Herberman et al. 1984).

Lymphoid Versus Nonlymphoid Targets

Initial studies describing murine NK cells were done with lymphoma cells as targets (Kiessling et al. 1975, Herberman et al. 1975, Sendo et al. 1975, Zarling et al. 1975, Kiessling and Wigzell 1979, Herberman and Holden 1978, Roder et al. 1981). Similarly, in our own and other studies on the identification of the NC effectors, nonlymphoid tumor targets were used that were derived mostly from chemically induced fibrosarcomas (Stutman et al. 1978, 1980b, 1981, Paige et al. 1978, Burton 1980, Burton et al. 1981, Lust et al. 1981). Although never intended as such, the resulting association between NK-lymphoid and NC-nonlymphoid became so widespread throughout the literature and, inadvertently, became so established that some investigators defined the type of effector cells based only on the morphology or anchorage dependency of the target cells under study. Our own studies have shown that such a "target preference" is no longer tenable (Lattime et al. 1983a). When a large number of lymphoid and nonlymphoid tumors, both spontaneous and induced, were tested, they fell within three main categories: (1) targets that were exclusively NK sensitive and were lysed by a resting or activated Qa-5$^+$ NK cell, (2) targets that were exclusively NC sensitive and were lysed by a resting or an augmented Qa-5$^-$ NC cell, and (3) targets that were sensitive to both NK and NC cells. In the third category, most of the tumors are lysed by Qa-5$^-$ NC cells and by a superimposed Qa-5$^+$ NK component that is usually manifested after augmentation by IFN inducers (Lattime et al. 1983a, Lattime and Stutman 1983). Most of the nonlymphoid tumors tested belonged in the third category (Lattime et al. 1983a). Furthermore, although NC cells are negative for most of the murine NK markers when negative selection is used (Stutman et al. 1980b, Lattime et al. 1981), NC targets, such as the WEHI-164, are also lysed by cells that bear NK surface markers when positive selection is used (Kumar et al. 1985). For example, positively selected Mac-1$^+$ NK cells induced in the peritoneal cavity of mice after *Listeria* infection, which are also Qa-5$^+$ and asialo GM-1$^+$, can kill both Yac-1 and WEHI-164 targets in long-tem assays (Holmberg and Ault 1984). On the other hand, it is highly probable that not everything that kills WEHI-164 is necessarily an NC cell, as we argued at the beginning of this essay for the NK cells. The fact that mast cells kill WEHI-164 targets (Ernst et al. 1985) is a good example of different cell types expressing similar "functions," as we argued for the variety of cells that can kill the NK-prototypic targets, rather than an indication that NC cells are mast cells.

In summary, almost all of the targets derived from nonlymphoid tumors in mice and humans are susceptible to lysis by NK, NC, or AK cells, and there is no basis for the claim of tumor type specificity for any given NCMC effector cell. We insist on this point because, unfortunately, the view that NK cells kill lymphoid and NC cells kill nonlymphoid tumors still dominates. For example, during the discussion of a paper on the effects of opioid peptides on NK activity (Cohn 1975), it was argued that since the Kaposi's tumor was a "sarcoma" it should be a target for NC and not for NK cells!

Target Recognition

The actual target structures that are recognized by NK or NC cells are still undefined. However, it is interesting to note that when the murine prototype NK (Yac-1) and NC (WEHI-164) targets were studied for their capacity to cross-react in unlabeled target inhibition of lysis; each of the NK and the NC targets could inhibit the other's lysis (Stutman et al. 1980b, Lattime et al. 1981, 1982c, see also Collins et al. 1981, Patek et al. 1983, Lin et al. 1983, note that what appear to be NC cells are called NK cells in the paper by Collins et al.). This would suggest shared as well as individual recognition determinants.

Based on the hypothesis that NC and NK cells could recognize surface glycoproteins on target cells via lectinlike receptors, it was shown that monosaccharides at low concentrations (20–50 mM) could inhibit NC and NK killing, with no interference in killing by alloimmune cytotoxic T cells (Stutman et al. 1980a). This observation has been confirmed on murine NK cells (Brunda et al. 1983, which additionally reveals blocking of macrophage-mediated killing, Gorczynski et al. 1983) and in human NK cells (MacDermott et al. 1981, Forbes et al. 1981, Vose et al. 1983, Ortaldo et al. 1984c, Ortaldo and Herberman 1984, Haubeck et al. 1985). Furthermore, the same type of monosaccharides that could inhibit direct lysis by murine NK cells (Stutman et al. 1980a) could also inhibit lysis of NK-susceptible targets via a soluble mediator released by mouse NK cells (Wright and Bonavida 1981). The mechanism of the sugar-mediated inhibition of NK and NC lysis is still undefined and appears not to involve actual recognition steps (Vose et al. 1983, Ortaldo et al. 1984c). It is worth noting that 6-phosphate forms of the sugars produced the best inhibition, which suggests that the action could be on some form of receptor-mediated endocytosis at the target level (Forbes et al. 1981), perhaps related to internalization of soluble mediators of lysis (Wright and Bonavida 1981). However, the exclusive involvement of 6-phosphate residues has also been questioned (Haubeck et al. 1985). The actual patterns of inhibition of NK-, NC-, and macrophage-mediated killing by the monosaccharides are complex and show variations between targets, in some cases with broad inhibitions by many sugars and in others with more restricted patterns, especially with D-mannose preference (Stutman et al. 1980a, Brunda et al. 1983). The murine studies also show that freshly generated allosensitized cytotoxic T cells are not affected by the sugars (Stutman et al. 1980a, Palladino et al. 1983); however an NK- and NC-like pattern of blocking by sugars was observed with cytotoxic T cell cloned lines (Palladino et al. 1983), which points again to similarities between fresh NK cells and cloned T cell lines (Brooks et al. 1982, 1983a,b). Studies on human cells have also shown that sugars could inhibit NK killing without affecting conventional T cell killing (MacDermott et al. 1981). In summary, although the sugar-inhibition studies have not clarified the "antigenic" structures on the targets, they have pointed to some peculiar aspects of the killing process that are common to NK, NC, macrophage, and cytotoxic T cell lines but are not shared by conventional cytotoxic T cells.

Ontogeny and Genetics

In murine studies, some marked differences among strains in distribution of activity and, possibly, in genetic control have been described for NK and NC cells. However, regardless of the strain, there is a strong influence of genes distal to the D end of the H-2 region for both NK and NC cells (Stutman et al. 1978, 1980b, 1981, Stutman and Cuttito 1980, 1981, 1982, Kiessling and Wigzell 1979, Clark and Harmon 1980, Roder et al. 1981, Clark et al. 1981, Lattime et al. 1982b). Most notably, a number of mouse strains express low or no NK activity while showing normal NC activity (Stutman and Cuttito 1980, 1981, 1982, Clark et al. 1981, Lattime et al. 1982b). Mouse strains can be separated into three groups according to NK activity: (1) those that have significant NK activity against Yac-1 targets and the activity is augmentable by IFN and IFN inducers, (2) those that have low or no NK activity that is augmentable by IFN and IFN inducers, such as the prototypic low NK A/J strain or mice homozygous for the beige mutation (Lattime et al. 1982b), and (3) those that have low or no NK activity that is not augmentable by IFN and IFN inducers, such as the PL/J and SJL/J strains (Lattime et al. 1982b) and mice homozygous for the moth-eaten (me/me) mutation (Stutman O and Lattime EC unpublished data). As mentioned above, these mouse strains with partial or total NK cell deficiencies all manifest significant NC cell activity (Paige et al. 1978, Lattime et al. 1982b, Stutman O and Lattime EC unpublished data). One interesting point is that the NK deficiency in beige mice shows different behavior regarding augmentation by IFN inducers or lymphokines, depending on the background strain that expresses the mutation. Thus, beige mice in the C57BL/6 background have low NK activity augmentable by lymphokines, while NK activity in beige mice in the SJL/J background is not augmentable (Stutman O and Lattime EC unpublished data).

NK and NC cells also differ in their ontogeny and in their presence in adult and older animals. While resting NK cell activity in the spleen develops at approximately three to four weeks of age and declines to low levels in adult mice (Herberman and Holden 1978, Kiessling and Wigzell 1979, Roder et al. 1981), spleen NC cell activity is present at birth or within the first week of life and remains at constant levels for the entire lives of the mice (Stutman et al. 1978). The rapid decline in NK cell activity (Herberman and Holden 1978) may be somewhat deceiving, since no such age-related decline of NK activity is observed in murine peripheral blood lymphocytes (Lanza and Djeu 1982, Stutman O, Lattime EC, Yron I unpublished data).

Surface Phenotype of NC and NK Cells

One important difference between murine NK and NC cells is the fact that while a variety of surface markers appear to be preferentially expressed on NK cells, NC cells are consistently negative for most of those markers (Stutman et al. 1978, 1980b, 1981, Paige et al. 1978, Lattime et al. 1981, 1982b, 1983a,b, Burton 1980, Lust et al. 1981). It is worth stressing that all of these studies used negative selection (lysis of cells with antibodies and complement) and reached such conclusions when it was observed that the cell depletions had either no effect or produced enrichment of the activity under study. NC cells even have a low expression of H-2 histocompatibility antigens (Burton 1980, Stutman et al. 1980b, 1981, Lattime et al. 1981). Indeed, one method for enrichment of NC cells from spleen preparations is to treat them with the appropriate anti–H-2 reagents and complement, which produces enrichment of NC in the minority of cells (5–10% of the population) that are not lysed by the treatment (Burton 1980, Stutman et al. 1980b). However, by positive selection with the fluorescence-activated cell sorter, we have found NC activity in spleen cells with both low and high H-2 expression (Bykowsky MJ and Stutman O unpublished data). The T-200 determinant can also be detected on NC as well as NK cells (Lattime and Stutman 1983, Djeu et al. 1983). Accordingly, NC cells are not "null," but they certainly lack or have very low amounts of most of the surface antigens that are usually expressed on NK cells. Positive selection with NK 1.1 antibodies showed some NC-like activity in the "positive" fractions (Kumar et al. 1985). Positive selection with Mac-1 has also produced populations capable of killing both Yac-1 and WEHI-164 (Holmberg and Ault 1984). Since the Mac-1 $^+$ NK cells have been obtained after in vivo boosting with *Listeria* and can kill a variety of NK-resistant targets (Holmberg and Ault 1984), they may represent an in vivo counterpart of the AK cells discussed below that are capable of killing both NK and NC targets.

The most used surface markers in the murine NK studies are as follows: (1) Thy-1 (a fraction of NK cells are Thy-1 $^+$; see Mattes et al. 1979, Minato et al. 1981), (2) Qa-2 (Koo et al. 1980, Lattime et al. 1981), (3) Qa-5 (Chun et al. 1979, Lattime et al. 1981, Minato et al. 1981), (4) NK-1.1 and 1.2 (or 2.1., since there are some questions concerning allelism versus separate genes) (Glimcher et al. 1977, Burton 1980, Burton et al. 1981, 1982, Pollack and Emmons 1982), and (5) the ganglioside asialo-GM-1 (Kasai et al. 1980). Ly-5 was considered to be an NK marker (Kasai et al. 1979; Minato et al. 1981) but is apparently a determinant expressed on most hematopoietic cells (Scheid and Triglia 1979) and part of the polymorphic T-200 surface glycoproteins (Omary et al. 1980). We have used Qa-5 extensively as a differential marker between NC (Qa-5 $^-$) and NK (Qa-5 $^+$) in negative selection, especially since Qa-5 is expressed both in resting and in activated NK cells (Chun et al. 1979, Minato et al. 1981, Lattime et al. 1981). As mentioned above, NK cells induced after *Listeria* infection and selected for positivity with the Mac-1 marker kill both Yac-1 and WEHI-164 targets in long-term assays and have the following surface phenotypes: Qa-5 $^+$, asialo GM-1 $^+$, LFA-1 $^+$, Ly-5.1 $^+$, and NK 1.2 $^+$ (30% of these are also Thy-1 $^+$). NK cells are negative for Lyt-1, Lyt-2, and other Mac antigens, as well as for Leu-7 and Leu-11 markers of human NK subsets (Holmberg and Ault 1984). Some complications have recently arisen regarding the putative NK surface markers, since the surface phenotype of cloned NK cells and cloned cytotoxic T cells appear to be similar; both cloned cell types express Thy-1, Qa-5, NK 1.1. or 1.2/2.1, asialo-GM-1 and Ly-5 (Brooks et al. 1982, 1983a,b). As Brooks et al. (1983a) indicate, the only two markers that may differentiate between NK and cytotoxic T cell clones are Lyt-2, which is preferentially expressed on the T lines (although some of the NK lines are Lyt-2 $^+$) and the ganglioside asialo-GM-2, which is preferentially expressed on NK cloned lines and not on cytotoxic T lymphocytes (CTL) (Dennert et al. 1982, Brooks et al. 1982, 1983a,b).

The human studies show the same ambiguities as the murine ones, and surface markers detected on cells with NK activity or large granular morphology are also expressed on other cell types, especially T lymphocytes, monocytes, and myeloid cells (Timonen 1983, Hercend et al. 1983, Ortaldo and

Herberman 1984). For example, of eight cloned NK cell lines, all had different phenotypes when tested for expression of T1, T3, T4, T8, T11, T12, Mol, and HNK-1/Leu-7; some of them had surface phenotypes identical to cytotoxic T cell clones (Hercend et al. 1983). As was the case in the murine studies, periodic claims of some "exclusive" serologic markers for NK cells have been made in the human studies (Timonen 1983, Ortaldo and Herberman 1984).

Lineage

The issue of lineage of NK and NC in mice (as well as in humans) still remains undefined. The main problem is the variety of the surface markers expressed on NK cells; this includes surface markers characteristic of T, monocyte-macrophage, and myeloid cell lineages. Some thoughts on this problem were reported by Stutman (1982) and Stutman and Lattime (1983). At present, we are inclined to think of NK-like activity (the capacity to lyse NK-susceptible targets in vitro) as being a property of cells within different lineages, and the property may be expressed at certain stages of their development. This may occur preferentially with cells in the T, monocyte-macrophage, and granulocyte (including basophilic and mast cell) lineages, and the stages that express activity may be, in some instances, transitory. Thus, we favor a view of "horizontal" lineage cutting across several different "vertical" lineages, rather than placing NK cells in either an independent special lineage or on a branch of a defined cellular lineage. This concept is clearly testable, and it may well explain the peculiar surface phenotype of murine and human NK and AK effector cells, some of the morphologic granular features of the effectors, and the results obtained with a variety of monoclonal antibodies tested on human NK cells (see studies on pages 31 to 99 in Herberman 1982, also Ortaldo et al. 1981, where marked serologic heterogeneity and variability is described in the large granular lymphocyte population enriched for NK cells). In humans, the serologic analysis of NK cells shows that markers of the T, myeloid, and monocytic lineages are detected (Timonen 1983, Ortaldo and Herberman 1984). In addition, the surface phenotype may be variable, especially after culture (Ortaldo et al. 1981).

Since human activated B cells also express the Tac antigen, which defines the receptor for interleukin (IL) 2 (Tsudo et al. 1984), it is obvious that speculations on the T lineage relation of NK cells based on the IL 2 effects should be made with some care. The same comment can be made about the papers that will inevitably appear in the near future and will describe the presence (or the absence) of either the surface heterodimer of the T cell receptor or of rearranged genes coding for the receptor chains in some cell line capable of killing NK-susceptible targets. Our view of such findings would be simply that some

T cells can display NK activity, if the results are positive. It is highly probable that the lineage "conflict" is actually derived from the issue discussed in our section about the problems with NCMC.

NC Equivalents in Humans

The question of NC equivalents in man remains unresolved (see Stutman 1982 for further comment). In addition to some of our examples (Stutman 1982) based on studies utilizing anchorage-dependent targets in human studies, a recent publication described a monoclonal antibody that detects in man a natural effector cell that lyses anchorage-dependent targets but that does not affect conventional NK cells capable of lysing K-562 targets (Rola-Pleszczynski and Lieu 1983). Whether such a reagent indeed detects the human NC equivalent awaits further analysis. It is worth saying that the cells defined by this monoclonal antibody, as is the case with murine NC cells (Lattime et al. 1982a), are not affected by IFN (Lieu et al. 1984).

NK and NC Morphology

The identification of the LGL as a population that was enriched for NK activity in man (Saksela et al. 1979b, Timonen et al. 1981, de Landazuri et al. 1981), mice (Luini et al. 1981, Kumagai et al. 1982, Itoh et al. 1982), and rats (Reynolds et al. 1981) has resulted in a tendency to equate NK activity to LGL. Most of the studies in humans now concentrate on the activity of LGL in blood. However, it is clear from those same studies that, although there is indeed an enrichment of NK activity in the fractions containing LGL, there is also significant cytotoxic activity in fractions with low LGL content (de Landazuri et al. 1981). The fractions with high LGL content but with low cytotoxicity indicate that NK cells can bind to the targets but do not have the full lytic capacity. The low LGL fractions with more than expected lytic activity usually are not discussed. The demonstration that cells enriched for LGL have NK cell activity has developed into an "all NK cells are LGL" notion and has resulted in studies that use only the LGL fractions and discard the rest. This type of preselection may result in the loss of valuable information regarding non-LGL NK cell activities. In the early murine studies showing NK effector-target binding, the electron micrographs of the effector-target conjugates did not indicate an exclusive role of LGL in the murine system, since most of the bound effectors shown in the micrographs did not exhibit a granular structure (Roder et al. 1978). Conversely, murine cytolytic T cell clones consistently showed a marked granular structure (Engers et al. 1980, Brooks et al. 1983a,b) as did cloned murine NK cells (Dennert et al. 1982, Brooks et al. 1982, 1983b). To complicate things further, a cloned NK cell line has been defined, based on ultrastructure and surface immunoglobulin

(Ig) E receptor expression, as being related to the basophil series (Galli et al. 1982), and NK-like cell lines with LGL morphology have recently been obtained from cultures of murine thymus cells (Born et al. 1983). Thus, it is possible that the LGL morphology may be related to a peculiar stage of readiness for lysis that is shared by different cell types. On the other hand, large granular Leu-3$^+$ and T4$^+$ cells that can bind to NK-susceptible targets but do not kill them, even when boosted with IFN, and that may have other immunologic functions have been described in humans (Velardi et al. 1985).

Our studies have shown that NK and NC activities in murine cells from the peritoneal cavity (Lattime et al. 1982d) and spleen (Paige et al. 1978) are separable by sedimentation at unit gravity. These activities are the function of small to intermediate-size lymphocytes. In peritoneal washings, this separation technique produced excellent resolution for NK, NC, and cytotoxic macrophages (Lattime et al. 1982d).

In sum, although the description of the LGL as the main representative of NK activity in certain tissues has been extremely important in defining some of the characteristics of NK cells, especially in the human studies, it seems probable that they could still reflect a subpopulation of NCMC. Whether the peculiar granular structure is an intrinsic property of NK cells or whether it is related to separation procedures, culture conditions, long-term propagation in culture, granulocytic lineage, activation for rapid lysis, or any combination of these needs further study to determine. On the other hand, to argue that murine NK cells can produce glycogen-rich and mucus-secreting cells in culture based only on morphology (the cells are NK because they are LGL) and some suggestive lysis of the feeder layers (Ginsburg et al. 1983) seems a good example of the LGL dogma.

REGULATION OF NCMC BY LYMPHOKINES

In this section we will comment on the effects of various preparations containing IL 2 and other lymphokines on the growth and function of NCMC effector cells. We will discuss the effects observed with IL 2 and IL 3 on NK and NC cells and comment briefly on IFN. There are two reasons for this: firstly, that there is an overabundance of descriptions of the augmentation of NK activity by crude or pure preparations of IFN in humans and experimental animals (for example see pages 505, 525, 529, 549, 569, 581, 593, 609, 633, 645, 687 in Herberman 1980 and pages 349, 355, 361, 369 in Herberman 1982a for the effects of IFN on NK cells, mostly human studies) and secondly, that IFN or IFN inducers have no detectable effects on NC cells, which are the main focus of our own studies (Lattime et al. 1982a, 1983a,b, Lattime and Stutman 1983). A recent abstract indicates that a possible human equivalent of the murine NC cell is also unaffected by IFN (Lieu et al. 1984).

Alpha, beta, or gamma IFN can augment NK activity after brief exposure in vitro, and a variety of in vivo agents that augment NK activity seem to have a final common pathway related to their capacity to induce IFN production (Trinchieri and Santoli 1978, Gidlund et al. 1978, Senik et al. 1979, Djeu et al. 1979, Ortaldo and Herberman 1984). It has been clearly shown in humans and rodents that the effects of IFN on NK activity can be attributed to four interacting mechanisms: (1) the increase of the fraction of NK cells that form conjugates with the target cells, (2) the increase of the fraction of bound effector cells that kill the targets, (3) the improvement of the kinetics of lysis, and (4) a favoring of effector recycling (for a good example of the four stages see Saksela et al. 1979a, Targan and Dorey 1980, Silva et al. 1980, Timonen et al. 1981, Ullberg and Jondal 1981, Reynolds et al. 1982, to cite but a few). It is worth noting that not all types of IFN have these effects, and some types of human alpha IFN, while having potent antiproliferative and antiviral effects, have no NK-augmenting activities (Ortaldo et al. 1984a). Similarly, not all LGL-like cells that form conjugates with NK-susceptible targets without killing them can be activated into killer cells with IFN (Velardi et al. 1985).

From all of these studies, a linear model for in vitro development of NK activity has emerged; it includes: (1) an *undefined progenitor* cell that does not bind or kill targets and that may or may not have some distinctive cell surface antigen, (2) a *recognizable precursor or pre-NK cell* that can bind to the target, but is incapable of lysis and that bears some distinctive cell surface antigen (although one may question how "distinctive" most NK markers are), (3) the *NK effector cells* that can bind and lyse the targets and may or may not express LGL morphology, and (4) the *activated or augmented NK cell* that, as a result of the action by augmenting agents, such as IFN, binds to targets and kills more efficiently with more rapid kinetics and is also capable of more efficient recycling (see almost any review on NK cells for further details). However, it is worth mentioning that in most of these models, there is no direct evidence that one cell type actually gives rise to a functionally different cell type, as described above (see Ortaldo and Herberman 1984 for further comments, see Velardi et al. 1985 for a good example).

The observation of Henney et al. (1981) that IL 2 could augment murine NK activity after 24-hour pulse treatments and that it could synergize with IFN provided an important clue on the nature of NK regulation. Although the preparations of IL 2 were not pure (albeit IFN free) the actual role of IL 2 was demonstrated by removing the augmenting activity after absorption with IL 2 receptor–bearing T cells, as well as by neutralization with a monoclonal antibody against IL 2 (Henney et al. 1981). One previous study showed that cultivation of nude or normal mouse spleen cells for three days in IL 2–containing supernatants produced only a marginal effect on NK activities (Orn et al. 1980). However, there is agreement that in addition to the capacity to produce long-term lines and clones of NK-like cells, IL 2–containing materials augment NK activity of murine cells after short in vitro pulse treatments in mice (Kuribayashi et al. 1981, Minato et al. 1981, Handa et al. 1983, Kawase et al. 1983, Lattime et al. 1983b, Olabuenaga et al. 1983, Suzuki et al. 1983, Weigent et al. 1983). Some studies also report augmentation of NK activity even after in vivo administration of IL 2–containing material (Hefeneider et al. 1982). Similar in vitro studies using human cells have also shown augmentation of NK activity by IL 2 of varying degree of purity, including recombinant IL 2 (see for example Timonen et al. 1982, Domzig and Stadler 1982, Domzig et al. 1983, Ortaldo et al. 1984b, Lanier et al. 1985, Rook et al. 1985).

Although there is agreement about the fact that augmentation occurs, there are questions concerning the mechanism of augmentation, especially direct versus indirect effects of the IL 2–containing materials on NK activity. The indirect effects of IL 2 would be mediated by an IL 2–dependent lymphokine other than the IL 2 itself. The demonstration that IL 2 preparations of varying purity could induce gamma IFN production by murine NK cells, using either NK clones (Handa et al. 1983) or spleen cells (Kawase et al. 1983), and that antibodies to gamma IFN could block the in vitro enhancement of murine and human NK cells by IL 2 (Weigent et al. 1983) led to the belief that IL 2 enhances NK activity primarily through the induction of gamma IFN as the actual augmenting factor (Weigent et al. 1983, Kawase et al. 1983, Ortaldo et al. 1984b). On the other hand, studies with human cells show that antibodies against IL 2 can abrogate NK activity in vitro and that such an effect is reversed by the addition of IL 2 but not by IFN (Domzig et al. 1983).

Murine or human partially purified IL 2 could induce the production of gamma IFN by nylon-nonadherent mouse spleen cells after 24 hours of incubation (Kawase et al. 1983). However, a plastic-adherent cell (macrophage?) was required for the IL 2–triggered gamma IFN production. The plastic-adherent cell could be replaced by a supernatant obtained from adherent cells that were incubated for 24 hours with IL 2–containing preparations. IFN production and NK augmentation were independent of T (or Thy-1$^+$) cells and could be detected in nude mouse spleen cells, as well as in the NK-deficient beige mouse (Kawase et al. 1983). The initial study by Henney et al. (1981), using murine spleen cells pulse treated for 24 hours with the IL 2–containing material, showed two other findings: (1) that IL 2 plus IFN produced an additive augmentation of NK activity, and (2) that IL 2 alone in various degrees of purification produced two types of effects. These effects were the prevention of the spontaneous decay of NK cells in culture (this peculiarity of the murine NK cell was first described by Herberman et al. in 1975 and is not shared by other animals) and the augmentation of NK activity above control levels, which ranged from 50–300%. Based on the IL 2 remaining in the cultures after treatment with monoclonal anti–IL 2 antibodies (Henney et al. 1981, Kuribayashi et al. 1981), which was still detectable but had no augmenting effects on NK activity, one of us postulated that while T cells may require low levels of IL 2 for proper function, NK cells may require much higher concentrations of IL 2 (Stutman 1981b). Such a high dose dependency was also observed in the effects of IL 2 on NK augmentation in mice (Kawase et al. 1983) and in humans (Ortaldo et al. 1984b, Schmidt et al. 1985). The additive effect of IL 2 and IFN could also be interpreted as a result of each factor acting directly on a phenotypically different NK cell sub-set (Thy-1$^-$ Qa-5$^+$ for IFN and Thy-1$^+$ Qa-5$^+$ for IL 2), as proposed by Minato et al. (1981). However, other studies (Chun et al. 1979, Kawase et al. 1983) show that IL 2–mediated NK augmentation can be induced in Thy-1$^-$ populations. This implies that the compartments suggested by Minato et al. (1981) are probably the consequence of the NK-like activity being shared by different cell types rather than actual NK subsets. This is especially true since NK-like activity can also be induced on T cells by cultivation in high doses of IL 2–containing materials (Brooks 1983, Brooks et al. 1983b, Teh and Yu 1983). Similarly, human thymocytes can be induced to bind and kill NK-targets either when cultivated in IL 2 and stimulator lymphoblastoid lines (Torten et al. 1982) or directly after culture in semipurified IL 2 (Toribio et al. 1983). The NK-like effector cells in this study are derived from the T-3$^+$ population of thymocytes (Toribio et al. 1983). Comparable results have been obtained with murine thymocytes (Born et al. 1983). Finally, high concentra-tions of IL 2–containing supernatants converted specific cloned cytotoxic T cells into NK-like effectors, and such conversion was IL 2 dose depen-dent and reversible (Brooks 1983, Brooks et al. 1983a). In summary, IL 2–containing materials seem to be able to produce NK-like behavior under certain in vitro conditions and especially at high concentrations, on cells clearly within the T cell lineage. Whether such effects are actually mediated by IL 2 proper or by other factors needs further study. It is obvious that many of these studies could fall within the AK category, although in this section we primarily tried to discuss experiments that used fresh NK cells pulse treated with IL 2 for 24 hours or less. It is worth repeating here (see also section on "Lineage") that neither the IL 2 effects on NK activity nor the fact that some T cells can display NK-like activity should be considered as evidence for es-tablishing the lineage of the NCMC effectors.

Our own studies showed that IL 2–containing supernatants, which are IL 3 and IFN free, can augment both NK and NC activity in spleen cells after 24-hour pulse treatments (Lattime et al. 1983b). IL 3 (semipurified; kindly pro-vided by Dr. J. Ihle) (Ihle et al. 1982) had no effect on NK activity but clearly augmented NC activity (Lattime et al. 1983b). The IL 2–mediated augmenta-tion of NK was a combination of prevention of the culture-induced decay of NK activity, as well as an augmentation above the levels of killing produced by fresh NK cells and was mediated by Qa-5$^+$ cells (Lattime et al. 1982a,

1983b, Lattime and Stutman 1983). Since NC cells are stable in short-term culture (Paige et al. 1978), the effects of IL 2 and IL 3 clearly represent augmentation above the control levels (Lattime et al. 1983b). The effects on NC cells show two interesting aspects. One is that IL 2 probably acts directly on the NC cells, since the argument that augmentation is mediated by IFN does not apply to this system because IFN and IFN inducers have no detectable effects on NC cells (Lattime et al. 1982a, 1983b). The second aspect is that a different and complex lymphokine, IL 3, which has no effect on NK cells, can augment NC activity in vitro (Lattime et al. 1983b) and also permits the long-term growth of cell lines that lyse NC susceptible targets (Djeu et al. 1983). Although a detailed discussion of IL 3 is beyond the scope of this chapter, it is apparent that from a lymphokine that earlier appeared to have predominant activity on T cells (Ihle et al. 1982), IL 3 has evolved into a multispecific colony-stimulating factor–like molecule with effects on both early stem cells and on committed precursors of a variety of hematopoietic lineages (Ihle et al. 1983). IL 3 is produced by activated T cells, by some T lymphomas, and by some myeloid tumors, such as WEHI-3 (Ihle et al. 1982). The cDNA for murine IL 3 has been recently cloned and expressed, and mRNA for IL 3 was isolated from both a T lymphoma and WEHI-3 (Fung et al. 1984). At the T cell level, the production of IL 2 and IL 3 by Lyt-1$^+$ Lyt-2$^-$ murine T cells, in response to alloantigens, cannot be dissociated, and production of both lymphokines seems to be triggered simultaneously by the same stimulus and produced by the same T cell (Miller and Stutman 1983). This lengthy comment is included here in an attempt to avoid conclusions about the lineage of NC cells based on the described effects of IL 3 on certain cell populations, such as mast cells (Ihle et al. 1983).

The studies with human NK cells (mostly as LGL) also support the possibility of both direct and indirect (via gamma IFN) effects of IL 2 on the function and growth of NK cells (Timonen et al. 1982, Domzig and Stadler 1982, Domzig et al. 1983, Weigent et al. 1983, Vose and Bonnard 1983, Abo et al. 1983, Ortaldo et al. 1984b, Ortaldo and Herberman 1984, Lanier et al. 1985, Rook et al. 1985). Studies using the anti-Tac monoclonal antibody, which detects the human IL 2 receptor (Leonard et al. 1982), have shown that IL 2–triggered proliferation of Leu-7$^+$ (Abo et al. 1983) or of LGL-enriched populations (Ortaldo et al. 1984b) requires expression of IL 2 receptor and is inhibited by anti-TAC. They also show that IL 2–mediated augmentation of NK cell activity after short pulse treatments with IL 2 appears to be independent of TAC expression, since it is not affected by anti-Tac antibodies (Ortaldo et al. 1984b, Lanier et al. 1985). Whether the latter effect is mediated by an IL 2 receptor–independent pathway or actually by low-affinity IL 2 receptors, which are poorly inhibited by anti-Tac, as described by Robb et al. (1984), needs further study. All of these studies used purified or recombinant

IL 2. All Leu-11$^+$ cells appear capable of response to IL 2, while only the Leu-7$^+$ Leu-11$^+$, and not the Leu-7$^+$ Leu-11$^-$, cells are responsive to augmentation by IL 2 (Lanier et al. 1985). One study suggests that exogenous IL 2 induces gamma IFN production by LGL and that the augmenting effect is due to the IFN, since anti-IFN could inhibit augmentation (Ortaldo et al. 1984b). However, two other studies have shown that anti-gamma IFN antibodies did not affect the IL 2–dependent augmentation of NK activity (Rook et al. 1985, Lanier et al. 1985). Thus, based on its kinetics and lack of inhibition by anti-IFN, it was concluded that the augmentation of NK activity in normal NK cells or NK cells obtained from patients with acquired immune deficiency syndrome is mediated directly by IL 2 and is independent of gamma IFN (Rook et al. 1985). Conversely, Ortaldo et al. (1984b) postulate that the mechanism for NK cell boosting by IL 2 is by "direct interaction" with LGL that produce gamma IFN, which is then the activating agent, and that such direct interaction is independent of accessory cells and IL 2 receptors (compare with the murine studies by Kawase et al. 1983). A recent study compared the role of IL 2 and IL 2 receptors on cloned NK cell lines (Schmidt et al. 1985). When compared to T cell clones, the NK clones showed lower densities of IL 2 receptor regardless of their surface phenotype (some are T3$^+$ T8$^+$) and required a ten times higher dose of recombinant IL 2 for proliferation, and blocking with anti-TAC showed that IL 2 is both necessary and sufficient for NK proliferation. Conversely, only the T3$^+$ NK clones could be induced to express IL 2 receptors after stimulation by anti-T11 antibodies (Schmidt et al. 1985).

Culture-Induced Cells with NCMC-Like Activities

One of the reasons for including the in vitro culture–induced NCMC-like effectors is that this heterogeneous group of cells can certainly kill the prototypic NK susceptible targets, in addition to a variety of other targets. The main property that these effectors have in common is that their activities are detected in cultures of cells "alone," cells cultured with IL 2–containing supernatants, or cells in mixed lymphocyte cultures with allogeneic normal lymphoid or tumor stimulators. In the first two cases, the cytotoxic activity appears spontaneously, and in the third case, AK activity is superimposed on the specific T cell component and has a reactivity that is different from the immunizing antigen. (For examples of spontaneous cytotoxicity see Levy et al. 1979, Thorn 1980, Burton et al. 1978, Burton 1980; for fetal calf serum (FCS)–induced cytotoxicity see Zielske and Golub 1976, Levy et al. 1979, Thorn 1980, Lattime and Stutman 1985; for in vivo priming with FCS and subsequent culture in FCS-containing medium see Golstein et al. 1978; for cultured cells with poly I acid see Dorfman et al. 1982.) All of the cited studies show generation of cytotoxicities that are usually mediated by a T-like cell (or Thy-1 $^+$ cell in the murine studies) that can kill a variety of targets, including NK-susceptible and resistant, as well as some syngeneic normal cells. (For examples of the activation of cytotoxic effector cells with IL 2–containing materials in the absence of further stimulation see Kedar et al. 1982, Teh and Yu 1983 for murine studies and Grimm et al. 1982, 1983 for human studies.) Both the murine and human effectors appear as a somewhat special type of T cell, different from conventional T and from NK cells. The human studies designate the phenomenon lymphokine-activated killers (LAK) and suggest that IL 2 alone (as semipurified material) but neither IFN nor IL 1 is sufficient for the direct activation of the cells (Grimm et al. 1983). In both cases, a wide variety of targets are lysed by these effector cells (see especially Kedar et al. 1982, Grimm et al. 1982, 1983; for effectors induced in mixed lymphocyte cultures see Seeley and Golub 1978, Seeley et al. 1979, Jondal and Targan 1978, Zarling et al. 1978, Poros and Klein 1978, Callewaert et al. 1978, Paciucci et al. 1980, Lopez-Botet et al. 1982, Shain et al. 1982, Macphail et al. 1984, to cite just a few of these studies). One common feature of all of the mixed culture–induced effectors is that the cytotoxicities obtained have a much broader spectrum of reactivity than the antigenicities of the stimulating cells in the culture and certainly include the capacity to kill an extended spectrum of NK and NC susceptible targets, as well as some NK-resistant targets. It is generally agreed, especially in the mixed allogeneic cultures, that the anomalous component is superimposed on the specific cytotoxic T cell component and that the mixed cultures induce a heterogeneous population of specific T and less-specific and anomalous cytotoxic effectors. The specific T and the less-specific anomalous components are mediated by different effector cells, as has been shown in some of the aforementioned studies. In some studies, removal of the Lyt-2 $^+$ cells that give rise to the specific T cell component responding to the alloantigens produces a marked increase in the AK compartment (Macphail et al. 1984).

Several studies on NK activation certainly seem to fall into the AK category. For example, the observation that resting human NK cells proliferate and develop a variety of activation antigens (HLA-DR, the antigen 4F-2, transferrin receptors, and Tac) after six days in culture with IL 2–containing material (London et al. 1985). In a study of actual AK development by IL 2, it was observed that the precursors of AK are in the Leu-11 $^+$ population, which per se has the highest resting NK activity, and that such cells lacked Leu-7, Leu-3, and Leu-4 (Itoh et al. 1985). As we indicated previously, cloned NK cells grown in IL 2–containing materials have complex phenotypes that range from NK-like to those of conventional cytotoxic T cells (Hercend et al. 1983, Schmidt et al. 1985).

In summary, in both animal and human studies, the induction of NCMC-like activity in culture has three main properties: (1) it is mediated by a T-like cell (consistently Thy-1 $^+$ in all of the murine studies cited, regardless of the generation procedure used), which in most cases can be dissociated from the specific cytotoxic T cell component or from conventional NK cells, (2) the effector cells generated have a broad reactivity that includes NK-susceptible and NK-resistant targets (also NC-susceptible targets in the murine studies) and in most cases reactivity against a variety of malignant and normal syngeneic targets, such as Con A– or LPS-induced blasts, and lymphoblastoid lines, and (3) the presence of FCS and other activating factors, such as IL 2 or alloantigens, are absolute requirements for the in vitro induction. Probably the most pertinent interpretation for many of these results is that proposed by Klein (1982), who regards them as part of the polyclonally activated T cell repertoire. Our own version of all of this is that the AK-type reactivity may represent the in vitro expression of stages of differentiation of T cells, which may be normally expressed during either renewal or responses to antigen, and it supports the views of Claesson and Miller (1985) that both allogeneic and syngeneic specificities can be expressed by the same cytotoxic T cell.

The possibility that IL 2 levels may affect the type of specificities obtained was suggested by one of us (Stutman 1981b) and corroborated experimentally by Brooks (1983), who showed that high levels of IL 2–containing supernatants could change the surface phenotype and target specificity of cloned cytotoxic T cells to that of NK-like cells. Such dose dependency was also observed in human studies using LGL-enriched populations, and it showed that IL 2–mediated activation occurred only at high doses (Ortaldo et al. 1984b). Our own results indicate that in the simple model of culture-induced NK-like cells that are cultured alone in FCS for a few days, the observed level of NK activity correlates with the levels of IL 2 present in the cultures, which in turn is also dependent on expression of self class II antigens (Lattime et al. 1985). Since the different models of culture-induced NCMC effectors probably produced different levels of IL 2 and other lymphokines, it is possible that the variations in the "repertoire" of the different effectors could be related to such concentration effects (Stutman 1981b).

CONCLUSION

Owing to space limitations (this chapter has turned out to be rather long) and to a reluctance to delve into the description of the "real" functions of NCMC and its multiple effectors, we will conclude with some brief comments on the possible in vivo role of NCMC as an antitumor defense mechanism. As we indicated at the beginning, there is agreement that NK cells may be important in controlling experimental and spontaneous blood-borne metastases, in the sense that conditions in which NK cells are decreased usually favor metastatic spread (Gorelik et al. 1979, 1982, Hanna 1980, Hanna and Fidler 1981, Hanna and Burton 1981, Talmadge et al. 1981, to cite but a few; for some critical comments on some of these experiments see Stutman 1983a,b). The increased local growth of transplanted tumors in NK-deficient animals has also been suggestive of an in vivo role for NK cells (Kiessling and Wigzell 1979, Roder et al. 1981; see also pages 1105 and 1121 in Herberman 1980 and pages 1323, 1331, 1339, 1347, 1353, 1359, and 1369 in Herberman 1982a; for criticisms on conclusions reached about transplanted tumors see Stutman 1981a, 1983a,b, 1985). Finally, the role of NK cells as a surveillance mechanism preventing tumor development is, at present, highly questionable (Stutman 1983a,b, 1984a,b,c, 1985), although it has been predicted that NK cells could "rescue" immunologic surveillance (Bloom 1982, Roder et al. 1981, Herberman 1983). In a variety of murine models of induced and spontaneous lymphoid and nonlymphoid tumor development in mice with low NK activity that we studied, no clear relationship between NK cell activity and increased risk for tumor development was observed (Stutman 1983a,b, 1984a,b,c). This observation prompted one of us to write that ". . . either immunological surveillance in its strict definition is not mediated by NK cells or is a very restricted phenomenon which, by a stroke of chance, does not apply to any of the experimental models selected . . ." (Stutman 1983b p. 1205). The models selected were: (1) spontaneous lymphoma-leukemia (and other tumors) in NK low strains, (2) T cell leukemia (and skin tumor) development after methylcholanthrene exposure in NK low strains, (3) T cell leukemia development after methyl-nitrosourea in NK low strains, and (4) lymphoma and other tumor development after transplacental or postpartum (different ages) administration of ethyl-nitrosourea (ENU) and urethane to NK low strains (Stutman 1983a,b, 1984a,c, Stutman O unpublished data). It is worth noting that ENU, at all dosage levels and times of administration, has no depressive activity on NK cells (Stutman 1983a,b, 1984a,c). Furthermore, the reverse situation is also true in a model of B lymphoma induction by treatment of nude mice with anti-mu chain of Ig antibodies, in which the lymphomas appear in the presence of an intact or augmented NK compartment in high NK mouse strains (Stutman 1983a,b, 1984a,b). It is obvious that extreme care must be taken in extrapolating these results to clinical situations or in transforming them into general views. An example of the danger could be the NK deficiencies in patients with the X-linked lymphoproliferative syndrome. When initially observed, it was hailed as evidence that the increased risk for lymphoma development in such patients was due to the NK deficiency (Sullivan et al. 1980); however, it was later shown that the NK deficiency in such patients was a consequence of the lymphoid proliferation, rather than its permissive factor (Seeley et al. 1982). This sobering fact is certainly a good note on which to end this chapter.

ACKNOWLEDGMENT

The experimental work described in this text was supported by National Institutes of Health grants CA-08748 and CA-15988 and American Cancer Society grant IM-188. Dr. Lattime is a Leukemia Society Scholar. This text was completed May 1, 1985.

REFERENCES

Abo T, Miller CA, Balch CM, Cooper MD. 1983. Interleukin 2 receptor expression by activated HNK-1+ granular lymphocytes: A requirement for their proliferation. J Immunol 131:1822–1826.

Abrams SI, Brahmi Z. 1984. Compared mechanisms of tumor cytolysis by human natural killer cells and activated polymorphonuclear leukocytes. J Immunol 123:3192–3196.

Abruzzo LV, Rowley DA. 1983. Homeostasis of the antibody response immunoregulation by NK cells. Science 222:581–585.

Babior BM, Parkinson DW. 1982. The NK cell: A phagocyte in lymphocyte's clothing? Nature 298:511–512.

Bean MA, Bloom BR, Herberman RB, et al. 1975. Cell-mediated cytotoxicity for bladder carcinoma: Evaluation of a workshop. Cancer Res 35:2902–2913.

Becker S, Fenyo EM, Klein E. 1976. The "natural killer" cell in the mouse does not require H-2 homology and is not directed against type or group-specific antigens of murine C viral proteins. Eur J Immunol 6:882–887.

Bennett M, Baker EE. 1977. Marrow-dependent cell function in early stages of infection with lysteria monocytogenes. Cell Immunol 33:203–210.

Bennett M, Baker EE, Eastcott JW, Kumar V, Yonkosky D. 1976. Selective elimination of marrow precursors with the bone-seeking isotope 89Sr: Implications for hemopoiesis/lymphopoiesis/viral leukemiogenesis and infection. J Reticuloendothel Soc 20:71–87.

Biron CA, Welsh RM. 1982. Activation and role of natural killer cells in virus infections. Med Microbiol Immunol 170:155–172.

Bloom BR. 1982. Natural killers to rescue immune surveillance? Nature 300:214–215.

Born W, Ben-Nun A, Bamberger U, et al. 1983. Killer-cell lines derived from mouse thymus, resembling large granular lymphocytes and expressing natural killer-like cytotoxicity. Immunobiology 165:63–77.

Brooks CG. 1983. Reversible induction of natural killer cell activity in cloned murine cytotoxic T lymphocytes. Nature 305:155–158.

Brooks CG, Kuribayashi K, Sale GE, Henney CS. 1982. Characterization of five cloned murine cell lines showing high cytolytic activity against YAC-1 cells. J Immunol 128:2326–2335.

Brooks CG, Burton RC, Pollack SB, Henney CS. 1983a. The presence of NK alloantigens on cloned cytotoxic T lymphocytes. J Immunol 131:1391–1395.

Brooks CG, Urdal DL, Henney CS. 1983b. Lymphokine-driven "differentiation" of cytotoxic T-cell clones into cells with NK-like specificity: Correlations with display of membrane macromolecules. Immunol Rev 72:43–72.

Brunda MJ, Wiltrout RH, Holden HT, Varesio L. 1983. Selective inhibition by monosaccharides of tumor cell cytotoxicity mediated by mouse macrophages, macrophage-like cell lines and natural killer cells. Int J Cancer 31:373–379.

Burton RC. 1980. Alloantisera selectively reactive with NK cells: Characterization and use in defining NK cell classes. *In* Herberman RB, ed., Natural Cell-Mediated Immunity Against Tumors. Academic Press, New York, pp. 19–35.

Burton RC, Chism SE, Warner NL. 1978. In vitro induction and expression of T cell immunity to tumor associated antigens. Contemp Top Immunobiol 8:69–106.

Burton RC, Bartlett SP, Kumar V, Winn HJ. 1981. Studies on natural killer (NK) cells: II. Serologic evidence for heterogeneity of murine NK cells. J Immunol 127:1864–1868.

Burton RC, Bartlett SP, Winn HJ. 1982. Alloantigens specific for natural killer cells. *In* Herberman RB, ed., NK Cells and Other Natural Effector Cells. Academic Press, New York, pp. 105–112.

Bykowsky MJ, Lattime EC, Stutman O. 1985. Susceptibility to lysis by natural cytotoxic (NC) cells is independent of target cell cycle (Abstract). Fed Proc 44:1525.

Callewaert DM, Lightbody JJ, Kaplan J, Jaroszewski J, Peterson WD, Rosenberg JC. 1978. Cytotoxicity of human peripheral lymphocytes in cell-mediated lympholysis, antibody-dependent cell-mediated lympholysis and natural cytotoxicity assays after mixed lymphocyte culture. J Immunol 121:81–85.

Campbell PA. 1976. Immunocompetent cells in resistance to bacterial infections. Bacteriological Reviews 40:284–313.

Chernyakhovskaya IY, Slavina EG, Svet-Moldavsky GJ. 1970. Antitumor effect of lymphoid cells activated by interferon. Nature 238:71–72.

Chun M, Pasanen V, Hammerling U, Hammerling GF, Hoffmann MK. 1979. Tumor necrosis serum induces a serologically distinct population of NK cells. J Exp Med 150:426–431.

Claesson MH, Miller RG. 1985. Functional heterogeneity in allospecific cytotoxic T lymphocyte clones: II. Development of syngeneic cytotoxicity in the absence of specific antigenic stimulation. J Immunol 134:684–690.

Clark EA, Harmon RC. 1980. Genetic control of natural cytotoxicity and hybrid resistance. Adv Cancer Res 31:227–285.

Clark EA, Shultz LD, Pollack SB. 1981. Mutations in mice that influence natural killer (NK) cell activity. Immunogenetics 12:601–613.

Cohen IR, Wekerle H. 1973. Regulation of autosensitization: the immune activation and specific inhibition of self recognizing thymus-derived lymphocytes. J Exp Med 137:224–238.

Cohen IR, Globerson A, Feldman M. 1971. Autosensitization in vitro. J Exp Med 133:834–845.

Cohn M. 1985. Discussion. *In* Guillemin R, Cohn M, Melnechuk T, eds., Neural Modulation of Immunity. Raven Press, New York, p. 160.

Collins JL, Patek PA, Cohn M. 1981. Tumorigenicity and lysis by natural killers. J Exp Med 153:89–106.

de Landazuri MO, Lopez-Botet M, Timonen T, Ortaldo J, Herberman RB. 1981. Human large granular lymphocytes spontaneous and interferon-boosted NK activity against adherent and nonadherent tumor cell lines. J Immunol 127:1380–1383.

Dennert G, Yogeeswaren G, Yamata S. 1981. Cloned cell lines with natural killer activity: Specificity, function and cell surface markers. J Exp Med 153: 545–556.

Djeu JY, Heinbaugh JA, Holden HT, Herberman RB. 1979. Augmentation of mouse natural killer activity by interferon and interferon inducers. J Immunol 122:175–181.

Djeu JY, Lanza E, Pastore S, Hapel AJ. 1983. Selective growth of natural cytotoxic but not natural killer effector cells in interleukin-3. Nature 306:788–791.

Domzig W, Stadler BM. 1982. The relation between human natural killer cells and interleukin 2. *In* Herberman RB, ed., NK Cells and Other Natural Effector Cells. Academic Press, New York, pp. 409–414.

Domzig W, Stadler BM, Herberman RB. 1983. Interleukin 2 dependence of human natural killer (NK) cell activity. J Immunol 130:1970–1973.

Dorfman N, Winkler D, Burton RC, Kossayda N, Sabia P, Wunderlich J. 1982. Broadly reactive murine cytotoxic cells induced in vitro under syngeneic conditions. J Immunol 129:1762–1769.

Engers HD, Collavo D, North M, et al. 1980. Characterization of cloned murine cytolytic T cell lines. J Immunol 125:1481–1486.

Ernst PB, Petit A, Lee TGE, Befus AD, Bienenstock J. 1985. Mast cell mediated cytotoxicity resembles natural cytotoxic (NC) activity (Abstract). Fed Proc 44:584.

Fischer DG, Hubbard WJ, Koren HS. 1981. Tumor cell killing by freshly isolated perpheral blood monocytes. Cell Immunol 58:426–435.

Forbes JT, Bretthauer RK, Oeltmann TN. 1981. Mannose 6-, fructose 1-, and fructose 6-phosphates inhibit human natural cell mediated cytotoxicity. Proc Natl Acad Sci USA 78:5797–5801.

Fung MC, Harpel AJ, Ymer S, et al. 1984. Molecular cloning of cDNA for murine IL-3. Nature 307:233–237.

Galli SJ, Dvorak AM, Ishizaka T, et al. 1982. A cloned cell with NK function resembles basophils by ultrastructure and expresses IgE receptors. Nature 298:288–290.

Gidlund M, Orn A, Wigzell H, Senik A, Gresser I. 1978. Enhanced NK cell activity in mice injected with interferon and interferon inducers. Nature 273:759–761.

Ginsburg H, Ben-David E, Kinarty A, et al. 1983. Murine interleukin-2 generates glycogen-rich and mucus-secreting NK cells. Immunology 49:571–583.

Glimcher L, Shen FW, Cantor H. 1977. Identification of a cell-surface antigen selectively expressed on the natural killer cell. J Exp Med 145:1–9.

Golstein P, Luciani MF, Wagner H, Rollinghoff M. 1978. Mouse T cell-mediated cytolysis specifically triggered by cytophylic xenogeneic serum determinants: A caveat for the interpretation of experiments done under "syngeneic" conditions. J Immunol 121:1533–1538.

Gomard E, Leclerc JC, Levy JP. 1974. Spontaneous antilymphoma reaction of pre-leukemia AKR mice is a non-T killing. Nature 150:671–673.

Gorelik E, Fogel M, Feldman J, Segal S. 1979. Differences in resistance to metastatic tumor cells and cells from local tumor growth to cytotoxicity of natural killer cells. JNCI 63:1397–1404.

Gorczynski RM, Kennedy M, Chang MP, MacRae S. 1983. Recognition specificities, development and possible biological function of natural killer cells in the mouse: I. Spleen focus forming assay for natural killer activity and analysis of lectin-like recognition structures on the surface of murine natural killer cells. Cell Immunol 80:335–348.

Gorelik E, Wiltrout RH, Okumura J, Habu S, Herberman RB. 1982. Role of NK cells in the control of metastatic spread and growth of tumor cells in mice. Int J Cancer 30:107–112.

Greenberg AH, Playfair JHL. 1974. Spontaneous arising cytotoxicity to the P-815 mastocytoma in NZB mice. Clin Exp Immunol 10:99–110.

Grimm EA, Mazumder A, Zhang HZ, Rosenberg SA. 1982. Lymphokine-activated killer cell phenomenon: Lysis of natural killer-resistant fresh solid tumor cells by interleukin 2–activated autologous human peripheral blood lymphocytes. J Exp Med 155:1823–1841.

Grimm EA, Robb RJ, Roth JA, et al. 1983. Lymphokine-activated killer cell phenomenon: III. Evidence that IL-2 is sufficient for direct activation of peripheral blood lymphocytes into lymphokine activated killers. J Exp Med 158:1356–1361.

Gupta S. 1980. Natural killer cells—Immunologist's fancy? Gastroenterology 78:865–867.

Handa K, Suzuki R, Matsui H, Shimizu Y, Kumagai K. 1983. Natural killer (NK) cells as a responder to interleukin-2 (IL-2): II. IL-2 induced interferon gamma production. J Immunol 130:988–992.

Hanna N. 1980. Expression of metastatic potential of tumor cells in young nude mice is correlated with low levels of natural killer cell–mediated cytotoxicity. Int J Cancer 26:675–680.

Hanna N, Burton RC. 1981. Definitive evidence that natural killer (NK) cells inhibit experimental tumor metastasis in vivo. J Immunol 127:1754–1758.

Hanna N, Fidler IJ. 1981. Relationship between metastatic potential and resistance to natural killer cell–mediated cytotoxicity in three murine tumor systems. JNCI 66:1183–1190.

Hansson M, Kiessling R. 1983. Reactivity of natural killer cells against normal target cells. Clinics in Immunology and Allergy 3:495–506.

Harfast B, Andersson T, Stejskal V, Perlmann P. 1977. Interactions between human lymphocytes and paramyxovirus-infected cells: Adsorption and cytotoxicity. J Immunol 119:1132–1137.

Hatcher FM, Kuhn RE. 1982. Natural killer (NK) cell activity against extracellular forms of Trypanosoma cruzi. *In* Herberman RB, ed., NK Cells and Other Natural Effector Cells. Academic Press, New York, pp. 1091–1097.

Haubeck HD, Kolsch H, Imort M, Hasilik A, Von Figura K. 1985. Natural killer cell-mediated cytotoxicity does not depend on recognition of mannose 6-phosphate residues. J Immunol 134:65–69.

Hefeneider SH, Henney CS, Gillis S. 1982. In vivo interleukin-2 induced augmentation of natural killer cell activity. *In* Herberman RB, ed., NK Cells and Other Natural Effector Cells. Academic Press, New York, pp. 421–426.

Hellstrom KE, Hellstrom I. 1974. Lymphocyte-mediated cytotoxicity and blocking serum activity to tumor antigens. Adv Immunol 18:209–277.

Hellstrom KE, Hellstrom I, Sjogren HO, Warner GA. 1971. Cell-mediated immunity to human tumor antigens. *In* Amos DB, ed., Progress in Immunology I. Academic Press, New York, pp. 940–949.

Henney CS, Kuribayashi K, Kern DE, Gillis S. 1981. IL-2 augments natural killer cell activity. Nature 291:335–338.

Herberman RB, ed. 1980. Natural Cell-Mediated Immunity Against Tumors. Academic Press, New York, 1309 pp.

Herberman RB, ed. 1982a. NK Cells and Other Effector Cells. Academic Press, New York, 1546 pp.

Herberman RB. 1982b. Natural killer cells and their possible relevance to transplantation biology. Transplantation 34:1–7.

Herberman RB. 1983. Possible role of natural killer cells in host resistance against tumors and other diseases. Clinics in Immunology and Allergy 3: 479–494.

Herberman RB, Holden HT. 1978. Natural cell-mediated immunity. Adv Cancer Res 27:305–377.

Herberman RB, Nunn ME, Lavrin DH. 1975. Natural cytotoxic reactivity of mouse lymphoid cells against syngeneic and allogeneic tumors: I. Distribution of reactivity and specificity. Int J Cancer 16:216–229.

Herberman RB, Nunn ME, Holden HT, Staal S, Djeu JY. 1977. Augmentation of natural cytotoxic reactivity of mouse lymphoid cells against syngeneic and allogeneic target cells. Int J Cancer 19:555–564.

Herberman RB, Mason L, Ortaldo JR. 1984. Studies on the possible relationship of NC cells to mouse NK cells. In Hoshino T, Koren HS, Uchida A, eds., Natural Killer Activity and Its Regulation. Excerpta Medica, Amsterdam, pp. 16–21.

Hercend T, Meuer S, Reinherz EL, Schlossman SF, Ritz J. 1982. Generation of a cloned NK cell line derived from the "null cell" fraction of human peripheral blood. J Immunol 129:1299–1305.

Hercend T, Reinherz EL, Meuer S, Schlossman SF, Ritz J. 1983. Phenotypic and functional heterogeneity of human cloned natural killer cell lines. Nature 301:158–160.

Holmberg LA, Ault KA. 1984. Characterization of natural killer cells induced in the peritoneal exudate of mice infected with Listeria monocytogenes: A study of their tumor target specificity and their expression of murine differentiation antigens and human NK-associated antigens. Cell Immunol 89:151–168.

Ihle JN, Lee JC, Hapel AJ. 1982. Interleukin 3: Biochemical and biological properties and possible roles in the regulation of immune responses. Lymphokines 6:239–262.

Ihle JN, Keller J, Orszolan S, et al. 1983. Biological properties of homogeneous interleukin 3: I. Demonstration of WEHI-3 growth factor activity, mast cell growth factor activity, P cell stimulating factor activity, colony stimulating factor activity and histamine-producing cell-stimulating factor activity. J Immunol 131:282–287.

Itoh K, Suzuki R, Umezu Y, Hanaumi K, Kumagai K. 1982. Studies of murine large granular lymphocytes: II. Tissue, strain and age distribution of LGL and LAL. J Immunol 129:295–400.

Itoh K, Tilden AB, Kumagai K, Balch CM. 1985. Leu 11+ lymphocytes with natural killer (NK) activity are precursors of recombinant interleukin 2 (rIL-2)–induced activated killer (AK) cells. J Immunol 134:802–807.

Jondal M, Targan S. 1978. In vitro induction of cytotoxic effector cells with spontaneous killer cell specificity. J Exp Med 147:1621–1636.

Karre K, Seeley JK. 1979. Cytotoxic Thy-1.2 positive blasts with NK-like target selectivity in murine mixed lymphocyte cultures. J Immunol 123:1511–1518.

Kasai M, Leclerc JM, Shen FW, Cantor H. 1979. Identification of Ly 5 on the surface of natural killer cells in normal and athymic inbred mouse strains. Immunogenetics 8:153–159.

Kasai M, Iwamori M, Nagai Y, Ilumura K, Tada T. 1980. A glycolipid on the surface of mouse natural killer cells. Eur J Immunol 10:175–180.

Kawase I, Brooks CG, Kuribayashi K, et al. 1983. Interleukin 2 induces gamma-interferon production: Participation of macrophages and NK-like cells. J Immunol 131:288–292.

Kedar E, Ikejiri BL, Gorelik E, Herberman RB. 1982. Natural cell-mediated cytotoxicity in vitro and inhibition of tumor growth in vivo by murine lymphoid cells cultured with T cell growth factor (TCGF). Cancer Immunol Immunother 13:14–23.

Kiessling R, Klein E, Wigzell H. 1975. "Natural killer" cells in the mouse: I. Cytotoxic cells with specificity for mouse Moloney leukemia cells: Specificity and distribution according to genotype. Eur J Immunol 5:112–117.

Kiessling R, Wigzell H. 1979. An analysis of murine NK cells as to structure/ function and biological relevance. Immunol Rev 44:165–208.

Klein E. 1982. Lymphocyte-mediated lysis of tumor cells in vitro: Antigen-restricted clonal and unrestricted polyclonal effects. Springer Semin Immunopathol 5:147–159.

Koo G, Jacobson J, Hammerling G, Hammerling U. 1980. Antigenic profile of murine natural killer cells. J Immunol 125:1003–1006.

Koren HS, Herberman RB. 1983. Natural killing—Present and future (Summary of a workshop on natural killer cells). JNCI 70:785–786.

Kumagai K, Itoh K, Suzuki R, Hinuma S, Saitoh F. 1982. Studies of murine large granular lymphocytes: I. Identification as effector cells in NK and K cytotoxicities. J Immunol 129:388–394.

Kumar V, Luevano E, Bennett M. 1979. Hybrid resistance to EL-4 lymphoma cells: I. Characterization of natural killer cells that lyse EL-4 cells and their distinction from marrow dependent natural killer cells. J Exp Med 150:531–547.

Kumar V, Hackett J, Lipscomb M, Bennett M, Koo G. 1985. Studies of purified NK-1.1+ natural killer (NK) cells (Abstract). Fed Proc 44:1525.

Kunkel LA, Welsh RM. 1981. Metabolic inhibitors render resistant target cells sensitive to natural killer cell-mediated lysis. Int J Cancer 27:73–79.

Kuribayashi K, Gillis S, Kern DE, Henney CS. 1981. Murine NK cell cultures: Effects of IL-2 and interferon on cell growth and cytotoxic reactivity. J Immunol 126:2321–2327.

Lanier LL, Benike CJ, Phillips JH, Engelman EG. 1985. Recombinant interleukin 2 enhanced natural killer cell-mediated cytotoxicity in human lymphocyte subpopulations expressing the Leu 7 and Leu 11 antigens. J Immunol 134:794–801.

Lanza E, Djeu JY. 1982. Age-independent natural killer activity in murine peripheral blood. *In* Herberman RB, ed., NK Cells and Other Natural Effector Cells. Academic Press, New York, pp. 335–340.

Lattime EC, Stutman O. 1983. Natural cell mediated cytotoxicity against tumors in mice. Survey and Synthesis of Pathology Research 2:57–68.

Lattime EC, Stutman O. 1985. The generation of culture activated killer cells (AK) is interleukin-2 dependent and requires self-Ia recognition. Int J Cancer 35:535–542.
Lattime EC, Pecoraro GA, Stutman O. 1981. Natural cytotoxic cells against solid tumors in mice: III. A comparison of effector cell antigenic phenotype and target cell recognition structures with those of NK cells. J Immunol 126: 2011–2014.
Lattime EC, Pecoraro GA, Cuttito MJ, Stutman O. 1982a. Solid tumors are killed by NK and NC cell populations: Interferon inducing agents do not augment NC cell activity under NK activating conditions. In Herberman RB, ed., NK Cells and Other Natural Effector Cells. Academic Press, New York, pp. 179–186.
Lattime EC, Pecoraro GA, Stutman O. 1982b. Natural cytotoxic cells against solid tumors in mice: IV. Natural cytotoxic (NC) cells are not culture activated natural killer (NK) cells. Int J Cancer 30:471–477.
Lattime EC, Pecoraro GA, Stutman O. 1982c. Target cell recognition by natural killer and natural cytotoxic cells. In Herberman RB, ed., NK Cells and Other Natural Effectors. Academic Press, New York, pp. 713–718.
Lattime EC, Pelus LM, Stutman O. 1982d. Enrichment and characterization of effector populations mediating NK, NC, ADCC and spontaneous macrophage cytotoxicity in murine peritoneal exudate cell preparations. In Herberman RB, ed., NK Cells and Other Natural Effector Cells. Academic Press, New York, pp. 193–199.
Lattime EC, Pecoraro GA, Cuttito MJ, Stutman O. 1983a. Murine nonlymphoid tumors are lysed by a combination of NK and NC cells. Int J Cancer 32: 523–528.
Lattime EC, Pecoraro GA, Stutman O. 1983b. The activity of natural cytotoxic (NC) cells is augmented by interleukin 2 and interleukin 3. J Exp Med 157: 1070–1075.
Leonard WJ, Depper JM, Uchiyama T, Smith KA, Waldmann TA, Greene WC. 1982. A monoclonal antibody that appears to recognize the receptor for human T cell growth factor: Partial characterization of the receptor. Nature 300: 267–269.
Levy RB, Shearer GM, Kim JJ, Asofsky RM. 1979. Xenogeneic serum-induced murine cytotoxic cells: I. Generation of effector components specific for self and allogeneic target cells. Cell Immunol 48:276–287.
Lieu H, Girard M, Rola-Pleszcynski M. 1984. Human natural cytotoxic (NC) cells are distinguishable from natural killer (NK) cells by target cell affinity, membrane markers and sensitivity to biological response modifiers (Abstract). Fed Proc 43:1805.
Lin Y, Collins JL, Patek PQ, Cohn M. 1983. An analysis of the sensitivity of somatic cell hybrids to natural killer cell and natural cytotoxic cell-mediated lysis. J Immunol 131:1154–1159.
Lohmann-Matthes ML, Domzig W, Roder J. 1979. Promonocytes have the functional characteristics of natural killer cells. J Immunol 123:1883–1886.
London L, Perussia B, Trinchieri G. 1985. Induction of proliferation in vitro of resting human natural killer cells: Expression of surface activation antigens. J Immunol 134:718–727.
Lopez C, Kirkpatrick D, Fitzgerald PA, et al. 1982. Studies of the cell lin-

eage of the effector cells that spontaneously lyse HSV-1 infected fibroblasts (NK(HSV-1)). J Immunol 129:824–828.

Lopez-Botet M, Silva A, Rodriguez J, de Landazuri MO. 1982. Generation of 'T' cell blasts with NK-like activity in human MLC cellular precursors, IL-2 responsiveness and phenotype expression. J Immunol 129:1109–1115.

Luini W, Boraschi D, Alberti S, Aleotti A, Tagliabue A. 1981. Morphological characterization of a cell population responsible for natural killer activity. Immunology 43:663–668.

Lust JA, Kumar V, Burton RC, Bartlett SP, Bennett MC. 1981. Heterogeneity of natural killer cells in the mouse. J Exp Med 154:306–317.

MacDermott RP, Kienker LJ, Bertovich MJ, Muchmore AV. 1981. Inhibition of spontaneous but not antibody-dependent cell-mediated cytotoxicity by simple sugars: Evidence that endogenous lectins may mediate spontaneous cell-mediated cytotoxicity. Immunology 44:143–152.

Macphail S, Paciucci PA, Stutman O. 1984. Phenotypic heterogeneity of anti-syngeneic tumor killer cells (ASTK) generated in allogeneic mixed lymphocyte reactions. J Immunol 123:3205–3210.

Mahdavi V, Periasamy M, Nadal-Ginard V. 1982. Molecular characterization of two myosin heavy chain genes expressed in the adult heart. Nature 297:659–664.

Mattes MJ, Sharrow SO, Herberman RB, Holden HR. 1979. Identification and separation of Thy 1 positive mouse spleen cells active in natural cytotoxicity and antibody-dependent cell-mediated cytotoxicity. J Immunol 123:2851–2860.

McCoy JL, Herberman RB, Rosenberg EB, Donnelly FC, Levine PH, Alford C. 1973. ^{51}Chromium-release assay for cell-mediated cytotoxicity of human leukemia and lymphoid tissue-culture cells. Natl Cancer Inst Monogr 37:59–67.

Miller RA, Stutman O. 1983. Limiting dilution analysis of T helper cell heterogeneity: A single class of T cell makes both IL-2 and IL-3. J Immunol 130:1749–1753.

Minato N, Reid L, Bloom BR. 1981. On the heterogeneity of murine natural killer cells. J Exp Med 154:750–762.

Moller G, ed. 1979. Immunol Rev 44:1–165.

Nabel G, Allard WJ, Cantor H. 1982. A cloned cell line mediating natural killer cell function inhibits immunoglobulin secretion. J Exp Med 156:658–663.

Nogueira N, Cohn ZA. 1979. Trypanosoma cruzi in vitro induction of macrophage microbicidal activity. J Exp Med 148:288–300.

Olabuenaga SE, Brooks CC, Gillis S, Henney CS. 1983. Interleukin-2 is not sufficient for the continuous growth of cloned NK-like cytotoxic cell lines. J Immunol 131:2386–2391.

Oldham RK. 1983. Natural killer cells: Artifact to reality: An odyssey in biology. Cancer Metastasis Rev 2:323–336.

Omary B, Trowbridge IS, Scheid M. 1980. Target-effector interaction in the human and murine natural killer system. J Exp Med 150:471–481.

Orn A, Gidlund M, Ojo E, et al. 1980. Factors controlling the augmentation of natural killer cells. In Herberman RB, ed., Natural Cell Mediated Immunity Against Tumors. Academic Press, New York, pp. 581–592.

Ortaldo JR, Herberman RB. 1984. Heterogeneity of natural killer cells. Annual Review of Immunology 2:359–394.

Ortaldo JR, Sharrow SO, Timonen T, Herberman RB. 1981. Determination of surface antigens on highly purified human NK cells by flow cytometry with monoclonal antibodies. J Immunol 127:2401–2409.

Ortaldo JR, Herberman RB, Harvey C, et al. 1984a. A species of human alpha interferon that lacks the ability to boost natural killer activity. Proc Natl Acad Sci USA 81:4926–4929.

Ortaldo JR, Mason AT, Gerard JP, et al. 1984b. Effects of natural and recombinant IL 2 on regulation of IFN-gamma production and natural killer activity: Lack of involvement of the TAC antigen for these immunoregulatory effects. J Immunol 133:779–783.

Ortaldo JR, Timonen TT, Herberman RB. 1984c. Inhibition of activity of human NK and K cells by simple sugars: Discrimination between binding and post-binding events. Clin Immunol Immunopathol 31:439–443.

Paciucci PA, Macphail S, Zarling JM, Bach FH. 1980. Lysis of syngeneic solid tumor cells by alloantigen stimulated mouse T and non-T cells. J Immunol 124:370–375.

Paige CJ, Feo Figarella E, Cuttito MJ, Cahan A, Stutman O. 1978. Natural cytotoxic cells against solid tumors in mice: II. Some characteristics of the effector cells. J Immunol 121:1827–1835.

Palladino MA, Lattime EC, Pecoraro GA, Stutman O, Oettgen HF. 1983. Characterization of IL-2–dependent cytotoxic T-cell clones: III. Inhibition of killing activity by monosaccharides. Cell Immunol 76:286–294.

Patek PA, Collins JL, Cohn M. 1983. Evidence that cytotoxic T cells and natural cytotoxic cells use different lytic mechanisms to lyse the same targets. Eur J Immunol 13:433–436.

Pollack SB, Emmons SL. 1982. Anti-NK 2.1: An activity of NZB anti-BALB/c serum. *In* Herberman RB, ed., NK Cells and Other Natural Effector Cells. Academic Press, New York, pp. 113–118.

Poros A, Klein E. 1978. Cultivation with K562 cells leads to blastogenesis and increased cytotoxicity with changed properties of the active cells when compared to fresh lymphocytes. Cell Immunol 41:240–255.

Pross HF, Baines MG. 1982. Studies of human natural killer cells: I. In vivo parameters affecting normal cytotoxic function. Int J Cancer 29:383–390.

Reynolds CW, Timonen T, Herberman RB. 1981. Natural killer (NK) cell activity in the rat: I. Isolation and characterization of the effector cells. J Immunol 127:282–287.

Reynolds CW, Timonen TT, Holden HT, Hansen CT, Herberman RB. 1982. Natural killer cell activity in the rat: Analysis of effector cell morphology and effects of interferon on natural killer cell function in the athymic (nude) rat. Eur J Immunol 12:577–582.

Robb RJ, Greene WC, Rusk CM. 1984. Low and high affinity cellular receptors for interleukin 2: Implications for the level of Tac antigen. J Exp Med 160:1126–1146.

Roder J, Kiessling R, Biberfeld P, Andersson B. 1978. Target-effector interaction in the natural killer (NK) cell system: II. The isolation of NK cells and studies on the mechanism of killing. J Immunol 121:2509–2517.

Roder JC, Lohmann-Matthes ML, Domzig W, Wigzell H. 1979. The beige mutation in the mouse: II. Selectivity of the natural killer (NK) cell defect. J Immunol 123:2174–2181.

Roder JC, Karre K, Kiessling R. 1981. Natural killer cells. Prog Allergy 28: 66–159.

Roder JC, Helfand SL, Werkmeister J, McGarry R, Beaumont TJ, Duwe A. 1982. Oxygen intermediates are triggered early in the cytolytic pathway of human NK cells. Nature 298:569–571.

Rodriguez AM, Santoro F, Afchin D, Bazin H, Capron A. 1981. Trypanosoma cruzi infection in B cell deficient rats. Infect Immun 31:524–529.

Rola-Pleszczynski M, Lieu H. 1983. Human natural cytotoxic lymphocytes: Definition by a monoclonal antibody of a subset which kills an anchorage-dependent target cell line but not the K-562 cell line. Cell Immunol 82: 326–333.

Rook AH, Hooks JJ, Quinnan GV, et al. 1985. Interleukin 2 enhances the natural killer cell activity of acquired immunodeficiency syndrome patients through a gamma-interferon–independent mechanism. J Immunol 134:1503–1507.

Rosenberg EB, Herberman RB, Levine PH, Halterman RH, McCoy JL, Wunderlich JR. 1972. Lymphocyte cytotoxicity reactions to leukemia-associated-antigens in identical twins. Int J Cancer 9:648–658.

Saksela E, Timonen T, Cantell K. 1979a. Human natural killer cell activity is augmented by interferon via recruitment of pre-natural killer cells. Scand J Immunol 10:257–266.

Saksela E, Timonen T, Ranki A, Hayry P. 1979b. Morphological and functional characterization of isolated effector cells responsible for human natural killer activity to fetal fibroblasts and to cultured cell line targets. Immunol Rev 44:71–123.

Scheid MP, Triglia D. 1979. Further description of the Ly-5 system. Immunogenetics 9:423–433.

Schmidt RE, Hercend T, Fox DA, et al. 1985. Human natural killer clones differ from T cell clones in regard to activation by interleukin 2 and the T11 antigen complex (Abstract). Fed Proc 44:596.

Seeley JK, Golub SH. 1978. Studies on cytotoxicity generated in human mixed lymphocyte cultures: I. Time course and target spectrum of several distinct concomitant cytotoxic activities. J Immunol 120:1415–1422.

Seeley JK, Masucci G, Poros A, Klein E, Golub SH. 1979. Studies on cytotoxicity generated in human mixed lymphocyte cultures: II. Anti-K-562 effectors are distinct from allospecific CTL and can be generated from NK-depleted T cells. J Immunol 123:1303–1311.

Seeley JK, Bechtold T, Purtilo DT, Lindsten T. 1982. NK-deficiency in x-linked lymphoproliferative syndrome. In Herberman RB, ed., NK cells and Other Natural Effector Cells. Academic Press, New York, pp. 1211–1218.

Sendo F, Aoki T, Boyse EA, Buafo CK. 1975. Natural occurrence of lymphocytes showing cytotoxic activity to BALB/c radiation-induced leukemia RLoL cells. JNCI 55:603–609.

Senik A, Gresser I, Maury C, Gidlund M, Orn A, Wigzell H. 1979. Enhancement by interferon of natural killer cell activity in mice. Cell Immunol 44:186–200.

Shain B, Holt CA, Lilly F. 1982. Lack of specificity for viral and H-2 antigens by anomalous T killer cells generated in murine leukocyte cultures. J Immunol 129:722–729.

Shustik C, Cohen IR, Schwartz RS, Latham-Griffin E. 1976. T lymphocytes with promiscuous cytotoxicity. Nature 263:699–701.

Silva A, Bonavida A, Targan S. 1980. Mode of action of interferon-mediated modulation of natural killer cytotoxic activity: Recruitment of pre-NK cells and enhanced kinetics of lysis. J Immunol 125:479–484.

Stutman O. 1981a. Immunological surveillance and cancer. *In* Waters H, ed., The Handbook of Cancer Immunology. Garland STPM, New York, pp. 1–25.

Stutman O. 1981b. NK cells, antitumor surveillance and interleukins. Immunology Today 2:205–208.

Stutman O. 1982. Natural cell-mediated cytotoxicity against tumors in mice. *In* Serrou B, Rosenfeld C, Herberman RB, eds., Human Cancer Immunology vol 4: Natural Killer Cells. Elsevier Biomedical Press, Amsterdam, pp. 205–223.

Stutman O. 1983a. The immunological surveillance hypothesis. *In* Herberman RB, ed., Basic and Clinical Tumor Immunology. Martinus Nijhoff, Boston, pp. 1–81.

Stutman O. 1983b. Current evidence for immunological surveillance against tumors in mice and possible role of NK and NC cells. *In* Yamamura Y, Tada T, eds., Progress in Immunology V. Academic Press, Tokyo, pp. 1195–1207.

Stutman O. 1984a. Natural anti-tumor resistance in immune-deficient mice. *In* Sordat B, ed., Immune-deficient Animals. S. Karger, Basel, pp. 30–39.

Stutman O. 1984b. High incidence of lymphomas in nude mice treated with anti-mu antibodies but with normal or high NK activity. *In* Hosino T, Koren HS, Uchida A, eds., Natural Killer Activity and Its Regulation. Excerta Medica, Amsterdam, pp. 384–388.

Stutman O. 1984c. Tumor development in mouse strains with low NK activity. *In* Hosino T, Koren HS, Uchida A, eds., Natural Killer Activity and Its Regulation. Excerpta Medica, Amsterdam, pp. 389–393.

Stutman O. 1985. Immunological Surveillance Revisited. *In* Mitchell M, Reif A, eds., Immunity to Cancer. Academic Press, New York, pp. 323–342.

Stutman O, Cuttito MJ. 1980. Genetic influences affecting natural cytotoxic (NC) cells in mice. *In* Herberman RB, ed., Natural Cell-Mediated Immunity Against Tumors. Academic Press, New York, pp. 431–442.

Stutman O, Cuttito MJ. 1981. Normal levels of natural cytotoxic cells against solid tumors in NK-deficient beige mice. Nature 290:254–257.

Stutman O, Cuttito MJ. 1982. Genetic control of NC activity in the mouse: Three genes located in chromosome 17. *In* Herberman RB, ed., NK Cells and Other Natural Effectors. Academic Press, New York, pp. 281–289.

Stutman O, Lattime EC. 1983. Natural cytotoxic cells against tumour in mice. Clinics in Immunology and Allergy 3:507–521.

Stutman O, Paige CJ, Feo Figarella E. 1978. Natural cytotoxic cells against solid tumors in mice: I. Strain and age distribution and target cell susceptibility. J Immunol 121:1819–1826.

Stutman O, Dien P, Wisun RE, Lattime EC. 1980a. Natural cytotoxic cells against solid tumors in mice: Blocking of cytotoxicity by D-mannose. Proc Natl Acad Sci USA 77:2895–2898.

Stutman O, Feo Figarella E, Paige CJ, Lattime EC. 1980b. Natural cytotoxic (NC) cells against solid tumors in mice: General characteristics and comparison to natural killer (NK) cells. *In* Herberman RB, ed., Natural Cell-Mediated Immunity Against Tumors. Academic Press, New York, pp. 187–229.

Stutman O, Lattime EC, Feo Figarella E. 1981. Natural cytotoxic (NC) cells against solid tumors in mice: A comparison with natural killer (NK) cells. Fed Proc 40:55–60.

Sullivan JL, Byron KS, Brewster FE, Purtilo DT. 1980. Deficient natural killer cell activity in x-linked lymphoproliferative syndrome. Science 210.543–545.

Suzuki R, Handa K, Itoh K, Kumagai K. 1983. Natural killer (NK) cells as a responder to interleukin 2 (IL-2): I. Proliferative response and establishment of cloned cells. J Immunol 130:981–987.

Takasugi M, Mickey MR, Terasaki PI. 1973. Reactivity of lymphocytes from normal persons on cultured tumor cells. Cancer Res 33:2898–2902.

Talmadge JE, Meyers KM, Prieur DJ, Starkey JR. 1981. Role of NK cells in tumor growth as metastasis in beige mice. Nature 284:622–624.

Targan S, Dorey F. 1980. Interferon activation of pre-spontaneous killer (pre-SK) cells and alteration in kinetics of lysis of both "pre-SK" and active SK cells. J Immunol 124:2157–2161.

Teh HS, Yu M. 1983. Activation of nonspecific killer cells by interleukin 2-containing supernatants. J Immunol 131:1827–1833.

Thorn RM. 1980. Murine T cell mediated cytotoxicity against syngeneic and allogeneic cell lines induced by fetal calf serum. Cell Immunol 54:203–214.

Timonen T. 1983. Characteristics of fresh and cultured natural killer cells. Clinics in Immunology and Allergy 3:465–477.

Timonen T, Ortaldo JR, Herberman RB. 1981. Characteristics of human large granular lymphocytes and relationship to natural killer and K cells. J Exp Med 153:569–582.

Timonen T, Ortaldo JR, Stadler BM, Bonnard GD, Sharrow SO, Herberman RB. 1982. Cultures of purified human natural killer cells: Growth in the presence of interleukin 2. Cell Immunol 72:178–185.

Toribio ML, de Landazuri MO, Lopez-Botet M. 1983. Induction of natural killer-like cytotoxicity in cultured human thymocytes. Eur J Immunol 13:964–969.

Torten M, Sidell N, Golub SH. 1982. IL-2 and stimulator lymphoblastoid cells will induce human thymocytes to bind and kill K562 targets. J Exp Med 156:1545–1550.

Trinchieri G, Santoli D. 1978. Anti-viral activity induced by culturing lymphocytes with tumor-derived or virus transformed cells: Enhancement of human natural killer cell activity by interferon and antagonistic inhibition of susceptibility of target cells to lysis. J Exp Med 148:1314–1332.

Tsudo M, Uchiyama T, Uchino H. 1984. Expression of Tac antigen on activated normal human B cells. J Exp Med 160:612–617.

Ullberg M., Jondal M. 1981. Recycling and target binding capacity of human natural killer cells. J Exp Med 153:615–628.

Velardi A, Grossi CE, Cooper MD. 1985. A large subpopulation of lymphocytes with T helper phenotype (Leu3/T4+) exhibits the property of binding to NK cell targets and granular lymphocyte morphology. J Immunol 134:58–64.

Vose BM, Bonnard GD. 1983. Limiting dilution analysis of the frequency of T cells and large granular lymphocytes proliferating in response to interleukin 2: The effects of lectin on the proliferative frequency and cytotoxic activity of cultured lymphoid cells. J Immunol 130:687–693.

Vose BM, Harding M, White W, Moore M, Gallagher J. 1983. Effect of simple sugars on natural killing: Evidence against the involvement of a lectin-like mechanism in target recognition. Clin Exp Immunol 51:517–524.

Weigent DA, Stanton GJ, Johnson HM. 1983. IL-2 enhances natural killer cell activity through induction of gamma interferon. Infect Immun 41:992–997.

Welsh RM, Hallenbeck LA. 1980. Effect of virus infection on target-cell susceptibility to natural killer cell-mediated lysis. J Immunol 124:2491–2497.

Wright SC, Bonavida B. 1981. Selective lysis of NK-sensitive target cells by a soluble mediator released from murine spleen cells and human peripheral blood lymphocytes. J Immunol 126:1516–1521.

Zarling J, Nowinski RC, Bach FH. 1975. Lysis of leukemia cells by spleen cells from normal mice. Proc Natl Acad Sci USA 72:2780–2789.

Zarling JM, Robins HI, Raich PC, Bach FH, Bach ML. 1978. Generation of cytotoxic T lymphocytes to autologous human leukemia cells by sensitization to pooled allogeneic normal cells. Nature 274:269–271.

Zielske JV, Golub SH. 1976. Fetal calf serum-induced blastogenic and cytotoxic responses of human lymphocytes. Cancer Res 36:3842–3850.

IMMUNOLOGICAL APPROACHES
TO CANCER THERAPY

Symposium on Fundamental Cancer Research, Vol. 38.
© 1986 by The University of Texas System Cancer Center.

16. The Immunobiology of B Cell Lymphoma: Clonal Heterogeneity as Revealed by Anti-idiotype Antibodies and Immunoglobulin Gene Probes

Ronald Levy,* Timothy Meeker,* James Lowder,*
Shoshana Levy,* Kristiaan Thielemans,*† Roger A. Warnke,‡
Michael L. Cleary,‡ and Jeffrey Sklar‡

*Departments of *Medicine/Oncology and ‡Medicine/Pathology, Stanford
University, Stanford, California 94305*

Human B cell lymphomas are considered to be monoclonal cell populations that are derived from a single original transformed cell. This notion is based on analyses of karyotypes (Rowley 1978, Klein 1983) X chromosome–linked enzymes (Friedman and Fialkow 1976, Fialkow et al. 1973), and immuno-globulin (Ig) protein expression (Warnke and Levy 1980) of the tumor cell population. Assuming that these tumors are monoclonal, we have produced antibodies directed against the idiotypic determinants of the cell surface Ig of a series of cases of human B cell malignancy. We have used these antibodies as diagnostic monitoring reagents, as therapeutic agents, and as probes for the biology of the disease. Diagnostic and therapeutic trials show that anti-idiotype antibodies have clinical utility. However, their role in the management of these diseases remains to be defined. We find that some human B cell malignancies are composed of two populations of cells, each with its unique Ig idiotype and distinct Ig gene rearrangements. In addition, we find that within a given clone there is heterogeneity in the expressed Ig variable (V) region sequence because of somatic mutations.

MATERIALS AND METHODS

Patients

The patients selected for this study had lymphoid malignancy that contained cell surface Ig, tumor tissue accessible for biopsy, no evidence of serum para-protein, and a projected life expectancy of greater than one year. Biopsies

†Current address for Kristiaan Thielemans: Afdeling Hematologie/Immunologie, Vrije Universiteit Brussel, Brussels, Belgium.

were performed to obtain tumor tissue and cells for immunologic analysis (Warnke and Levy 1980, Loken and Herzenberg 1975) and for the production and screening of anti-idiotype antibodies. At least one monoclonal anti-idiotype antibody was produced for each patient. During the time antibodies were being prepared, the patients' clinical statuses were monitored. Prior to inclusion in therapeutic trials, the patients were reevaluated. They were required to have disease that was objectively measurable. Repeat biopsies were obtained to confirm the continued reactivity of the tumor with the anti-idiotype antibodies.

Production of Antibodies

Considerable effort was devoted to streamlining the antibody production procedures. Two different strategies were developed. One involved hybridizing human tumor cells to either mouse myeloma cells (Levy and Dilley 1978) or to human lymphoblastoid cell lines (Handley and Royston 1982). Such hybrids secreted the tumor-derived Ig, which could be isolated in pure form and used to immunize mice. The other strategy involved immunizing mice directly with the human tumor cells. In both cases antibody-secreting hybridomas were produced from the immunized mice and screened for anti-idiotype specificity. When the mice were immunized with pure protein, the frequency of anti-idiotype–producing hybridomas was approximately 15%. When they were immunized with whole tumor cells, the frequency was approximately 1% (Thielemans et al. 1984). The antibodies were used in immunofluorescence and immunoperoxidase procedures on tumor cells and tissues. They were also used in immunoassays to measure idiotype protein in the sera of the patients. For therapeutic trials, the antibody-producing hybridoma cells were injected into mice, and large quantities of antibody were purified from the resulting ascites fluid (Miller et al. 1982).

Analysis of Ig DNA

High molecular weight DNA was purified from 10^6 to 10^7 cells. DNA was digested with restriction enzymes, and the resulting fragments were separated by electrophoresis in agarose gels. Separated DNA fragments were transferred out of the gels onto activated nylon membranes (Southern 1975). Membranes were hybridized with ^{32}P-radiolabeled DNA fragments specific for the heavy-chain joining region (J_H), the heavy-chain constant region (C_μ), and the constant regions of the kappa (C_κ) and lambda (C_λ) light-chain genes (Cleary et al. 1984).

Antibody Therapy

Patients were premedicated with acetaminophen and diphenhydramine. Antibody doses of less than 10 mg were diluted in 250 ml of 5% albumin. Larger doses of antibody were diluted in normal saline. Antibody infusions were performed over 4–24 hours. During periods of therapy, patients' physical examination, blood cell counts, chemistry screening panel, urinalysis, and creatinine clearance were evaluated. Serum samples were collected immediately before, immediately after, one hour after, and four hours after each dose. Radiographs were repeated as indicated. Accessible tumors (blood, bone marrow, lymph nodes, or pleural effusions) were sampled to document tumor penetration by antibody.

RESULTS AND DISCUSSION

Individuality of B Cell Tumors

Hybridomas producing antibodies that reacted only with the Ig from the patient's tumor but not with normal Ig or that from several unrelated patients were chosen. Subsequent testing was performed on tissue sections and cell suspensions of normal tonsil. Examples were found of antibodies that seemed specific when tested on isolated proteins that did react with cells in the normal tonsil. Other examples were found that were specific on isolated proteins but failed to react with the same target on cell membranes. Both of these types of antibodies were discarded.

Seventeen different anti-idiotype antibodies were used to search for idiotypic cross-reaction among lymphoma patients. Each of these 17 antibodies reacted only with its respective tumor and not with any of the other 16. To expand the power of the analysis, the 17 antibodies were pooled and used to screen a prospective series of 300 additional lymphoma cases. It had previously been determined that the 17-fold dilution resulting from pooling did not diminish the reactivity of any of the antibodies with their respective tumor targets. Moreover, this pool of 17 antibodies gave no reaction with normal tonsil cell populations. When this pool of 17 was tested on 300 additional lymphoma patients using flow cytometry on cell suspension and using immunoperoxidase on frozen tissue sections, no positive reactions were detected. Therefore, we conclude that the frequency of idiotypic identity between B cell tumors from different patients must be extremely low. It is still possible, however, that antibodies could be selected by a less rigid screen that would allow for cross-reaction between different tumors.

TABLE 16.1. *Anti-Idiotype Therapy*

Patient	Tumor Immuno-Phenotype	Pre-therapy Serum Id (µg/ml)	Mouse Isotype	Highest Single Dose (mg)	Peak Mouse Serum Level (µg/ml)	Total Dose (mg)	Duration of Therapy (days)	Anti-mouse*	Binding to Tumor	Response	Toxicity
PK	μ, λ	5	IgG2b	120	18	400	27	None	LN + PBL + BM +	CR	None
FS	μ, κ	400	IgG1	560	50	1,530	17	(20)		PR	Fever, chills, dyspnea, rash
BL	μ, κ	243	IgG1	900	50	2,101	18	None	PBL + LN −	NR	Fever, chills, dyspnea, thrombocytopenia
RD	μ, λ	0.10	IgG1	600	330	1,993	57	None	ND	PR	None
BJ	μ, κ	0.02	IgG2b	800	107	2,492	29	(17)	LN +	MR	Fever, chills, thrombocytopenia
CJ	μ, κ	2.20	IgG1	700	136	3,079	40	(24)	PBL +	PR	Fever, rigor, thrombocytopenia
CP	μ, λ	0.01	IgG1	730	269	3,080	21	(13)	LN +	NR	Fever, rigor, rash, neutropenia
CG	μ, κ	0.01	IgG1	600	242	3,173	38	None	LN + PBL + BM +	PR-MR	Mild chills
TG	μ, λ	3.26	IgG2a	800	270	1,775	21	(10)		NR	Fever, chills, hypotension azotemia, facial palsy
KL	μ, λ	0.01	IgG1 IgG2a IgG2b	600†	230	600	7	None	ND	NE	None
PE	μ, κ	14.5	IgG2a	783	240	3,183	42	None	ND	CR-PR	None

*Value in parentheses is day of therapy on which anti-mouse reaction was first detected.

†200 mg of each isotype.

Id = idiotype; LN = lymph node; PBL = peripheral blood lymphocytes; BM = bone marrow; CR = complete remission; PR = partial remission; MR = minimal response; NR = no response; NE = not evaluable; ND = not done.

Idiotype Protein in the Sera of Lymphoma Patients

The sera of eight patients with "nonsecreting" B cell lymphomas were tested for the presence of circulating idiotype protein. None of these patients had elevated levels of total serum IgG or IgM, as determined by radial immunodiffusion. No paraproteins could be detected by immunoelectrophoresis. A two-sided enzyme-linked immunoabsorbent assay was designed with a sensitivity limit of 10 ng/ml. A series of patients displayed a wide spectrum of serum idiotype levels (Table 16.1). These levels showed no correlation with the histologic type of lymphoma. However, within the assessment of a given patient, serial measurements have been found to mirror tumor burden, as judged by standard clinical evaluations. In selected patients, we isolated idiotypic Ig from the serum by immunoabsorption on anti-idiotype covalently linked to a solid phase. By this procedure, we could calculate that, for the patients with the highest serum idiotype levels (BL, FS, and PE), as much as 60% of their total circulating IgM was derived from the malignant clone.

Clinical Trial

Eleven patients were selected for a therapeutic trial of monoclonal anti-idiotype antibody (Table 16.1). All had disease that was objectively evaluable. Eight had follicular lymphoma, one had diffuse large cell lymphoma, one had diffuse poorly differentiated small and large cell lymphoma, and one had prolymphocytic leukemia. Ten of these patients had previously been treated with, and had failed, multiple courses of chemotherapy and radiotherapy. One patient received prior therapy with interferon only. No steroids or cytotoxic agents were administered to any patient from one month before therapy and until the trial and follow-up were complete.

Plasmapheresis was used to reduce serum idiotype levels in patients PK, FS, and BL. In the latter two patients, who had serum idiotype levels in excess of 200 μg/ml, three whole-volume plasma exchanges on successive days resulted in a reduction of serum idiotype to 10–20% of the initial levels. No further reduction was obtained by continued plasmapheresis, and after cessation of the procedure, the serum idiotype returned to the baseline level over several days. These two patients were maintained on plasmapheresis during the entire trial of antibody administration. The dose of anti-idiotype antibody required to achieve an excess in the serum varied with each patient according to the level of idiotype protein, the tumor burden, and the sites of tumor involvement. During the course of therapy, 5 of the 10 evaluable patients developed antibody responses against the mouse Ig. This occurred from 10–30 days after the initiation of therapy. This response was most dramatic in patient CP, the only patient who had not received prior immunosuppressive therapies. After anti-mouse antibody was present, significant levels of mouse antibody could not be achieved and clinical responses were not seen. In the absence of an immune response or serum idiotype, there was very little toxicity observed, but in the presence of either one, fever, chills, and dyspnea were regularly seen. These symptoms usually subsided when infusion was slowed and temporarily stopped.

The most dramatic antitumor effect occurred in the first patient, whose case was previously reported (Miller et al. 1982). He has remained in complete, unmaintained remission for 3 1/2 years, with no evidence of return of serum idiotype or idiotype-positive cells in bone marrow and blood. Five of the nine evaluable patients have had clinically significant but partial or temporary responses. All responses began between 8 and 16 days after the initiation of therapy. Two patients received a second course of therapy resulting in stabilization of growing disease but no regression. The causes for the different results in these patients can only be speculated upon at the present time, but they could include differences in antibody class, antibody affinity, idiotype targets, serum idiotype levels, host responses, and tumor heterogeneity.

Genetic Heterogeneity in Malignant B Cell Populations

During the course of these studies, we unexpectedly identified several patients whose lymphomas contained two cell populations, each with a different idiotype (Sklar et al. 1984). The heterogeneity of these tumor populations became apparent in different ways. One patient with diffuse well-differentiated lymphocytic lymphoma was immediately suspected of having more than one cell population because he had both κ- and λ-positive cells. In three other patients with nodular poorly differentiated lymphocytic lymphoma, tissue immunoperoxidase and cell fluorescent analysis disclosed that the anti-idiotype antibody made for each of them reacted with a subpopulation of the tumor cells, even though in each of these cases the entire tumor population expressed IgM κ.

The genetic basis of the heterogeneity in these cases was proved by cell separation studies and DNA analysis. The anti-idiotype antibodies were used with the fluorescence-activated cell sorter to divide the cells into reactive and unreactive populations. DNA was isolated from each population, cut with restriction endonuclease, and analyzed by the Southern blot procedure with probes for the heavy- and light-chain genes. In each of these cases, we were able to show that the two cell populations had rearranged different Ig genes. The two clones in one case of nodular lymphoma appeared to have a common origin since they had the same heavy-chain gene rearrangement but different light-chain gene rearrangements. None of the patients who had two genetically distinct clones received therapy with antibodies.

A different type of genetic heterogeneity was uncovered during therapy with anti-idiotype antibody (Meeker et al. 1985). In four of the patients who achieved partial remission, subsequent biopsies showed tumor cell populations that no longer reacted with the antibodies even though they continued to express the same type of heavy- and light-chain products in the same density on the cell surface. In each of these cases, DNA analysis showed that the new cell populations were derived from the original clone, since they had rearranged the same heavy- and light-chain genes. Presumably, subtle mutations in the V regions had occurred and were selected for growth under the influence of the antibody treatment. This hypothesis has now been confirmed in one case by determining the nucleotide sequence of the heavy-chain V-region genes.

Clearly, both types of genetic variation seen here—biclonality and clonal evolution—can complicate attempts to use anti-idiotype antibodies for therapy. Neither complication is insurmountable, however. For instance, we have been able to produce antibodies that react with the idiotype of second clones. More interesting is the implication of these findings for the biology of these tumors. Do these separate clones have their origin in a common stem cell or do they represent a multihit induction of malignancy? Are they separate clones or are they evolved descendants controlled or selected by the host immune mechanisms, such as idiotype networks? These will be the subjects of future investigation.

REFERENCES

Cleary ML, Chao J, Warnke R, Sklar J. 1984. Immunoglobulin gene rearrangement as a diagnostic criterion of B cell lymphoma. Proc Natl Acad Sci USA 81:593–597.

Fialkow PJ, Klein E, Klein G, Clifford P, Singh S. 1973. Immunoglobulin and glucose-6-phosphate dehydrogenase as markers of cellular origin in Burkitt lymphoma. J Exp Med 139:89–102.

Friedman JM, Fialkow PJ. 1976. Cell marker studies of human tumorigenesis. Transplant Rev 28:17–33.

Handley HH, Royston I. 1982. A human lymphoblastoid B cell line useful for generating immunoglobulin-secreting human hybridomas. *In* Mitchell MS, Oethgen HF, eds., Hybridomas in Cancer Diagnosis and Treatment. Raven Press, New York, pp. 125–132.

Klein G. 1983. Specific chromosomal translocations and the genesis of B cell–derived tumors in mice and man. Cell 32:311–315.

Levy R, Dilley J. 1978. Rescue of immunoglobulin secretion from human neoplastic lymphoid cells by somatic cell hybridization. Proc Natl Acad Sci USA 75:2411–2415.

Loken MR, Herzenberg LA. 1975. Analysis of cell populations with a fluorescence-activated cell sorter. Ann NY Acad Sci 254:163–171.

Meeker T, Lowder J, Cleary ML, Warnke R, Sklar J, Levy R. 1985. Emergence of idiotype variants during therapy of B cell lymphoma with anti-idiotype antibodies. N Engl J Med 312:1658–1665.

Miller RA, Maloney DG, Warnke R, Levy R. 1982. Treatment of B cell lym-

268

RONALD LEVY ET AL.

phoma with monoclonal anti-idiotype antibody. N Engl J Med 306:517–522.

Rowley JD. 1978. Chromosome studies in malignant lymphoma. *In* Levy R, Kaplan HS, eds., Malignant Lymphomas. UICC Technical Report Series, vol 37. International Union Against Cancer, Geneva, pp. 71–95.

Sklar J, Cleary ML, Thielemans K, Gralow J, Warnke R, Levy R. 1984. Biclonal B cell lymphoma. N Engl J Med 311:20–27.

Southern EM. 1975. Detection of specific sequences among DNA fragments separated by gel electrophoresis. J Mol Biol 98:503–517.

Thielemans K, Maloney DG, Meeker T, et al. 1984. Strategies for production of monoclonal anti-idiotype antibodies against human B cell lymphomas. J Immunol 133:495–501.

Warnke R, Levy R. 1980. Detection of T and B cell antigens with hybridoma monoclonal antibodies: A biotin-avidin-horseradish peroxidase method. J Histochem Cytochem 28:771–776.

Symposium on Fundamental Cancer Research, Vol. 38.
© 1986 by The University of Texas System Cancer Center.

17. Immunorestoration

Robert A. Good and Neena Kapoor*

Oklahoma Medical Research Foundation, Oklahoma City, Oklahoma 73104

Methods of restoring immune function began with treatment of patients with agammaglobulinemia and used injections of gammaglobulin that, because of persistent problems of aggregation, had to be given intramuscularly to avoid anaphylactoid reactions (Dwyer 1984). This approach has not been entirely satisfactory for many reasons, but substitution gammaglobulin therapy has improved in recent years with the availability of preparations of gamma-globulin that can be administered intravenously (Barandun et al. 1962, Pirofsky 1984). These preparations are well tolerated and improve the management of patients with antibody deficiency syndromes (Pirofsky 1984, Barandun et al. 1968, Cunningham-Rundles et al. 1983), although untoward reactions may occasionally be observed (Day et al. 1984).

Cellular engineering to correct primary immunodeficiencies began when the analysis of lymphoid development revealed that stem cells in human fetal liver or bone marrow could develop into two separate lymphoid populations (Good 1957) under influences of the thymus (T cells). The lymphoid populations develop into B cells in birds under the influence of the bursa of Fabricius (Cooper et al. 1965, 1966). In mammals, the B cell development takes place in the fetal liver or bone marrow. Patients born with T and B lymphocyte developmental defects had their severe combined immunodeficiency syndromes (SCID) completely corrected by bone marrow transplantation, using a matched sibling donor to assure the best possible histocompatibility match (Gatti et al. 1968, Good 1969). Such transplants have now been used in approximately 100 SCID patients to correct what seems to be at least six different forms of the syndrome (Good 1981).

This same approach has also been applied to the reconstruction of hematopoietic tissues, lymphoid tissues, and lymphoid functions to successfully treat patients whose lymphoid and hematopoietic tissues have been destroyed

*Current address for Drs. Good and Kapoor: Department of Pediatrics, University of South Florida All Children's Hospital, St. Petersburg, Florida 33701

by total body irradiation or profound chemical myeloablation for various malignancies or to correct congenital metabolic and hematopoietic disorders. More than 40 otherwise lethal diseases are already being cured by this method (Good 1982, Good et al. 1983, Thomas 1981, Krivit et al. 1984, Pahwa et al. 1978).

Thymus transplantations and fetal liver plus thymus transplantations have also been used to correct immunodeficiency diseases when a matched sibling donor is not available (Pahwa et al. 1977, O'Reilly et al. 1980). These alternative approaches to bone marrow transplantation have achieved impressive results in correcting immune functions. Unfortunately, they are not always readily available and have not been as reliable as the matched sibling donor bone marrow transplants. Bone marrow transplants have also been taken from major histocompatibility complex (MHC)–matched donors who are close relatives (Dupont et al. 1979) and, in a few instances, from MHC-matched donors from large donor panels from the general population (Hobbs 1981).

More recently, marrow transplantation across major histocompatibility barriers in experimental animals has been accomplished without graft-versus-host reaction (GVHR) by using bone marrow that has been purged of T lymphocytes, postthymic T precursors, and also thymus-influenced pre–T cells. Acute GVHR is avoided and long-surviving chimeras are produced (Muller-Rucholtz et al. 1976, Sprent et al. 1975, Onoe et al. 1980, Krown et al. 1981). Mice prepared in this way often have significant immunologic deficiencies attributable to failure of the essential interactions between T lymphocyte accessory cells and B lymphocytes of donor origin. Late wasting or runting disease (Rayfield and Brent 1983, Longley et al. 1984) has been avoided when donors have been treated or if marrow from donors carrying the nu/nu athymic genetic composition was used (Himeno and Good 1985, Ikehara et al. 1985a)

In man, if haploidentical donors are employed, the late wasting and runting disease and also immunodeficiencies are often avoided by using techniques that purge the bone marrow of unwanted immunocompetent or committed precursors of thymocytes. With these findings as background data, several methods have been developed to correct SCID and other primary immunodeficiencies when matched sibling donors are not available. The first of these was the lectin-purging technique developed by Reisner and Kapoor in our laboratory (Reisner et al. 1981,1983). This method that was developed for use in humans was an adaptation of a technique developed first for mice by Reisner et al. (1978) at the Weizmann Institute in Rehovot, Israel, then for monkeys in our laboratory (Reisner et al. 1983), and finally used for humans. The method involves a lectin separation technique first with soybean agglutinin and then with two cycles of E-rosetting, which effectively purges bone marrow of cells that initiate GVHR (Reisner et al. 1981,1983). Using this purged haploidentical marrow, transplantation has permitted full correction of SCID when an

MHC-matched sibling donor is not available. Experience to date comprises some 60 bone marrow transplantations to treat children with SCID without matched sibling donors. In approximately one-half of these SCID recipients given haploidentical purged bone marrow transplants, the immunorestoration has been quite complete. Another one-fourth of such patients achieved T cell corrections, but failed to obtain full B cell function. These patients can be maintained in good health by treatment with intravenous immunoglobulin. Graft-versus-host disease has not been a problem, but failure of bone marrow to engraft or loss of the correcting transplant has been an annoying difficulty in some cases. Thus far, monoclonal antibody purging of bone marrow, which has been so effective in eliminating acute GVHR (Onoe et al. 1982) in mice is just being perfected for preparation for human haploidentical bone marrow transplantations for effective immunorestoration (Parkman R personal communication 1985). Furthermore, in humans, a single cycle of E-rosetting coupled with cyclosporin treatment of the recipient has also been used with some success to permit haploidentical bone marrow transplantation. Purging of T cells from the marrow using antibody coupled to the toxic molecule ricin is being tested (Filipovich et al. 1980).

We have a glimpse of the potential for successful treatment through cellular engineering, which can be seen from testing already under way in experimental animals. This testing shows the possibility of preventing and effectively treating many different autoimmune diseases (Himeno and Good 1985) introducing genes for resistance to viruses with oncogenic potential (Wustrow et al. 1985) preventing juvenile diabetes (Ikehara et al. 1985b) and treating and preventing inborn errors of metabolism (Ikehara S unpublished data). Approximately 5,000 bone marrow transplantations from allogeneic donors have been carried out since 1968, when we first introduced the MHC-matched sibling donor methodology for human marrow transplantation. We anticipated that during 1985 and 1986, as many as 5,000 bone marrow transplantations will be done. This must be considered only a beginning in the development of immunologic and hematopoietic restoration using principles of cellular engineering.

ACKNOWLEDGMENT

This research was aided by March of Dimes grant 1-789 and National Institutes of Health grants AI-22360 and AG-05628.

REFERENCES

Barandun S, Kistler P, Jeunet F, Isliker H. 1962. Intravenous administration of human γ-globulin. Vox Sang 7:157.
Barandun S, Riva G, Spengler GA. 1968. Immunologic deficiency: Diagnosis,

forms and current treatment. *In* Bergsma D, ed., Immunological Deficiency Disease in Man. March of Dimes, White Plains, New York, pp 40–52.

Cooper MD, Peterson RDA, Good RA. 1965. Delineation of the thymic and bursal lymphoid systems in the chicken. Nature 205:143–146.

Cooper MD, Peterson RDA, South MA, Good RA. 1966. The function of the thymus system and the bursa system in the chicken. J Exp Med 123:75–102.

Cunningham-Rundles C, Smithwick E, Siegal FP, et al. 1983. Use of intravenous pH 4.0 treated gammaglobulin in humoral immunodeficiency diseases. *In* Wedgewood RJ, Rosen FJ, Paul NW, eds., Primary Immunodeficiency Diseases. Alan R. Liss, Inc., New York, pp. 201–203.

Day NK, Good RA, Wahn V. 1984. Adverse reactions in selected patients following intravenous infusions of gammaglobulin. Am J Med 76:25–32.

Dupont B, O'Reilly RJ, Pollack MS, Good RA. 1979. Use of HLA genotypically different donor in bone marrow transplantation. Transplant Proc 11:219–224.

Dwyer JM. 1984. Thirty years of supplying the missing link: History of gamma globulin therapy for immunodeficient states. Am J Med 76(Suppl):46–52.

Filipovich AM, Ramsay NKC, McGlave P, et al. 1980. Mismatched bone marrow transplantation at the University of Minnesota: Use of related donors other than HLA, MLC identical siblings and T cell depletion. *In* Gale RP, ed., Recent Advances in Bone Marrow Transplantation. Alan R. Liss, Inc. New York, pp. 757–768.

Gatti RA, Meuwissen HJ, Allen HD, Hong R, Good RA. 1968. Immunological reconstitution of sex-linked lymphopenic immunological deficiency. Lancet 2:1366–1369.

Good RA. 1957. Morphological basis of the immune response and hypersensitivity. *In* Felton HM, ed., Host Parasite Relationship in Living Cells. Charles C Thomas, Springfield, Illinois, pp. 68–161.

Good RA. 1969. Immunologic reconstitution: The achievement and its meaning. Hosp Pract 4:41–47.

Good RA. 1981. Anticipating the exciting future of immunology. *In* Bralow SP, ed., Basic Research and Clinical Medicine. Hemisphere Publishing Corporation, New York, pp. 125–209.

Good RA. 1982. Towards safer marrow transplantation. N Engl J Med 306:421–423.

Good RA, Kapoor N, Reisner Y. 1983. Bone marrow transplantation: An expanding approach to treatment of many diseases. Cell Immunol 82:36–54.

Himeno K, Good RA. 1985. Marrow transplantation across major histocompatibility barriers to prevent autoimmune diseases in inbred mice (Abstract). Fed Proc 44:3201.

Hobbs JR, Barrett AJ, Chambers D, et al. 1981. Reversal of clinical features of Herler's disease and biochemical improvement after treatment by bone-marrow transplantation. Lancet 2:709–712.

Ikehara S, Good RA, Takao N, et al. 1985a. Rationale for bone marrow transplantation in treatment of autoimmune diseases. Proc Natl Acad Sci USA 82:2483–2487.

Ikehara S, Ohtsuki M, Good RA, et al. 1985b. Prevention of type I diabetes in NOD mice by allogenic bone marrow transplantation. Proc Natl Acad Sci USA 82:7743–7747.

Krivit W, Pierpont ME, Ayaz K, et al. 1984. Bone marrow transplantation in the Maroteaux-Lamy syndrome (Mucopolysaccharidosis type VI): Biochemical and clinical status 24 months after transplantation. N Engl J Med 311:1606–1611.

Krown SE, Coico R, Scheid MP, Fernandes G, Good RA. 1981. Immune function in fully allogeneic mouse bone marrow chimeras. Clin Immunol Immunopathol 19:268–283.

Longley RE, Dorn AK, Good RA. 1984. Immunodeficiency in leukemia free B6-AKR chimeras (Abstract). Fed Proc 43:1982.

Muller-Rucholtz W, Wattge HU, Muller-Hermelink HK. 1976. Bone marrow transplantation in rats across strong histocompatibility barriers by selective elimination of lymphoid cells in donor marrow. *In* Dupont B, Good RA, eds. Immunobiology of Bone Marrow Transplantation. Grune & Stratton, New York, pp. 189–193.

O'Reilly RJ, Pahwa R, Sorell M, et al. 1980. Transplantation of fetal liver and thymus in patients with severe combined immunodeficiencies. *In* Doria G, ed., The Immune System: Functions and Therapy of Dysfunction. Proceedings of the Serono Symposia, vol. 27. Academic Press, New York, pp. 241–253.

Onoe K, Fernandes G, Good RA. 1980. Humoral and cell-mediated immune responses in fully allogeneic bone marrow chimera in mice. J Exp Med 151:115–132.

Onoe K, Yasumizu R, Oh-Ishi T, et al. 1982. Specific elimination of the T lineage cells: Effects of in vitro treatment with anti-Thy 1 serum without complement on the adoptive cell transfer system. J Immunol Methods 49:315–322.

Pahwa R, Pahwa S, Good RA, Incefy GS, O'Reilly RJ. 1977. Rationale for combined use of fetal liver and thymus for immunologic reconstitution in patients with variants of severe combined immunodeficiency. Proc Natl Acad Sci USA 74:3002–3005.

Pahwa R, Pahwa S, O'Reilly R, Good RA. 1978. Treatment of the immunodeficiency diseases: Progress toward replacement therapy emphasizing cellular and macromolecular engineering. Springer Semin Immunopathol 1:355–405.

Pirofsky B. 1984. Intravenous immune globulin therapy in hypogammaglobulinemia: A review. Am J Med 76:53–60.

Rayfield LS, Brent L. 1983. Secondary mortality in fully allogeneic radiation chimeras is not caused by a delayed graft-versus-host reaction (GVHR). Transplant Proc 15:1454–1457.

Reisner Y, Itsicovitch L, Meshorer A, Sharon N. 1978. Hemopoietic stem cell transplantation using mouse bone marrow and spleen cells fractionated by lectins. Proc Natl Acad Sci USA 75:2933–2936.

Reisner Y, Kapoor N, Kirkpatrick D, et al. 1981. Transplantation for acute leukemia with HLA-A and B nonidentical parental marrow cells fractionated with soybean agglutinin and sheep red blood cells. Lancet 2:327–331.

Reisner Y, Kapoor N, Pollack S, et al. 1983. Use of lectins in bone marrow transplantation. *In* Advances in Bone Marrow Transplantation, Alan R. Liss, Inc., New York, pp. 355–387.

Sprent J, von Boehmer H, Nabholz N. 1975. Association of immunity and tolerance to host H-2 determinants in irradiated F^1 hybrid mice reconstituted with bone marrow cells from one parental strain. J Exp Med 142:321–331.

Thomas ED. 1981. Bone marrow transplantation. *In* Burchenal JH, Oettgen HF, eds., Cancer: Achievements, Challenges and Prospects for the 1980's. Grune & Stratton, New York, pp. 625–638.

Wustrow TPU, Katepodis N, Chester-Stock CC, Good RA. 1985. Prevention of leukemia and the increase of plasma levels of lipid bound sialic acid by allogeneic bone marrow transplantation in mice. Cancer Res 45:1097–1100.

THE WILSON S. STONE
AWARD LECTURE

Symposium on Fundamental Cancer Research, Vol. 38.

18. Development of Monoclonal Antibodies Reactive with the Product of the *neu* Oncogene

Jeffrey A. Drebin,* Victoria C. Link,*† David F. Stern,‡
Robert A. Weinberg,‡ and Mark I. Greene *†

*Department of Pathology, Harvard Medical School, and †Department of
Medicine, Tufts–New England Medical Center, Boston, Massachusetts
02111, and ‡Whitehead Institute for Biomedical Research, Massachusetts
Institute of Technology, Cambridge, Massachusetts 02142.*

Although the ability of some tumors to provoke an immune response in the syngeneic host has been documented for more than 30 years (Foley 1953, Prehn and Main 1957), the molecular basis of tumor antigenicity is poorly understood. While tumor antigens are potentially useful immunotherapeutic targets, there is no obvious reason why neoplastic cells should in fact display novel antigenic determinants. The presence of such structures on the neoplastic cell surface suggests that their expression may be linked in some way with the genetic changes that occur during carcinogenesis.

Recent studies in a number of laboratories have identified in spontaneous and chemically induced tumors and tumor cell lines activated cellular oncogenes capable of neoplastically transforming nonmalignant rodent cell lines following DNA transfection (Cooper 1982, Land et al. 1983). These activated oncogenes have been found exclusively in neoplastic tissues and are not found in normal tissues of the same individuals in which the tumors arose (Santos et al. 1984, Feig et al. 1984). Furthermore, molecular cloning and sequencing of several members of the *ras* oncogene family have demonstrated that the activation of the malignant potential of these oncogenes is caused by point mutations occurring at one of several critical sites; these changes result in the expression of a structurally altered oncogene product (Tabin et al. 1982, Der and Cooper 1983, Taparowsky et al. 1983, Yuasa et al. 1983). This finding has led to the suggestion that mutagenic activation of cellular oncogenes represents an important event in carcinogenesis. For the past several years we have been investigating the linkage between activation of cellular oncogenes and the expression of tumor antigens on the malignant cell surface. Recently, one such oncogene, which we call the *neu* oncogene (because it has been identified in the genomes of several rat neuroblastomas), has been studied in detail (Shih et al. 1981, Padhy et al. 1982, Schechter et al. 1984, Drebin et al. 1984a,b). Here we describe the development of a panel of monoclonal antibodies that react with cell surface domains of a protein encoded by the *neu* oncogene.

MATERIALS AND METHODS

Cell Culture Techniques

Cell lines were cultured in 100-mm tissue culture dishes (Costar, Cambridge, MA) and in 10 ml of Dulbecco's modified Eagle's medium (DMEM) (K. C. Biologicals, Lenexa, KS) supplemented with 10% fetal bovine serum, 1% penicillin-streptomycin-amphotericin B mixture (M.A. Bioproducts, Walkersville, MD), and 100 μg/ml of gentamycin sulfate (M.A. Bioproducts). Transformed cell lines were passaged twice weekly at a 1:20 dilution following release from the tissue culture dish surface with Trypsin-Versene (M.A. Bioproducts). Nontransformed cell lines were passaged in a similar fashion but at higher dilutions (1:30–1:50) to prevent the development of spontaneous transformants. Cell lines were maintained in a humidified air and 5% CO_2 incubator at 37°C and replaced from frozen stocks every two to three months.

Experimental Animals

C3H/HeJ mice and (C3H/HeJ × DBA/2J)Fl mice (C3D2 Fl mice) were obtained from Jackson Laboratories (Bar Harbor, ME). Inbred congenitally athymic BALB/c (nu/nu) mice were obtained from the National Cancer Institute animal colony at Frederick, MD. Immunocompetent mice were housed in the Cancer Research Animal Facility of the Department of Pathology, Harvard Medical School. Athymic mice were maintained in an animal isolator on sterile bedding and received autoclaved food and water. Animals used in this study were maintained in accordance with the guidelines of the Committee on Animals of the Harvard Medical School and those prepared by the Committee on Care and Use of Laboratory Animals of the Institute of Laboratory Animal Resources, National Research Council (DHEW publication number (NIH) 78–23, revised 1978).

Production of Hybridomas Secreting Monoclonal Antibodies

C3H/HeJ female mice were multiply immunized with intraperitoneal injections of *neu*-transformed NIH 3T3 cells emulsified in Freund's adjuvant. Mice whose sera reacted with p185 (by immunoprecipitation) and with cell surface determinants on *neu*-transformed cells (by immunofluorescence) were used to generate hybridomas. Mice were killed by cervical dislocation and their spleens were removed aseptically. Spleens were minced with forceps to produce a single cell suspension, filtered through nylon mesh to remove clumps, and treated with Tris–ammonium chloride to lyse erythrocytes. The immune splenocytes were centrifuged with aminopterin-sensitive NS-1 myeloma cells at a 7:1 ratio and were washed once in serum-free DMEM. After centrifugation at 1000 g, the medium was removed and the pellet of splenocytes and myeloma cells was gently resuspended by agitation. Room temperature phosphate-buffered saline (PBS) (0.3 ml) containing 40% polyethylene glycol 1600 (American Type Culture Collection, Rockville, MD) was added over one minute, and the cell suspension was warmed in a 37°C water bath for an additional minute. Fifteen milliliters of serum-free DMEM was added over a five-minute period, and the cells were centrifuged at 800 g.

The pellet was gently resuspended and mixed with 500 ml of hybrid selection medium (DMEM supplemented with 20% Zeta serum) (AMF Biologicals), 1 mM sodium pyruvate (GIBCO, Chagrin Falls, OH), 0.1 mM essential amino acids (GIBCO), 0.1 mM nonessential amino acids (GIBCO), 2 mM L-glutamine (GIBCO), 1% penicillin-streptomycin-amphotericin B mixture (M.A. Bioproducts), 100 μg/ml of gentamycin sulfate (M.A. Bioproducts), 10^{-4} M hypoxanthine (Sigma Chemical Co., St. Louis, MO), 4×10^{-7} M aminopterin (Sigma), and 1.6×10^{-5} M thymidine (Sigma). The fused cells in hybrid selection medium were distributed into 24-well plates (1 ml, containing roughly 2×10^5 splenocytes, per well), and plates were maintained in a humidified air and 10% CO_2 incubator at 37°C. The cultures were fed with 1 ml/well of hybrid selection medium 7 days after fusion and were examined for the presence of hybridomas on day 14.

Supernatants from wells containing growing hybridomas were screened for binding to cell line B104-1-1 by indirect immunofluorescence using the fluorescence-activated cell sorter (FACS) analysis as described below. Positive supernatants were subsequently tested for specificity by determining whether they bound to normal NIH 3T3 cells or to NIH 3T3 cells transformed by an H-*ras* oncogene. Hybridomas that appeared specific by these criteria were recloned three times at limiting dilution to ensure the presence of only a single clonal cell line.

Isotype Analysis of Monoclonal Antibodies

The heavy chain isotypes of the monoclonal antibodies characterized here were determined by double immunodiffusion in agar according to the method of Ouchterlony (Hudson and Hay 1980). Culture supernatants from hybridoma cell lines were concentrated 10-fold under nitrogen pressure by using an Amicon concentrator (Danvers, MA) and applied to wells cut in 5% agar gels cast on microscope slides. Isotype-specific anti-mouse immunoglobulin (Ig) antisera (Litton Bionetics, Kensington, MD) were placed in adjacent wells, and the slides were incubated in a humidified chamber at room temperature. Positive reactivity between a particular hybridoma supernatant and an isotype-specific antiserum was determined by the formation of a precipitin line within 24 hours.

FACS Analysis

Cells were removed from tissue culture dishes with buffered EDTA (Versene, M.A. Bioproducts) and washed twice in FACS medium (Hanks' balanced salt solution (GIBCO) supplemented with 2% fetal bovine serum, 0.1% sodium azide, and 10 mM Hepes). Cells (1×10^5 to 1×10^6) in 0.1 ml of FACS medium were incubated with antibody or control supernatant in a volume of 0.1 ml for one hour at 4°C. Cells were diluted in 2.5 ml of FACS medium centrifuged at 1000 g and washed twice more with 2.5 ml of FACS medium per wash. Following the final wash, the cell pellet was gently resuspended and cells were incubated with 0.1 ml of fluoroscein isothiocyanate (FITC)–conjugated rabbit anti-mouse IgG reactive with antibody heavy and light chains (Miles Laboratories, Elkhart, IN) diluted 1:20–1:50 in FACS medium for one hour at 4°C. Cells were diluted and washed as after the first incubation. The cell pellet was finally resuspended and the cells were fixed in 0.5–1.0 ml of 2% paraformaldehyde-PBS (188 mM NaCl, 20 mM PO_4, pH 7.2). In some experiments, samples were run on a Coulter Epics V cell sorter (85 channels/log unit fluorescence), while in others, samples were run on an Ortho 2150 Cytofluorograf (512 channels/log unit fluorescence) (Ortho Diagnostics, Raritan, NJ). Comparable results were obtained using the two machines, with the Ortho being slightly more sensitive. We routinely analyzed 10,000 cells/sample. Specific fluorescence was quantitated by converting to a linear scale and then subtracting the median fluorescence channel of cells stained with FITC-conjugated rabbit anti-mouse Ig alone (negative control) from the median fluorescence channel of cells stained with specific antibody followed by FITC-conjugated rabbit anti-mouse Ig (positive staining).

Purification of Monoclonal Antibodies

Hybridoma cells were washed free of serum and injected into irradiated (400 rad) C3D2 F1 mice to induce ascites. IgG2a monoclonal antibodies were purified from hybridoma ascitic fluid by sequential ammonium sulfate precipitation and protein A Sepharose chromatography. Ascitic fluid was gradually made 50% ammonium sulfate by the addition, at 4°C with stirring, of an equal volume of saturated ammonium sulfate. The solution was stirred for an additional 60 minutes to allow Ig to completely precipitate. The precipitate was collected by centrifugation at 15,000 g for 15 minutes and resuspended in PBS. The resulting Ig solution was dialyzed for 24 hours against PBS with at least three changes. It was clarified by centrifugation and passed over a protein A Sepharose column (Pharmacia, Uppsala, Sweden). The column was washed with normal saline until the optical density measured at 280 nm of the filtrate was less than 0.1. The bound Ig was then eluted with 3.5 M $MgCl_2$, dialyzed extensively against normal saline and then PBS, and filtered through a 0.45-μm filter. The antibody solution was concentrated using an Amicon concentrator under nitrogen pressure; the protein concentration was determined using the method of Bradford (1976) with bovine serum albumin as a standard, and the purified Ig was stored at -70°C.

IgG1 monoclonal antibodies were purified on DEAE-cellulose–Affi-Gel blue, according to the method of Bruck et al. (1982). Ig was ammonium sulfate–precipitated from ascitic fluid and dialyzed overnight in 10 mM NaCl, 20 mM Tris, pH 8.0. The solution was applied to a DEAE-cellulose–Affi-Gel blue column preequilibrated with 10 mM NaCl, and the column was washed with two column volumes of 10 mM NaCl, 20 mM Tris, pH 8.0. The column was then washed with two column volumes of 25 mM NaCl, 20 mM Tris, pH 8.0. Ig was eluted from the column with 50 mM NaCl, 20 mM Tris, pH 8.0. The eluted Ig was then dialyzed, filtered, concentrated, quantitated, and stored as described above for IgG2a antibodies.

Determination of Anchorage-independent Growth

Anchorage-independent growth capability was determined by assessing the colony-forming efficiency of cells suspended in soft agar. All colony-forming efficiency experiments were conducted using 60-mm tissue culture dishes. Agar underlayers consisted of 5 ml of 0.24% agarose RPMI-1640 supplemented with 10% fetal bovine serum, penicillin-streptomycin-amphotericin B mixture, and gentamycin. Overlayers contained 1×10^3 cells in 1 ml of 0.18% agarose RPMI-1640 supplemented with 10% fetal bovine serum, penicillin-streptomycin-amphotericin B mixture, and gentamycin. When antibody was added to soft agar cultures, it was incorporated into the top layer only. Cultures were fed at weekly intervals with 1 ml of DMEM containing 10% fetal bovine serum with antibiotics and the same amount of antibody that was added on day 0. On the day before colony counts were determined, the cultures were fed 1 ml of Hanks' balanced salt solution containing 1 mg/ml P-iodonitrotetrazolium violet (Sigma) to stain colonies. The next day, colonies < 0.5 mm were counted using a dissecting microscope and a calibrated template. Colonies were counted at 14 days. Each experimental group represented the mean of triplicate or quadruplicate samples.

Tumor Growth Assays

Tumor cells were released from tissue culture dishes with Trypsin-Versene and were washed three times in serum-free Hanks' balanced salt solution.

Cells were injected subcutaneously into the middorsum of BALB/c nude mice. Some animals received intraperitoneal injections of ascitic fluid containing anti-p185 antibody, while others received an isotype-matched control ascitic fluid, or Hanks' balanced salt solution. Growing tumors were measured using vernier calipers, and tumor area was calculated as the product of tumor length and width. Significance was determined by Student's t-test.

RESULTS

Preliminary studies, utilizing polyclonal antitumor antisera, of NIH 3T3 cells transformed by the *neu* oncogene suggested that these cells expressed cell surface antigenic determinants that were not found on normal NIH 3T3 cells or NIH 3T3 cells transformed by other oncogenes (Drebin et al. 1984a). We therefore attempted to produce monoclonal antibodies specific for these determinants, as described in Materials and Methods. To date, we have screened approximately 10,000 hybridomas for the production of monoclonal antibodies that specifically bind cell surface determinants on *neu*-transformed cells. We have identified five hybridomas that produce such antibodies; their names and the isotypes of their secreted antibodies are shown in Table 18.1. Also, as indicated in Table 18.1, immunoprecipitation analysis using these monoclonal antibodies has revealed that four of these antibodies precipitate a 185-kDa protein (p185) from *neu*-transformed NIH 3T3 cells (Drebin et al. 1984b, Stern DF, Drebin JA unpublished data). The ability of the other antibody (7.5.5) to precipitate p185 (or any other molecules) from *neu*-transformed NIH 3T3 cells is currently under investigation. It has recently been demonstrated that p185 is very likely the product of the *neu* oncogene (Schechter et al. 1984). Thus, we have produced a number of hybridomas secreting monoclonal antibodies that recognize cell surface domains of the *neu* oncogene product.

TABLE 18.1. *Isotypes of Monoclonal Antibodies Specifically Reactive with* **neu** *Transformed NIH 3T3 Cells*

Antibody	Isotype	Cell Surface Binding		Immuno- precipitation of p185
		B104-1-1	NIH 3T3	
DF7.5.5	IgG2b	+	−	N.T.
DF7.9.5	IgG1	+	−	+
DF7.16.4	IgG2a	+	−	+
DF7.16.5	IgM	+	−	+
DF7.21.2	IgG1	+	−	+

N.T. = not tested.

TABLE 18.2. *Expression of p185 on Murine and Rat Tumor Cell Lines*

Cell Line	Description	Immuno-fluorescence
NIH 3T3	Contact-inhibited mouse fibroblast	−
B104	Rat neuroblastoma	+
B104-2	1° Transfectant of B104 DNA	+
B104-1-1	2° Transfectant of B104 DNA	+ + + +
B104-1-2	2° Transfectant of B104 DNA	+
B103	Rat neuroblastoma	+
B103-1	1° Transfectant of B103 DNA	+ + +
B103-5	1° Transfectant of B103 DNA	+ +
B103-1-1	2° Transfectant of B103 DNA	+ +
B103-1-2	2° Transfectant of B103 DNA	+
XHT-1-1a	2° Transfectant of v-Ha-*ras* proviral DNA	−
RSV 3T3	RSV-transformed NIH 3T3	−
MSV 3T3	Moloney sarcoma virus–transformed NIH 3T3	−
HaSV 3T3	Harvey sarcoma virus–transformed NIH 3T3	−
PyD2	Polyoma virus–transformed mouse fibroblast	−
SVD2	SV40-transformed mouse fibroblast	−
S1509a	3-Methylcholanthrene–transformed mouse fibroblast	−

Cell surface p185 was quantitated by immunofluorescence flow cytometry as described in Materials and Methods. 1° and 2° indicate transfectants generated by passing the oncogene through one or two cycles of transfection in NIH 3T3 cells.

In order to confirm the linkage between the *neu* oncogene and the presence of cell surface p185, we performed live cell immunofluorescence flow cytometry assays, utilizing one of our p185-specific monoclonals, on murine cells transformed by a variety of agents. As shown in Table 18.2, p185 was found on 100% of the NIH 3T3 cell lines established by transfection of *neu* oncogenes. In contrast, p185 was not found on NIH 3T3 cells transformed by *mos*, *ras*, or *src* oncogenes or on murine fibroblasts transformed by polyoma, SV-40, or methylcholanthrene. The expression of p185 on several independent rat neuroblastomas, in which *neu* oncogenes have been detected by DNA transfection, is also indicated in Table 18.2. Thus the expression of cell surface p185, as detected by monoclonal antibody 7.16.4, appears to occur exclusively in cells containing rat *neu* oncogenes.

The phenomenon of antigenic modulation, in which a cell surface protein is removed from the cell as a result of antibody binding to it, has been described in a number of experimental systems (Boyse et al. 1967, Schreiner and Unanue 1977, Ritz et al. 1980). In an effort to determine whether p185 could be down-modulated as a result of binding an anti-p185 monoclonal antibody, we

JEFFREY A. DREBIN ET AL.

TABLE 18.3. *Antigenic Modulation of p185 Induced by Monoclonal Antibody 7.16.4*

Time (hours)	Surface p185 Expression (%)
0	100
+1	48
+2	34
+3	29

B104-1-1 cells were incubated with antibody 7.16.4 for varying amounts of time, and then were restained with antibody 7.16.4 followed by fluoresceinated rabbit anti-mouse immunoglobulin; cell surface fluorescence was quantitated by immunofluorescence flow cytometry as described in Materials and Methods.

cultured *neu*-transformed NIH 3T3 cells (cell line B104-1-1) with purified antibody 7.16.4 at 37°C for varying lengths of time, removed the cells from culture dishes, restained them with saturating amounts of antibody 7.16.4, and analyzed cell surface antibody-binding by indirect immunofluorescence, as quantitated on the Ortho Cytofluorograf. As shown in Table 18.3, incubation of cell line B104-1-1 in the presence of antibody 7.16.4 caused the rapid down-modulation of cell surface p185. Subsequent studies (Drebin JA, Link VC, Stern DF, Weinberg RA, Greene MI unpublished data) have shown that antibody-mediated down-modulation of cell surface p185 also results in the degradation of the protein, resulting in lower steady-state p185 levels. Thus, monoclonal anti-p185 antibodies appear to cause loss from the *neu*-transformed cell of the oncogene-encoded protein that may be responsible for the cell's malignant state.

A variety of in vitro characteristics distinguish neoplastic cells from non-neoplastic cells (Pollack et al. 1984). The single property most closely linked with the ability of cells to grow as tumors in vivo is their ability to form anchorage-independent colonies when suspended in agarose or methylcellulose (Freedman and Shin 1974). Since it appeared that incubation of *neu*-transformed cells with anti-p185 antibody caused loss from the cell of the p185 protein, we were interested in determining whether the addition of anti-p185 antibody to *neu*-transformed cells would cause these cells to revert to a less transformed phenotype, as measured by their ability to form anchorage-independent colonies. As shown in Table 18.4, all three anti-p185 monoclonal antibodies tested are able to inhibit the formation of anchorage-independent colonies by the *neu*-transformed NIH 3T3 cell line B104-1-1 by more than 75%. In contrast, a control IgG2a monoclonal antibody has no effect on the anchorage-independent growth of these cells (data not shown). Furthermore,

TABLE 18.4. *Effect on Monoclonal Anti-p185 Antibodies on the Anchorage-Independent Growth of* neu-*Transformed Cells*

Expt. No.	Cell Line	Antibody (Amount in μg)	Anchorage Independent Colonies	Suppression (%)
1	B104-1-1	—	61	—
	B104-1-1	7.16.4 (10)	1	98
	B104-1-1	7.9.5 (10)	9	85
	B104-1-1	7.21.2 (10)	15	75
2	B104-1-1	—	75	—
	B104-1-1	7.16.4 (1)	4	95
	B104-1-2	—	28	—
	B104-1-2	7.16.4 (1)	6	79
	RSV3T3	—	74	—
	RSV3T3	7.16.4 (1)	75	0

Cell lines B104-1-1 and B104-1-2 were transformed by transfection of *neu* oncogenes into NIH 3T3 cells. Cell line RSV 3T3 is a line of NIH 3T3 cells transformed by Rous sarcoma virus.

antibody 7.16.4 is able to inhibit the anchorage-independent growth of the independent *neu*-transformed NIH 3T3 cell line B104-1-2 to approximately the same degree as it does B104-1-1 cells, but it has no effect on the anchorage-independent growth of the *src*-transformed cell line RSV 3T3. Antibody 7.16.4 does not inhibit the adherent growth of *neu*-transformed cells in agar-free medium otherwise identical to that used for assaying anchorage-independent growth (data not shown). Thus, it does not exert toxic effects on the *neu*-transformed cells. Rather, it causes them to behave less like transformed cells and more like normal cells with respect to their ability to grow in the absence of anchorage.

The ability of anti-p185 monoclonal antibodies to inhibit the anchorage-independent growth of *neu*-transformed NIH 3T3 cells suggested that these antibodies might also be able to inhibit their tumorigenic growth in vivo. The result of a pilot study in which antibody 7.16.4 was injected into nude mice bearing B104-1-1 cell tumors is shown in Table 18.5. It is apparent that the antibody has a significant inhibitory effect on the tumorigenic growth of this *neu*-transformed NIH 3T3 cell line. We have subsequently found that this antibody has no effect on the tumorigenic growth of NIH 3T3 cells transformed by oncogenes unrelated to *neu* (data not shown). Thus, anti-p185 monoclonal antibodies are able to inhibit the neoplastic properties of *neu*-transformed NIH 3T3 cells in vivo as well as in vitro.

TABLE 18.5. *Interference with the Tumorigenic Growth of* neu-*Transformed Cells by Monoclonal Anti-p185 Antibody*

Day	Control Tumor Size (mm²)	Antibody-Treated Tumor Size (mm²)	Inhibition (%)
6	39.8 ± 3.1	20.9 ± 1.9	47
8	73.7 ± 10.6	27.0 ± 3.1	63
10	119.2 ± 12.3	27.3 ± 4.0	77
12	213.6 ± 20.1	37.6 ± 7.9	82
14	353.3 ± 22.9	47.5 ± 10.8	87

Groups of six BALB/c nude mice were inoculated subcutaneously with 1×10^6 neu-transformed NIH 3T3 cells (cell line B104-1-1) on day 0. Also on day 0, control mice received 1 ml of saline intraperitoneally, while antibody-treated mice received 1 ml of 7.16.4 ascites fluid intraperitoneally. Tumor size represents the mean ± standard error of the mean of the products of tumor length and width. The difference in tumor size between treated and control groups was significant on each day ($P < .001$).

DISCUSSION

Oncogenes capable of transforming normal rodent cell lines following DNA transfection have been identified in a significant fraction of human and animal tumors and tumor cell lines (Cooper 1982, Land et al. 1983). In addition, some tumors that do not contain activated oncogenes detectable by transfection experiments do contain cellular oncogenes that are chromosomally rearranged or transcriptionally activated (or both) (Taub et al. 1982, de Klein et al. 1982, Eva et al. 1982). Thus, abnormal oncogene expression and function may occur in many tumors. One oncogene active in transfection experiments was originally identified in a number of independently derived rat neuroblastomas (Shih et al. 1981); we refer to this gene as the *neu* oncogene. This oncogene is of particular interest because it appears to be distinct from the known retroviral oncogenes (Schechter et al. 1984), and it encodes a protein, p185, that displays certain domains on the cell surface (Drebin et al. 1984a).

　We have generated a panel of hybridomas that secrete antibodies reactive with cell surface domains of the p185 molecule and that immunoprecipitate p185 from metabolically labeled lysates of *neu*-transformed cells. These antibodies react with cell surface determinants found on all of the *neu*-transfected NIH 3T3 cell lines tested, but not with NIH 3T3 cell lines transformed by oncogenes unrelated to *neu*. They also bind to antigens on the rat neuroblastoma cell lines from which *neu* oncogenes were originally isolated.

　Culture of *neu*-transformed NIH 3T3 cells with monoclonal anti-p185 antibodies causes the rapid antigenic modulation of cell surface p185. There is also concomitant destruction of the modulated p185, so that cells cultured in the presence of antibody display lower total cellular p185 levels. Cells in which p185 is down-modulated by monoclonal antibodies are not killed by such treatment, but these cells do lose the phenotypic behavior that best distinguishes transformed cells from nontransformed cells, namely, the ability to form anchorage-independent colonies when suspended in agar. This effect occurs at low doses of antibody and is specific for cells transformed by *neu* oncogenes. Thus, it seems likely that the down-modulation of cellular p185 levels caused by monoclonal anti-p185 antibodies causes the cells to be unable to form anchorage-independent colonies.

At least one monoclonal anti-p185 antibody appears to be able to affect the neoplastic behavior of *neu*-transformed cells in vivo as well. When mice carrying tumors composed of *neu*-transformed NIH 3T3 cells are injected with antibody 7.16.4, the growth of these tumors is dramatically inhibited. It should be noted that each mouse was injected with a very large tumor cell dose and received a single injection of antibody. We are currently attempting to determine whether we can cure tumors composed of *neu*-transformed cells or merely inhibit their growth.

Studies from a number of laboratories have shown that monoclonal antibodies can inhibit tumor growth in vivo (Boss et al. 1983). Studies of antibodies raised against glycolipid antigens have suggested that IgG2a and IgG3 isotype murine monoclonal antibodies have the most dramatic antitumor activity (Herlyn and Koprowski 1982). It is thought that this activity is due to their ability to recruit a particular type of macrophage to perform antibody-dependent cell-mediated cytotoxicity (ADCC) (Adams et al. 1984). In contrast, antibodies raised against cellular receptors for certain growth factors appear to be able to inhibit tumor growth regardless of isotype, perhaps by interfering with growth factor binding (Trowbridge and Domingo 1981, Masui et al. 1984). It is important to note that antibody 7.16.4, used in the in vivo experiment described above is of the IgG2a isotype; we are currently attempting to determine whether antibody 7.16.4 is able to mediate ADCC. We are also studying our other p185 specific monoclonal antibodies in order to determine whether the ability of monoclonal antibodies directed at the p185 protein to inhibit tumor growth is dependent on the isotype of the antibody used. Regardless of the mechanism of antibody action, it is clear from the data presented here that monoclonal antibodies reactive with cell surface domains of the *neu* oncogene product are able to inhibit the tumorigenic growth of *neu*-transformed cells. Thus, the administration of monoclonal antibodies reactive with cell surface domains of oncogene-encoded proteins represents a potentially useful therapeutic approach to the treatment of malignancies caused by the activation of certain oncogenes.

ACKNOWLEDGMENT

We thank our colleagues for helpful discussion. This work was funded by grants from the National Institutes of Health and the American Cancer Society.

REFERENCES

Adams DO, Hall T, Steplewski Z, Koprowski H. 1984. Tumors undergoing rejection induced by monoclonal antibodies contain increased numbers of macrophages activated for a distinctive form of antibody-dependent cytolysis. Proc Natl Acad Sci USA 81:3506–3510.

Boss BD, Langman R, Trowbridge I, Dulbecco R, eds. 1983. Monoclonal Antibodies and Cancer. Academic Press, New York, 299 pp.

Boyse EA, Stockert E, Old LJ. 1967. Modification of the antigenic structure of the cell membrane by thymus-leukemia (TL) antibody. Proc Natl Acad Sci USA 58:954–959.

Bradford MM. 1976. A rapid and sensitive method for the quantitation of microgram quantities of protein using the principle of protein-dye binding. Anal Biochem 72:248–254.

Bruck C, Portetelle D, Glineur C, Bollen A 1982. One-step purification of mouse monoclonal antibodies from ascitic fluid by DEAE Affi-Gel blue chromatography. J Immunol Meth 53:313–319.

Cooper GM. 1982. Cellular transforming genes. Science 217:801–806.

de Klein A, van Kessel AG, Grosveld G, et al. 1982. A cellular oncogene is translocated to the Philadelphia chromosome in chronic myelocytic leukaemia. Nature 300:765–767.

Der CJ, Cooper GM. 1983. Altered gene products are associated with activation of cellular ras^k genes in human lung and colon carcinomas. Cell 32:201–208.

Drebin JA, Link VC, Stern DF, Weinberg RA, Greene MI. 1984a. Immune responses against transforming gene associated antigens. In Sercarz E, Cantor H, Chess L, eds., Regulation of the Immune System. Alan R. Liss Publishing Company, New York, pp. 919–928.

Drebin JA, Stern DF, Link VC, Weinberg RA, Greene MI. 1984b. Monoclonal antibodies identify a cell surface antigen associated with an activated cellular transforming gene. Nature 312:545–548.

Eva A, Robbins KC, Anderson PR, et al. 1982. Cellular genes analogous to retroviral onc genes are transcribed in human tumour cells. Nature 295:116–119.

Feig LA, Bast RC, Knapp RC, Cooper GM. 1984. Somatic activation of ras^k gene in a human ovarian carcinoma. Science 223:698–701.

Foley EJ. 1953. Properties of methylcholanthrene-induced tumors in mice of the strain of origin. Cancer Res 13:835–842.

Freedman V, Shin S. 1974. Cellular tumorigenicity in nude mice: Correlation with cell growth in semi-solid medium. Cell 3:355–358.

Herlyn D, Koprowski H. 1982. IgG2a monoclonal antibodies inhibit human tumor growth through interaction with effector cells. Proc Natl Acad Sci USA 79:4761–4765.

Hudson L, Hay FC. 1980. Practical Immunology. Blackwell Scientific Publications, London, pp. 117–121.

Land H, Parada LF, Weinberg RA. 1983. Cellular oncogenes and multistep carcinogenesis. Science 222:771–778.

Masui H, Kawamoto T, Sato JD, Wolf B, Sato G, Mendelsohn J. 1984. Growth inhibition of human tumor cells in athymic mice by anti-epidermal growth factor receptor monoclonal antibodies. Cancer Res 44:1002–1007.

Padhy LC, Shih C, Cowing D, Finkelstein R, Weinberg RA. 1982. Identification of a phosphoprotein specifically induced by the transforming DNA of rat neuroblastomas. Cell 28:865–871.

Pollack R, Chen S. Powers S, Verderame M. 1984. Transformation mechanisms at the cellular level. *In* Klein G, ed., Advances in Viral Oncology, vol. 4. Raven Press, New York, pp. 3–28.

Prehn RT, Main JM. 1957. Immunity to methylcholanthrene-induced sarcomas. JNCI 18:769–778.

Ritz J, Pesando JM, Notis-McConarty J, Schlossman SF. 1980. Modulation of human acute lymphoblastic leukemia antigen induced by monoclonal antibody *in vitro*. J Immunol 125:1506–1514.

Santos E, Martin-Zanca D, Reddy EP, Pierotti MA, Porta GD, Barbacid M. 1984. Malignant activation of a K-*ras* oncogene in lung carcinoma but not in normal tissue of the same patient. Science 223:661–664.

Schechter AL, Stern DF, Vaidyanathan L, et al. 1984. The *neu* oncogene: An *erbB*-related gene encoding a 185,000-M_r tumor antigen. Nature 312:513–516.

Schreiner GF, Unanue ER. 1977. Capping and the lymphocyte: Models for membrane reorganization. J Immunol 119:1549–1551.

Shih C, Padhy LC, Murray M, Weinberg RA. 1981. Transforming genes of carcinomas and neuroblastomas introduced into mouse fibroblasts. Nature 290:261–264.

Tabin CJ, Bradley SM, Bargmann CI, et al. 1982. Mechanism of activation of a human oncogene. Nature 300:143–149.

Taparowsky E, Shimizu K, Goldfarb M, Wigler M. 1983. Structure and activation of the human N-*ras* gene. Cell 34:581–586.

Taub R, Kirsch I, Morton C, et al. 1982. Translocation of the c-*myc* gene into the immunoglobulin heavy chain locus in human Burkitt lymphoma and murine plasmacytoma cells. Proc Natl Acad Sci USA 79:7837–7841.

Trowbridge IS, Domingo DL. 1981. Anti-transferrin receptor monoclonal antibody and toxin-antibody conjugates affect growth of human tumour cells. Nature 294:171–173.

Yuasa Y, Srivastava SK, Dunn CY, Rhim JS, Reddy EP, Aaronson SA. 1983. Acquisition of transforming properties by alternative point mutations within c-*bas/has* human proto-oncogene. Nature 303:775–779.

Contributors

Oreste Acuto
Division of Tumor Immunology
Dana-Farber Cancer Institute, and the
Department of Pathology
Harvard Medical School
Boston, Massachusetts 02115

Michael J. Bevan
Department of Immunology
Scripps Clinic and Research Foundation
La Jolla, California 92037

Thierry Boon
Ludwig Institute for Cancer Research,
and the Cellular Genetics Unit
Catholic University of Louvain
Brussels, Belgium

Kim Bottomly
Department of Pathology
Howard Hughes Medical Institute at
Yale University School of Medicine
New Haven, Connecticut 06510

Gary Cabirac
Department of Pathology and
  Laboratory Medicine
The University of Texas Health Science
  Center at Houston
Houston, Texas 77030

Thomas J. Campen
Division of Tumor Immunology
Dana-Farber Cancer Institute, and the
Department of Pathology
Harvard Medical School
Boston, Massachusetts 02115

Hsiu-Ching Chang
Division of Tumor Immunology
Dana-Farber Cancer Institute, and the
Department of Pathology
Harvard Medical School
Boston, Massachusetts 02115

Michael L. Cleary
Department of Medicine/Pathology
Stanford University
Stanford, California 94305

Patricia J. Conrad
Department of Pathology
Howard Hughes Medical Institute at
Yale University School of Medicine
New Haven, Connecticut 06510

Lynette Corbeil
Department of Veterinary Microbiology
  and Pathology
Washington State University
Pullman, Washington 99164

Carlo M. Croce
The Wistar Institute of Anatomy
  and Biology
Philadelphia, Pennsylvania 19104

Etienne De Plaen
Ludwig Institute for Cancer Research,
and the Cellular Genetics Unit
Catholic University of Louvain
Brussels, Belgium

Jeffrey A. Drebin
Department of Pathology
Harvard Medical School
Boston, Massachusetts 02115

Philippe Dubois
Laboratory of Microbial Immunity
National Institute of Allergy and
  Infectious Diseases
National Institutes of Health
Bethesda, Maryland 20205

Jan Erikson
The Wistar Institute of Anatomy
  and Biology
Philadelphia, Pennsylvania 19104

Isaiah J. Fidler
Department of Cell Biology
The University of Texas M. D. Anderson
  Hospital and Tumor Institute
  at Houston
Houston, Texas 77030

Patrick M. Flood
Department of Pathology
Howard Hughes Medical Institute at
Yale University School of Medicine
New Haven, Connecticut 06510

Philip Frost
Department of Cell Biology
  and Medicine
The University of Texas M. D. Anderson
  Hospital and Tumor Institute
  at Houston
Houston, Texas 77030

Robert A. Good
Department of Pediatrics
University of South Florida
All Children's Hospital
St. Petersburg, Florida 33701

Mark I. Greene
Department of Pathology
Harvard Medical School, and the
Department of Medicine
Tufts–New England Medical Center
Boston, Massachusetts 02111

Warner C. Greene
Metabolism Branch
National Cancer Institute
National Institutes of Health
Bethesda, Maryland 20205

Elizabeth A. Grimm
Surgical Neurology Branch
National Institute of Neurological and
  Communication Disorders and Stroke
National Institutes of Health
Bethesda, Maryland 20205

Jay Horowitz
Department of Pathology
Howard Hughes Medical Institute at
Yale University School of Medicine
New Haven, Connecticut 06510

Maureen Howard
Laboratory of Microbial Immunity
National Institute of Allergy and
  Infectious Diseases
National Institutes of Health
Bethesda, Maryland 20205

Steven K. Jacobs
Surgical Neurology Branch
National Institute of Neurological and
  Communication Disorders and Stroke
National Institutes of Health
Bethesda, Maryland 20205

Charles A. Janeway, Jr.
Deprtment of Pathology
Howard Hughes Medical Institute at
Yale University School of Medicine
New Haven, Connecticut 06510

Barry Jones
Department of Pathology
Howard Hughes Medical Institute at
Yale University School of Medicine
New Haven, Connecticut 06510

Neena Kapoor
Department of Pediatrics
University of South Florida
All Children's Hospital
St. Petersburg, Florida 33701

Jonathan Kaye
Department of Biology
University of California at San Diego
La Jolla, California 92093

Robert S. Kerbel
Department of Pathology
Queen's University
Kingston, Ontario, Canada K7L 3N6

Stanley J. Korsmeyer
Metabolism Branch
National Cancer Institute
National Institutes of Health
Bethesda, Maryland 20205

Margaret L. Kripke
Department of Immunology
The University of Texas M. D. Anderson
   Hospital and Tumor Institute
   at Houston
Houston, Texas 77030

Louis A. Lanza
Surgery Branch
National Cancer Institute
National Institutes of Health
Bethesda, Maryland, 20205

Edmund C. Lattime
Immunology Program
Memorial Sloan-Kettering
   Cancer Center
New York, New York 10021

Julian Leibowitz
Department of Pathology and
   Laboratory Medicine
The University of Texas Health Science
   Center at Houston
Houston, Texas 77030

Ronald Levy
Department of Medicine/Oncology
Stanford University
Stanford, California 94305

Shoshana Levy
Department of Medicine/Oncology
Stanford University
Stanford, California 94305

Victoria C. Link
Department of Pathology
Harvard Medical School, and the
Department of Medicine
Tufts–New England Medical Center
Boston, Massachusetts 02111

James Lowder
Department of Medicine/Oncology
Stanford University
Stanford, California 94305

Timothy Meeker
Department of Medicine/Oncology
Stanford University
Stanford, California 94305

Gilbert Melin
Surgical Neurology Branch
National Institute of Neurological and
   Communication Disorders and Stroke
National Institutes of Health
Bethesda, Maryland 20205

Peter C. Nowell
Department of Pathology and
  Laboratory Medicine
University of Pennsylvania
  School of Medicine
Philadelphia, Pennsylvania 19104

Dunia Ramarli
Division of Tumor Immunology
Dana-Farber Cancer Institute, and the
Department of Pathology
Harvard Medical School
Boston, Massachusetts 02115

Ellis L. Reinherz
Division of Tumor Immunology
Dana-Farber Cancer Institute, and the
Department of Medicine
Harvard Medical School
Boston, Massachusetts 02115

Jack A. Roth
Surgery Branch
National Cancer Institute
National Institutes of Health
Bethesda, Maryland 20205

Hans Dieter Royer
Division of Tumor Immunology
Dana-Farber Cancer Institute, and the
Department of Pathology
Harvard Medical School
Boston, Massachusetts 02115

Hans Schreiber
Department of Pathology
The University of Chicago
La Rabida–University of
  Chicago Institute
Chicago, Illinois 60649

Alan J. Schroit
Department of Cell Biology
The University of Texas M. D. Anderson
  Hospital and Tumor Institute
  at Houston
Houston, Texas 77030

Stewart Sell
Department of Pathology and
  Laboratory Medicine
The University of Texas Health Science
  Center at Houston
Houston, Texas 77030

Eileen Skaletsky
Department of Pathology
University of California at San Diego
La Jolla, California 92093

Jeffrey Sklar
Department of Medicine/Pathology
Stanford University
Stanford, California 94305

Uwe D. Staerz
Department of Immunology
Scripps Clinic and Research Foundation
La Jolla, California 92037

Peter Stein
Laboratory of Microbial Immunity
National Institute of Allergy and
  Infectious Diseases
National Institutes of Health
Bethesda, Maryland 20205

David F. Stern
Whitehead Institute for Biomedical
  Research
Massachusetts Institute of Technology
Cambridge, Massachusetts 02142

Hans J. Stauss
Department of Pathology
The University of Chicago
La Rabida–University of
  Chicago Institute
Chicago, Illinois 60649

David Strayer
Department of Pathology
Yale University
New Haven, Connecticut 06510

Osias Stutman
Immunology Program
Memorial Sloan-Kettering
 Cancer Center
New York, New York 10021

Kristiaan Thielemans
Afdeling Hematologie/Immunologie
Vrije Universiteit Brussel
Brussels, Belgium

John P. Tite
Department of Pathology
Howard Hughes Medical Institute at
Yale University School of Medicine
New Haven, Connecticut 06510

Yoshihide Tsujimoto
The Wistar Institute of Anatomy
 and Biology
Philadelphia, Pennsylvania 19104

Aline Van Pel
Ludwig Institute for
 Cancer Research, and the
Cellular Genetics Unit
Catholic University of Louvain
Brussels, Belgium

Carter Van Waes
Department of Pathology
The University of Chicago
La Rabida–University of
 Chicago Institute
Chicago, Illinois 60649

Françoise Vessière
Ludwig Institute for
 Cancer Research, and the
Cellular Genetics Unit
Catholic University of Louvain
Brussels, Belgium

Thomas A. Waldmann
Metabolism Branch
National Cancer Institute
National Institutes of Health
Bethesda, Maryland 20205

Roger A. Warnke
Department of Medicine/Pathology
Stanford University
Stanford, California 94305

Robert A. Weinberg
Whitehead Institute for Biomedical
 Research
Massachusetts Institute of Technology
Cambridge, Massachusetts 02142

Debra J. Wilson
Surgical Neurology Branch
National Institute of Neurological and
 Communication Disorders and Stroke
National Institutes of Health
Bethesda, Maryland 20205

Richard D. Wortzel
Department of Pathology
The University of Chicago
La Rabida–University of
 Chicago Institute
Chicago, Illinois 60649

Department of Scientific Publications
UT M. D. Anderson Hospital

Editorial Staff

CAROL A. KAKALEC: Monograph Editor
MELISSA G. BURKETT: Editorial Assistant
MARY E. DEISS: Word Processing

Index

recognition by anti-p185 antibody,
  282–285
90-kDa heterodimers. *See* T3-Ti
  molecular complex, Ti heterodimers
N-terminal amino acid sequencing of
  Ti_β subunit, 13–14

Oncogenes. *See also neu* oncogene
  in Burkitt's lymphoma, 79
  in chronic myelogenous leukemia,
    79–80
  point mutations in, 277, 286
  use as probes in study of B cell
    malignancies, 90–91

Phosphatidylserine, 189–194
Phospholipids
  recognition by macrophages, 187,
    188
Poxviruses
  classification of, 98–100

Rabbit fibroma virus, malignant. *See*
  Malignant rabbit fibroma virus
Red blood cells
  recognition by macrophages,
    187–193
    role of phosphatidylserine,
      189–193
  sickled human red blood cells
    recognition by peripheral blood
      monocytes, 193–194

Self and nonself recognition
  by macrophages, 183–184,
    200–201
  role of, in targeting nonspecific
    effector molecules, 45–46
Severe combined immunodeficiency
  syndromes, 25
  immunorestoration methods,
    269–271
Sézary leukemia, 72
Shope fibroma, 98
  Berry-Dedrick phenomenon, 103
  immunopathology of, 100–101
Shope fibroma viruses
  effects in vivo, 103–105
  genetic relationship with malignant

rabbit fibroma virus and
  myxoma, 102–108
in immunocompromised rabbits,
  107–108
microbiology, 98, 100
pathologic features, 100
strain differences, 107
Skin cancer, UV-induced
  immunology, 113–115
  suppressor cells
    origin of, 116–117
    role in carcinogenesis, 117–118
    specificity of, 115–116

T3
  modulated by anti-T3, 6
    effect on antigen recognition, 7
    effect on T4 and T8 clones, 7
T3 glycoprotein, 3, 4
  association with Ti clonotype, 9–12
T3-Ti molecular complex, 3–26
  characterization of, 9–12
  clonal T cell proliferation, 21–24
  implications for human disease,
    24–26
  Ti antigen receptors, 19
  Ti expression, surface, 20
  Ti heterodimers, 3–4, 63–64, 68
    T3-associated disulfide-linked,
      9–12, 19
  Ti molecules
    constant and variable domains
      of, 12–13
    peptide variability of, 12–13
  Ti_α subunit
    gene rearrangement during
      thymic ontogeny, 20
  Ti_β subunit
    amino acid sequencing of, 13–15
    combining sites, 17–18
    gene rearrangement during
      thymic ontogeny, 20
    genetic structure of, 13–19
    genomic organization of, 16–17
    homology between human and
      mouse clones, 14
    Kyte-Doolittle plot, 14, 15
    position of cysteine residues,
      15–16
    similarity to Ig system, 17–18